AF614704

Photodynamic Therapy in Dermatology

Michael H. Gold
Editor

Photodynamic Therapy in Dermatology

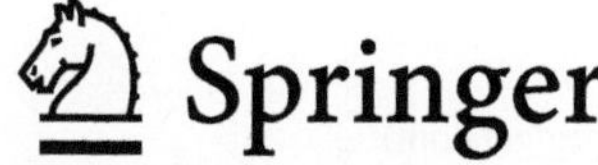

Editor
Michael H. Gold, MD
Dermatologic and Cosmetic Surgeon
Gold Skin Care Center
Tennessee Clinical Research Center
Nashville, TN
USA
and
Clinical Assistant Professor
Department of Dermatology
Vanderbilt University School of Medicine
and Vanderbilt University School of Nursing
Nashville, TN
USA
goldskin@goldskincare.com

ISBN 978-1-4419-1297-8 ISBN 978-1-4419-1298-5 (eBook)

DOI 10.1007/978-1-4419-1298-5

Springer New York Dordrecht Heidelberg London

Library of Congress Control Number: 2011923977

Printed on acid-free paper

Springer is part of Springer Science+Business Media (www.springer.com)

Preface

Photodynamic therapy (PDT) has truly found its place in dermatology and dermatologic surgery. Its utilization has increased steadily around the world and many investigators have contributed to the enormous amount of literature that can be found for the study of PDT. The path to utilization has basically taken two distinct routes: one that can be considered the United States model and one that can be considered the European model. These pathways have begun to intersect more and more over the past several years, and it is hoped that this textbook will be used as a major reference for those interested in PDT from a dermatology point of view in all corners of our world. PDT is truly global; although there are only two photosensitizers available in the United States, many more are available worldwide, with many clinicians utilizing PDT in different shapes and forms.

I have been very fortunate throughout my career to have worked alongside, been mentored by, and collaborated with many outstanding clinicians and scientists in dermatology. I am indebted to many, starting with my chairman during my residency, Dr. Henry Roenigk. Many outstanding teachers have paved the way for my career in dermatology, including Drs. William Caro, Ruth Frankel, June Robinson, and Jerome Garden. My fellow residents at Northwestern, most of whom are still my good friends, also contributed and still are contributing to our specialty in many exceptional ways. Drs. Amy Forman Taub, Morgan Magid, David Picascia, Dan Kaufman, Andrew Lazar, Richard Rubenstein, Neil Goldberg, and Kevin Pinski, to mention just a few, continue to motivate and push me to be involved in dermatology and always to strive for excellence. There are also my colleagues in the field and friends who have always been there for me, whom I am grateful to know, and with whom I consider it a privilege to work. I am also indebted to the contributors to this book and to Drs. David Goldberg, Mitch Goldman, and Mark Nestor. Others who have played an important part in my desire to learn more and more about PDT include Dr. Geoffrey Schulman and Paul Sowyrda.

I apologize to those whom I might have excluded unintentionally. I am also indebted to my family, my wife Cindee, and my children Ilissa and

Benjamin, who have endured my absence many nights when I was on the road, lecturing somewhere on the subjects I love. To my family and to my parents, thank you for making me the kind of doctor I have always dreamed of being.

Nashville, TN Michael H. Gold

Contents

Contributors

Surianti Binti Md Akir, BMedSc
Researcher, Department of Medicine (Dermatology), The University of Melbourne, Skin and Cancer Foundation, Carlton Victoria, Australia

Macrene Alexiades-Armenakas, MD, PhD
Assistant Clinical Professor, Department of Dermatology, Yale University School of Medicine;
Director and Founder, Dermatology and Laser Surgery Center, New York, NY, USA

Philipp Babilas, MD, PhD
Associate Professor, Department of Dermatology, Regensburg University Hospital, Regensburg, Germany

Robert Bissonnette, MD, FRCP
President, Innovaderm Research, Montreal, Canada

Peter Bjerring, MD, PhD
Professor, Department of Dermatology, Molholm Research, Molholm Hospital, Vejle, Denmark

Kaare Christiansen, MS
Medical Engineer, Department of Dermatology, Molholm Research, Molholm Hospital, Vejle, Denmark

Hannah C. de Vijlder, MD, MSc
Assistant Professor, Department of Dermatology, Erasmus Medical Center Rotterdam, Rotterdam, The Netherlands

Peter Foley, MD, FACD
Associate Professor, Department of Dermatology, Skin and Cancer Foundation, The University of Melbourne, Carlton, Victoria, Australia;
Department of Medicine (Dermatology), St Vincent's Hospital Melbourne, Fitzroy, Victoria, Australia

Amy Forman Taub, MD
Assistant Professor, Department of Dermatology, Northwestern University Medical School, Chicago, IL, USA;
Advanced Dermatology, Lincolnshire, IL, USA

Cara Garretson, MD
Cosmetic Fellow, Advanced Dermatology, Lincolnshire, IL, USA

Dore J. Gilbert, MD, LTC USAR
Associate Professor of Dermatology, University of California, Irvine, Ca.
Medical Director, Newport Dermatology and Laser Associates,
Newport Beach, CA, USA

Michael H. Gold, MD
Dermatologic and Cosmetic Surgeon, Gold Skin Care Center, Tennessee Clinical Research Center, Nashville, TN, USA;
Clinical Assistant Professor, Department of Dermatology, Vanderbilt University School of Medicine and Vanderbilt University School of Nursing, Nashville, TN, USA

Mitchel P. Goldman, MD
Medical Director, Goldman, Butterwick, Fitzpatrick and Groff Dermatology, La Jolla, CA, USA

Olle Larkö, MD
Professor, Consultant, Department of Dermatology, Sahlgrenska Academy, University of Gothenburg, Gothenburg, Sweden

George Martin, MD
Director, Dermatology and Laser Center of Maui, Kihei, HI, USA

H. A. Martino Neumann, MD, PhD
Profesor, Department of Dermatology, Erasmus Medical Center Rotterdam, Rotterdam, The Netherlands

Melanie Palm, MD, MBA
Associate, Surfside Dermatology, Encinitas, CA, USA

Ricardo Ruiz-Rodriguez, MD
Head, Department of Dermatology, Clínica Ruber of Madrid, Madrid, Spain;
Director, Clínica Dermatológica Internacional, Madrid, Spain

Carin Sandberg, MD, PhD
Consultant, Department of Dermatology, Sahlgrenska University Hospital, Gothenburg, Sweden

Rolf-Markus Szeimies, MD, PhD
Professor and Chair, Department of Dermatology and Allergology, Klinikum Vest Academic Teaching Hospital, Recklinghausen, Germany

Ann-Marie Wennberg, MD
Professor and Consultant, Department of Dermatology, Sahlgrenska University Hospital, Göteborg, Sweden

Brian Zelickson, MD
Adjunct Associate Professor, Director, Electron Microscopy Laboratory, Department of Dermatology, University of Minnesota, Minneapolis, MN, USA;
Zel Skin and Laser Specialists, Edina, MN, USA

1 History of Photodynamic Therapy

Michael H. Gold

Abstract

The history of photodynamic therapy (PDT) in medicine can be traced to the beginning of the twentieth century. Raab first reported, in 1900, that paramecia cells (*Paramecium caudatum*) were not affected when exposed to either acridine orange or a light source, but that they died within 2 h if exposed to both acridine orange and the light at the same time. PDT research turned to other potential photosensitizers following the initial reports, mainly those related to porphyrins. From these clinical investigations, the principles of PDT in human cancer cells had now been firmly established. PDT has truly become a global therapeutic option for many patients we treat in dermatology.

The history of photodynamic therapy (PDT) in medicine can be traced to the beginning of the twentieth century. Raab [1] first reported, in 1900, that paramecia cells (*Paramecium caudatum*) were not affected when exposed to either acridine orange or a light source, but that they died within 2 h if exposed to both acridine orange and the light at the same time. Acridine orange was used as a photosensitizer in this experiment and sensitized the paramecia cells to the effects of the light source. Von Tappeiner and Jodblauer [2], in 1904, first described the term *photodynamic effect* when they reported their experiment in which an oxygen-consuming reaction process in protozoa occurred after aniline dyes were applied with fluorescence. In 1905, Von Tappeiner and Jesionek [3] reported their experiences with topical 5% eosin. Topical 5% eosin was used as a photosensitizer with artificial light to successfully treat nonmelanoma skin cancers, lupus vulgaris, and condylomata lata in humans. It was postulated that the eosin, in a manner similar to the acridine orange studies, once incorporated into cells, could produce a cytotoxic reaction when exposed to a light source and oxygen. These studies, in 1905, were the first reports of PDT in human subjects and became the prototype for the future studies of PDT, in which a photosensitizer is applied to the skin, and in the presence of oxygen and an appropriate light source, can produce phototoxic reactions within the skin.

M.H. Gold (✉)
Dermatologic and Cosmetic Surgeon, Gold Skin Care Center, Tennessee Clinical Research Center, Nashville, TN, USA
and
Department of Dermatology, Vanderbilt University School of Medicine and Vanderbilt University School of Nursing, Nashville, TN, USA
e-mail: goldskin@goldskincare.com

M.H. Gold (ed.), *Photodynamic Therapy in Dermatology*,
DOI 10.1007/978-1-4419-1298-5_1,

Other Photosensitizers

PDT research turned to other potential photosensitizers following these initial reports, mainly those related to porphyrins. In 1911, Hausman et al. [4] reported their findings with the use of hematoporphyrin. They were able to successfully show that light-activated hematoporphyrin could photosensitize both guinea pigs and mice. In 1913, Meyer-Betz [5] self-injected hematoporphyrin and noticed that when the injected areas were exposed to a light source, they became swollen and painful. Unfortunately for the science of PDT and for himself, the phototoxic reaction in Meyer-Betz lasted for 2 months, which created difficulty for its regular use as a photosensitizer. In 1942, Auler et al. [6] reported that hematoporphyrin concentrated more in certain dermatologic skin tumors than in the surrounding tissues, and that, when fluoresced with light, the tumors were necrotic, demonstrating the photodynamic response of hematoporphyrin. Figge et al. [7] later reported that hematoporphyrin was also selectively absorbed into other cells, including embryonic, traumatized skin, and neoplastic areas.

Uses of Photodynamic Therapy

From these clinical investigations, the principles of PDT in human cancer cells had now been firmly established. A photosensitizer, which in this case was hematoporphyrin, could be absorbed and concentrated into the cancerous cells, and when activated by a proper light source and in the presence of oxygen, could be cytotoxic to these cells. In 1978, Dougherty et al. [8] presented their research with a new photosensitizer, known as hematoporphyrin purified derivative (HPD). HPD was a complex mixture of porphyrin subunits and by-products. Dougherty showed that HPD could be successfully used to treat cutaneous malignancies, with red light as the primary light source. Systemic HPD became the standard for PDT research, and a variety of medical uses emerged for PDT, both oncologic and non-oncologic. These medical uses are shown in Table 1.1.

Table 1.1 Uses of photodynamic therapy in dermatology

Actinic keratoses
Photodamage and associated actinic keratoses[a]
Bowen's disease
Superficial basal cell carcinoma
Superficial squamous cell carcinoma
Cutaneous T-cell lymphoma
Kaposi's sarcoma
Malignant melanoma
Actinic chelitis
Keratoacanthoma
Psoriasis vulgaris
Human papillomavirus
Molluscum contagiosum
Alopecia areata
Hirsutism
Acne vulgaris[a]
Sebaceous gland hyperplasia[a]
Hidradenitis suppurativa[a]

[a] Common indications for 5-aminolevulinic acid photodynamic therapy in the United States

Because of the unique nature of the skin and its accessibility for study with both natural light or artificial light sources, dermatological research became a prime focus for PDT research at this time. HPD, however, remained phototoxic in the skin for several months, making its practical use in dermatology difficult. In 1990, Kennedy et al. [9] changed the face of PDT forever when they introduced the first topical porphyrin derivative, known as aminolevulinic acid (ALA). This photosensitizer is known as a prodrug and is converted in the skin to its active form. They found that ALA could penetrate through the stratum corneum of the skin and be selectively absorbed by actinically damaged skin cells. They also described that ALA could be selectively absorbed by nonmelanoma skin cancer cells as well as the pilosebaceous units in the skin. Kennedy then described the PDT reaction of ALA. Once the ALA is applied to the skin, it is absorbed through the stratum corneum, and converted to it's active form, Protoporphyrin IX (PpIX).

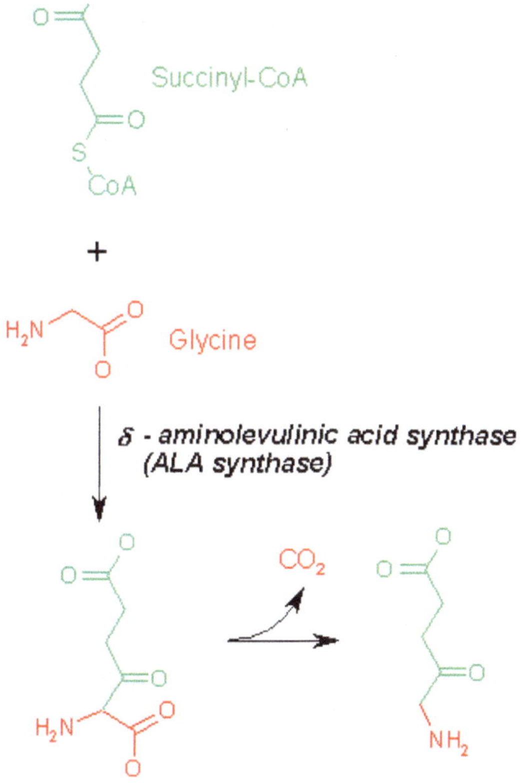

Fig. 1.1 PpIX absorption in vivo (mouse skin). *ALA* the natural precursor of PpIX in the heme pathway

ALA, the natural precursor of PpIX in the heme pathway, is shown in Fig. 1.1. ALA is the prodrug photosensitizing agent; PpIX is the photosensitizer. Research with PpIX originally focused on blue light in the US with ALA, while in Europe, much of the original work performed was with a red light source, and the methyl ester of ALA (MAL), to be described in more detail below. PpIX has since been shown to be photoactivated by a variety of lasers and light sources, as shown in Fig. 1.2. Figure 1.2 shows the absorption spectrum of PpIX, with peak absorption bands identified in both the blue light, known as the Soret Band, and red light spectrums. Smaller peaks of energy, in between these major absorption bands are also seen in Fig. 1.2, and these are important as sources of light to activate ALA and MAL, and have become very important to many as PDT moves further into the twenty-first century [10].

The heme biosynthetic pathway (Fig. 1.1) is maintained under a very close feedback loop apparatus, not allowing for buildup of heme or its precursors, such as PpIX, in tissues. Exogenous ALA forming PpIX is cleared from the body much more rapidly than its predecessor photosensitizer, HPD. Therefore, the potential for phototoxicity from ALA-induced PpIX is much reduced, only to days instead of several months. And, ALA penetrates only actinically damaged skin, thus increasing the specificity of ALA-PDT.

PDT has taken on two separate pathways, as noted in the Preface, since Kennedy's introduction of topically applied ALA. In the US, research has centered on 20% 5-ALA (Levulan® Kerastick™, Dusa Pharmaceuticals, Wilmington, MA) and its ability to treat AKs, photorejuvenation, inflammatory acne vulgaris, sebaceous gland hyperplasia, and hidradenitis suppurativa, among other entities. In Europe, research has centered on the methyl ester of 5-ALA, 16.8% MAL (Metvix® in Europe, Metvixia® in the US, Galderma Laboratories, Ft. Worth, TX), and its uses in treating nonmelanoma skin cancers and AKs. Interest in photorejuvenation and inflammatory acne vulgaris has seen a recent surge with MAL [10].

This textbook will explore the various photosensitizing drugs, the various indications for each drug, and the research which has been performed with the drugs, allowing the reader the opportunity to determine if PDT can play a vital role in their daily practice of dermatology. Each chapter and each of the authors have been chosen to bring their expertise to this project – I am confident we have achieved our goal.

PDT has truly become a global therapeutic option for many patients we treat in dermatology. The hope of this textbook was to bring to you, the reader, some of the brightest and best minds in the PDT field, from all over the world, and to utilize their strengths in presenting what we hope is, the most up-to-date and sophisticated PDT reference on the market.

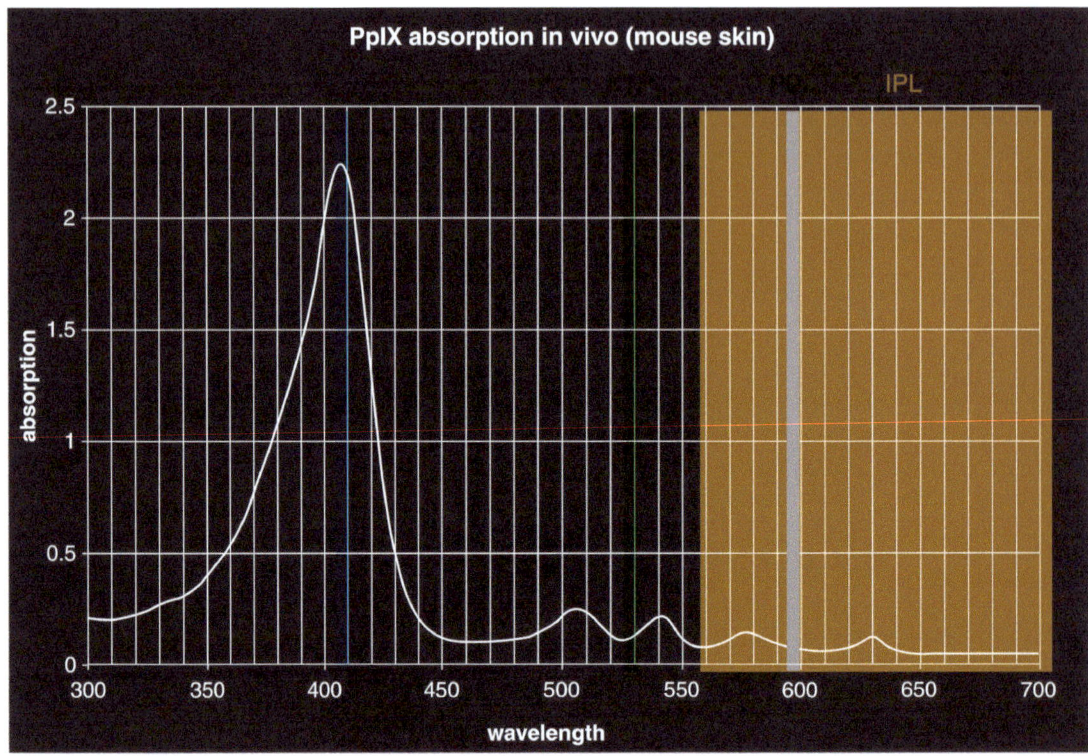

Fig. 1.2 The figure shows the absorption spectrum of PpIX, with peak absorption bands identified in both the blue light, known as the Soret Band and red light spectrums. Smaller peaks of energy, in between these major absorption bands are also seen, and these are important as sources of light to activate ALA and MAL

References

1. Raab O. Ueber die wirkung fluoreszierenden stoffe auf infusorien. Z Biol. 1900;39:524–6.
2. Von Tappeiner H, Jodblauer A. Uber die wirkung der photodynamischen (fluorescierenden) staffe auf protozoan und enzyme. Dtsch Arch Klin Med. 1904;80: 427–87.
3. Jesionek A, Von Tappeiner H. Behandlung der hautcarcinome nut fluorescierenden stoffen. Dtsch Arch Klin Med. 1905;85:223–7.
4. Hausman W. Die sensibilisierende wirkung des hamatoporphyrins. Biochem Zeit 1911;30:276–316.
5. Meyer-Betz F. Untersuchungen uber die bioloische (photodynamische) wirkung des hamatoporphyrins und anderer derivative des blut-und gallenfarbstoffs. Dtsch Arch Klin Med. 1913;112:476–503.
6. Auler H, Banzer G. Untersuchungen ueber die rolle der porphyrine bei geschwulstkranken menschen und tieren. Z Krebsforsch. 1942;53:65–8.
7. Figge FHJ, Weiland GS, Manganiello LDJ. Cancer detection and therapy. Affinity of neoplastic embryonic and traumatized tissue for porphyrins and metalloporphyrins. Proc Soc Exp Biol Med. 1948;68:640.
8. Dougherty TJ, Kaufman JE, Goldfarb A, Weishaupt KR, Boyle D, Mittleman A. Photoradiation therapy for the treatment of malignant tumors. Cancer Res. 1978;38:2628–35.
9. Kennedy JC, Pottier RH, Pross DC. Photodynamic therapy with endogenous protoporphyrin IX: basic principles and present clinical experiences. J Photochem Photobiol B. 1990;6:143–8.
10. Gold MH, Goldman MP. 5-Aminolevulinic acid photodynamic therapy: where we have been and where we are going. Dermatol Surg. 2004;30:1077–84.

Aminolevulinic Acid: Actinic Keratosis and Photorejuvenation

2

Melanie Palm and Mitchel P. Goldman

Abstract

ALA-PDT is a safe and effective treatment for nonhyperkeratotic lesions. Although FDA-approved for use with a blue light source, other laser and light sources have demonstrated promise in the treatment of actinic keratosis during PDT. Shorter incubation times maintain AK clearance rates but decrease the occurrence of phototoxic adverse events. With careful patient selection, ALA-PDT allows selective field treatment of precancerous skin lesions with improvement in overall photodamage. Patient satisfaction is high and cosmetic results can be excellent.

Aminolevulinic acid (ALA) was the first photosensitizer prodrug to be FDA-approved for use in topical photodynamic therapy (PDT). Since its approval over a decade ago, many aspects of ALA-PDT have been examined. Studies investigating the treatment of nonhyperkeratotic actinic keratosis (AK) with ALA-PDT have led to advances in treatment. Incubation times of ALA have decreased, multiple light sources have been used to elicit the reaction, and cosmetic benefits of treatment have been discovered. In the discussion that follows, background on ALA-PDT is provided. In addition, clinical studies regarding the treatment of AKs and photorejuvenation are summarized. Finally, a practical guide for treatment is provided for the reader to optimize treatment while avoiding common pitfalls of treatment.

M. Palm (✉)
Surfside Dermatology, Encinitas, CA, USA
e-mail: melanie.palm@gmail.com

Mechanism of PDT

PDT Mechanism of Action

PDT involves the activation of a photosensitizer by light in the presence of an oxygen-rich environment. Topical PDT involves the application of ALA or its methylated derivative (MAL) to the skin for varying periods of time. This leads to the conversion of ALA to protoporphyrin IX (PpIX), an endogenous photactivating agent. PpIX accumulates in rapidly proliferating cells of premalignant and malignant lesions [1], as well as in melanin, blood vessels, and sebaceous glands [2]. Upon activation by a light source and in the presence of oxygen, the sensitizer (PpIX) is oxidized, a process called "photobleaching" [3]. During this process, free radical oxygen singlets are generated, leading to selective destruction of tumor cells by apoptosis without collateral damage to surrounding tissues [4, 5]. Selective destruction of malignant cells is due in part to their reduced ferrochetalase activity, leading to

M.H. Gold (ed.), *Photodynamic Therapy in Dermatology*,
DOI 10.1007/978-1-4419-1298-5_2, © Springer Science+Business Media, LLC 2011

excessive accumulation of intracellular PpIX [6]. Recent in vitro research suggests that any remaining malignant cells following PDT have reduced survival [7]. A detailed explanation of the mechanism of action in PDT is found in Chap. 1.

ALA

δ-5-ALA is a hydrophilic, low molecular weight molecule within the heme biosynthesis pathway [1, 8]. ALA is considered a prodrug [9]. In vivo, it is converted to PpIX, a photosensitizer in the PDT reaction. In the United States, ALA is available as a 20% topical solution manufactured under the name Levulan Kerastick (DUSA Pharmaceuticals, Inc., Wilmington, MA). FDA-approved since 1999, Levulan is used for the treatment of nonhyperkeratotic AKs in conjunction with a blue light source, such as the Blu-U (DUSA, Wilmington, MA) [10]. It is supplied as a cardboard tube housing two sealed glass ampules, one containing 354 mg of δ-ALA hydrochloride powder and the other 1.5 mL of solvent [6]. The separate components are mixed within the cardboard sleeve just prior to use.

Esters of ALA are lipophilic derivatives of the parent molecule. Their chemical structure provides increased lipophilicity, allowing superior penetration through cellular lipid bilayers compared to ALA [2, 11]. MAL may offer better tumor selectivity [11–14] and less pain [14, 15] during PDT with less patient discomfort [15] compared to ALA.

Light Irradiation

No standardized guidelines for the "optimal irradiance, wavelength and total dose characteristics for PDT" exist according to the British Dermatology group and the American Society of Photodynamic Therapy Board [9, 16, 17]. However, certain laser and light sources are predictably chosen for PDT activation. Their wavelengths correspond closely with the four absorption peaks along the porphyrin curve. The Soret band (400–410 nm), with a maximal absorption at 405–409 nm, is the highest peak along this curve for photoactivating PpIX. Smaller peaks designated as the "Q bands" exist at approximately 505–510, 540–545, 580–584, and 630–635 nm [1, 2, 8]. There are advantages and disadvantages to exploiting the wavebands in either the Soret or Q bands for PDT. The Soret band peak is 10 to 20-fold larger than the Q bands, and blue light sources are often used to activate PpIX within this portion of the porphyrin curve, targeting lesions up to 2 mm in depth [14]. Longer wavelengths found within the Q bands produce a red light that penetrates more deeply (5 mm into the skin) but necessitates higher energy requirements [1, 8].

Light Sources

Light sources used in PDT can be categorized in a variety of ways, including incoherent versus coherent sources, or by color (and wavelengths) emitted. Incoherent light is emitted as noncollimated light and is provided through broadband lamps, light emitting diodes (LEDs), and intense pulsed light (IPL) systems. Noncoherent light sources are easy to use, affordable, easily obtained, and portable due to their compact size [18]. The earliest uses in PDT were filtered slide projectors that emitted white light [1]. Metal halogen lamps such as the Curelight (Photocure, Oslo, Norway, 570–680 nm) are often employed in PDT as they provide an effective light source in a time, power, and cost-effective manner [1, 19]. In Europe, the PDT 1200 lamp (Waldmann Medizintechnik, VS-Schwennigen, Germany) gained in popularity, providing a unit with high power density emitting a circular field of light radiation from 600 to 800 nm [12, 19]. Short arc, tunable xenon lamps have also been used, emitting light radiation from 400 to 1,200 nm [12]. The only widely available fluorescent lamp used in conjunction with PDT is the Blu-U (DUSA, Wilmington, MA) with a peak emittance at 417 ± 5 nm. LEDs provide a narrower spectrum of light irradiation, usually in a 20–50 nm bandwidth via a compact, solid, but powerful semiconductor [1, 20]. LEDs are simple to operate and are typically small in size, emitting light from the UV to IR portion of the electromagnetic spectrum [20]. However, the diminutive size of most LED panels necessitates multiple rounds of light illumination to treat larger areas. IPL is yet another source of incoherent light, emitting a radiation spectrum from approximately 500 to 1,200 nm [20]. Cutoff filters allow customization of the delivered wavelengths. This light source is particularly useful in photorejuvenation, targeting pigment, blood vessels, and even collagen.

Lasers provide precise doses of light radiation. As collimated light sources, lasers deliver energy to target tissues at specific wavelengths chosen to mimic absorption peaks along the porphyrin curve. Lasers used in PDT include the tunable argon dye laser (blue-green light, 450–530 nm) [12], the copper vapor laser-pumped dye laser (510–578 nm), long-pulse pulsed dye lasers (PDL) (585–595 nm), the Nd:YAG KTP dye laser (532 nm), the gold vapor laser (628 nm), and solid-state diode lasers (630 nm) [19]. Although laser sources allow the physician to delivery light with exact specifications in terms of wavelength and fluence, the fluence rate should be kept in the range of 150–200 mW/cm^2 to avoid hyperthermic effects on tissue [1, 14]. In fact, there is evidence to support that cumulative light dose of greater than 40 J/cm^2 can deplete all available oxygen sources during the oxidation reaction, making higher doses of energy during PDT unnecessary [3].

Clinical Applications

Actinic Keratoses

Background and Epidemiology

Actinic keratoses (AK) are a premalignant skin condition, comprising the third most common reason and 14% of all dermatology office visits [21, 22]. Approximately 4 million Americans are diagnosed with AKs annually [23], and according to one Australian study, 60% of Caucasian Australians aged 40 or older develop this condition [24]. The prevalence of AKs within the US population ranges from 11 to 26% with the highest incidence in southern regions and older Caucasian patients [25].

The concern for untreated AKs is their rate of transformation to cutaneous squamous cell carcinoma (SCC). A small percentage of SCC metastasizes [26], and this is more likely in higher risk areas, such as mucous membranes (e.g., lips) [27]. The reported conversion rate of AK to SCC varies widely, estimated as 0.025–16% per lesion per year [28–32]. AKs may be considered an in situ SCC [33, 34], with AK resting on the precancerous end of a spectrum that leads toward invasive SCC. It has been suggested that the AK/SCC continuum be graded as "cutaneous intraepithelial neoplasia," in a manner analogous to cervical malignancy. Further histopathologic evidence supports the link between AKs and SCC. Both lesions express tumor markers including the tumor suppressor gene p53 [35] and over 90% of biopsied SCCs have adjacent AKs within the examined histopathologic field [36].

Clinical Presentation and Diagnosis

AKs typically appear as 1–3 mm slightly scaly plaques on an erythematous base, often on a background of solar damage. They are often detected more easily through palpation than visual detection [37], due to their hyperkeratotic nature. The surrounding skin often shows signs of moderate to severe photodamage, including dyspigmentation, telangiectasias, and sallow coloration due to solar elastosis (Fig. 2.1). Individual AK lesions may converge, creating larger contiguous lesions. Most AKs are subclincial and not readily apparent to visual or palpable examination. The evidence for subclinical AKs is their fluorescence when exposed to ALA + Wood's lamp or a specialized CCD camera [38].

Although often asymptomatic, AKs may have accompanying burning, pruritus, tenderness, or bleeding [22]. Several variants of AK exist, including nonhyperkeratotic (thin), hyperkeratotic, atrophic, lichenoid, verrucous, horn-like (cutaneous horn), and pigmented variants [25]. AKs on the lip, most often occurring on the lower

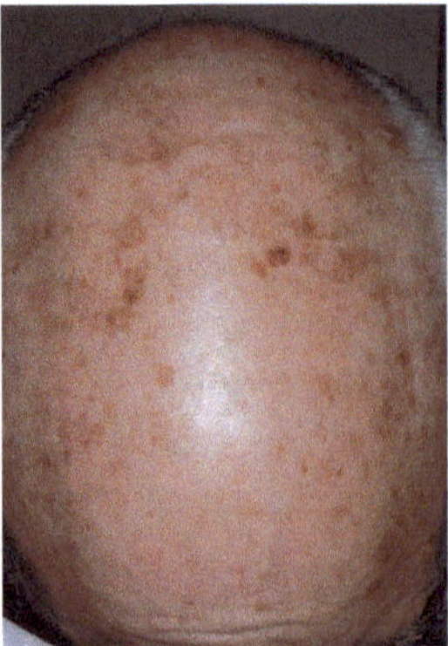

Fig. 2.1 Frontal scalp of a 71-year-old white male demonstrating moderate to severe photodamage. Numerous actinic keratoses characterized by erythematous scaly slightly elevated plaques are visible on a background of extensive solar lentigines

lip, are designated as actinic cheilitis [27]. As AKs often result from a long history of UV exposure, the lesions usually arise in heavily sun-exposed areas including the scalp, face, ears, lips, chest, dorsal hands, and extensor forearms [39]. Risk factors for AKs include fair skin (Fitzpatrick skin type I–III), history of extensive, cumulative sun exposure, increasing age, elderly males (due to UV exposure), history or arsenic exposure, and immunosuppression [21, 22].

Histopathology

Histopathologic examination of actinic keratoses is characterized by atypical keratinocytes and architectural disorder [22]. Early lesions demonstrate focal keratinocyte atypia originating at the basal layer of the epidermis and extending variably upward within the epidermis [40]. Hyperchromatic and pleomorphic nuclei and nuclear crowding characterize the cellular findings while architectural disorder is comprised of alternating ortho- and hyperkeratosis, hypogranulosis, and focal areas of downward budding in the basal layer of the epidermis [22, 25]. Solar elastosis is invariably present. Well-developed lesions may have apoptotic cells, mitotic figures, involvement of adnexal structures, lichenoid infiltrates, and a focal tendency toward full-thickness involvement (Fig. 2.2). Full-thickness atypia indicates transformation into SCC-in situ [25].

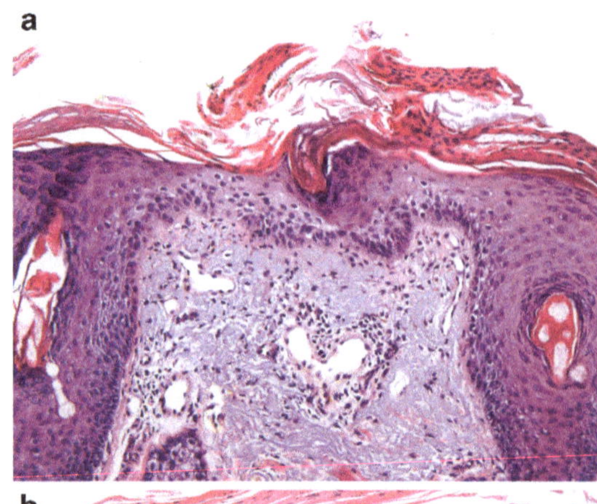

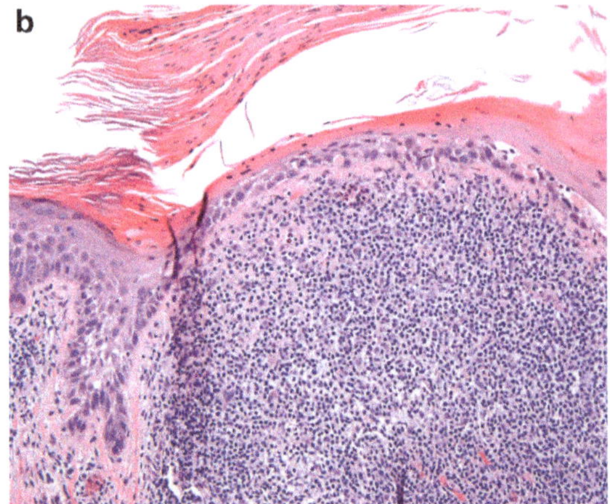

Fig. 2.2 (**a**) Histopathologic section of actinic keratosis stained with hematoxylin and eosin at 20× magnification. Lesion is characterized by alternating ortho- and hyperkeratosis with nuclear atypia and architectural disorder. Keratinocyte atypia approaches full-thickness in middle area of lesion. Note the gray, fragmented nature of the papillary dermis representing extensive solar elastosis. (**b**) Actinic keratosis, lichenoid variant. A brisk lympocytic infiltrate in the papillary dermis accompanies cytologic atypia of epidermal keratinocytes and marked architectural disorder. Numerous apoptotic cells are visible within the epidermis (Courtesy of Wenhua Liu, MD, Consolidated Pathology Consultants, Inc., Libertyville, IL)

Treatment Rationale

Treatment Options for AKs. Given the premalignant potential of AKs, and the metastatic potential of SCC, early treatment is paramount to preventing disease progression. Treatment options for AKs depend on a variety of factors including severity of involvement, duration or persistence of lesions, patient tolerability or desire for cosmesis, affordability/insurance coverage, and physician comfort with available treatment modalities [22, 32].

Although AKs can reliably be diagnosed by clinical examination alone [41], a low threshold for biopsy should be exercised on atypical lesions, or lesions not responsive to prior treatment.

While singular or few lesions may be approached with local, surgical treatment such as cryotherapy, curettage, excision, or dermabrasion, field treatment may be more appropriate when numerous lesions are identified. In addition, field therapy will treat subclinical AKs. Chemical peels, laser resurfacing, 5-fluorouracil (5-FU), topical diclofenac, topical retinoids, and topical immunomodulators (imiquimod) are all reasonable treatment options in addition to PDT.

A comparison of PDT to other field treatment options for AKs yields comparable clearance rates [42, 43]. In fact, a comparison of 100% clearance rates from phase III clinical trials reported complete AK clearance with ALA-PDT of 72%, comparable to 5-FU (72%), and superior to imiquimod (49%) and diclofenac (48%) [23]. A direct comparison study by Kurwa et al. [44] found comparable lesion area reduction rates between ALA-PDT (73%) and 5-FU (70%).

Advantages/Disadvantages of ALA-PDT for AKs

Clearance rates of AKs following PDT has ranged from 68 to 98% [45, 46]. Assuming near equivalent or even superior clearance rates of PDT compared to other field treatment options, PDT has several advantages in the treatment of AKs. Improvement of photodamage, superior cosmesis, and better patient satisfaction were documented in two studies by Szeimies et al. [43] and Goldman and Atkin [46]. Other procedures used for the clearance of AKs such as cryotherapy or chemical peels can result in hypopigmentation or even scarring [43, 47]. PDT, perhaps surprisingly to some, is a cost-effective means of treating AKs. Gold found ALA-PDT with a blue light source to be the least expensive treatment option for AKs compared to 5-FU, imiquimod, and diclofenac. In fact, ALA-PDT was approximately one-half the cost of a similar course of imiquimod for field AK treatment [23]. Additionally, PDT accomplished field treatment of precancerous lesions including subclinical ones [47].

Disadvantages of PDT are largely related to minor and expected adverse events following the procedure. Minor pain and erythema may occur during or following the procedure. Mild crusting and edema may occur, lasting up to 1 week. However, other treatment modalities for AKs have similar if not longer recovery periods. There are financial costs associated with the procedure. If PDT is performed for AK treatment and photorejuvenation, there is an associated out-of-pocket cost to the patient. The physician must also make an initial investment in the laser and light devices, although many of the light sources have multiple applications beyond PDT.

Treatment Results of ALA-PDT for AKs

Kennedy et al. [48], in 1990, was the first to exploit the use of topical 5-ALA in the treatment of nonmelanoma skin cancers. Using a 20% ALA compound and a filtered slide projector for a light source, a complete response rate of 90% was achieved in patients with AKs. Since this initial study, a variety of light sources have been investigated for use in PDT for the treatment of AKs. As the PDT reaction is activated from an emission spectra ranging from 400 to 800 nm [49], we have organized clinical studies according to the light source used. Table 2.1 provides a summary of peer-reviewed articles on the use of ALA-PDT in AK treatment.

Violet Light. A relatively recent study published by Dijkstra et al. [49] in 2001 investigated the use of violet light in ALA-PDT. The use of this emission spectrum was based on the premise that violet light was ten times more effective than red light in photosensitization with ALA [49]. A study population of 38 patients with varying skin conditions including BCC (2 patients with Gorlin–Goltz syndrome), Bowen's disease, and actinic keratoses were treated. A 20% ALA gel was applied to lesions for 8 hours under occlusion. Photoactivation followed using a lamp with a cold glass filter, emitting a spectrum of light between 400 and 450 nm. The sample size of AKs in this study was extremely small ($n=4$), making conclusions about violet light in ALA-PDT difficult. A clearance rate for the four AKs treated

Table 2.1 Published clinical studies on ALA-PDT for AKs

References	ALA preparation	Location of AKs	Incubation period (hours)	# Lesions treated (# patients)	Light source (wavelength in nm)	Response rate	Follow-up (months)
Kennedy et al. [48]	20% Emulsion	Not specified	3–6	10	Tungsten (>600)	90% CR	18
Wolf et al. [5]	20% Emulsion	Face and scalp	4–8	9	Tungsten, unfiltered	100% CR	3–12
Calzavara-Pinton et al. [1]	20% Cream	Face	6–8	50 (From pool of 85 patients with AKs, BCCs, SCCs, Bowen's)	Argon dye laser (630)	100% CR	24–36
Morton et al. [85]	20% Emulsion	Face and scalp	4	4	Xenon (630)	100% CR	12
Fijan et al. [86]	20% Emulsion	Not specified	20, Occluded	43 (9)	Halogen (570–690)	81% CR	3–20
Szeimies et al. [87]	10% Emulsion	Head, hands, arms	6, Occluded	36 (10)	Waldmann red lamp (580–740)	71% CR head	1
Fink-Puches et al. [61]	20% Emulsion	Head, neck, forearms, dorsal hands	4, Occluded	251 (28)	Halogen slide projector (300–800) with cutoff filters at 515, 530, 570, 610	71% CR	36
Fritsch et al. [54]	10% Ointment	Face and scalp	6, Occluded	(6)	Green lamp (543–548) vs. red Waldmann lamp (570–750)	100% CR for both green and red light	15
Jeffes et al. [56]	0–30% Emulsion	Face, scalp, trunk, extremities	3, Occluded	240 (40)	Argon dye laser (630)	91% CR face and scalp; 45% CR trunk and extremities	2
Karrer et al. [57]	20% Emulsion	Scalp, face	6, Occluded	200 (24)	Red light lamp (580–740) or PDL (585)	84% CR (red light) 79% CR (PDL)	1
Kurwa et al. [44]	20% Emulsion	Hands	4, Occluded	(14)	Metal halide lamp (580–740)	73% Lesion area reduction; comparable to 5-fluorouracil (5-FU)	6
Itoh et al. [58]	20% Emulsion, two or more sessions	Face, neck, extremities	4, Occluded	53 (10)	Red lamp (peak 630, range 600–700), excimer dye laser (630)	82% CR face and neck; 56% CR extremities	12
Dijkstra et al. [49]	20% Gel, two sessions	Unspecified	8, Occluded	4	Violet lamp (400–450)	50% CR	3–12
Jeffes et al. [42]	20% Solution	Face, scalp	14–18	70 (36)	Blue light (417)	85% CR	4

Markham and Collins [21]	% Concentration unspecified, cream	Scalp	4, Occluded	(4)	Red light (580–740)	75% CR	6
Varma et al. [59]	20% Ointment	Not specified	4, Occluded	127 (88 Patients with mixed diagnoses)	Waldmann red lamp (580–740)	77% CR after first, 99% after second, RR of 28%	6
Ruiz-Rodriguez et al. [65]	20% Emulsion	Face, scalp	4, Occluded	38	IPL (590–1,200)	76% CR one session; 91% CR two sessions	3
Alexiades-Amenakas and Geronemus [47]	20% Solution	Head, extremities, trunk	3 with Occlusion; 14–18 without occlusion	3,622 (36)	Long-pulsed PDL (595)	90–100% CR	8
Clark et al. [19]	20% Ointment	Not specified	4	23	Metal halide (590–730); Halogen lamp (570–680), diode laser (630)	91% CR	11
Goldman and Atkin [46]	20% Solution	Face, long-incubation PDT	15–20	(32)	Blue light (417)	94% CR of AKs; improved skin texture, pigmentation	3–6
Smith et al. [55]	20% Solution, two sessions	Face, scalp	1	(35)	Blue light (417) or PDL (595)	80% CR for blue light; 60% CR for PDL	1
Dragieva et al. [80]	20% Emulsion; transplant patients	Face, scalp	5, Occluded	32 (20)	Red light (580–740)	94% CR at 4 weeks; 72% at 48 weeks	12
Piacquadio et al. [52]	20% Solution, one to two sessions	Face, scalp	14–18	1,402 (243)	Blue (417)	91% CR one session; 83% CR two sessions	3
Touma et al. [6]	20% Solution	Face	1–3	(17)	Blue lamp (417)	87–94% CR	5
Gilbert [63]	20% Solution, 5-FU daily × 5 days pre-PDT	Face	0.5–0.75	(15)	IPL (560–1,200)	90% CR with combination therapy	12
Kim et al. [62]	20% Emulsion	Face	4, Occluded	12 (7)	IPL (555–950)	50%	3
Tschen et al. [41]	20% Solution, (one to two treatment sessions)	Face, scalp	14–18	968 (110)	Blue (417)	72–76% CR one session; 86% two sessions	12
Nakano et al. [17]	20% Cream (three treatment sessions)	Face	4, Occluded	(30)	Excimer dye laser (630)	100% CR in lesions <10 mm; 70% CR in lesions >10 mm diameter	12

with two sessions of PDT was 50% [49]. Although other lesions in the study had a more favorable clearance rate, further studies are needed to draw conclusions on the usefulness of violet light in PDT for precancerous skin lesions.

Blue Light. Perhaps the most popular emission spectrum used in the United States, blue light remains the only FDA-approved form of light for activating ALA (Fig. 2.3). As a result, numerous published studies exist on the use of blue light in ALA-PDT not only for the treatment of AKs, but also for other skin conditions responsive to this treatment modality. The relatively shorter wavelength of blue light only penetrates 1–2 mm but is potent in its photochemical effect, therefore blue light is often selected for the treatment of superficial lesions such as nonhyperkeratotic AK lesions [50].

In 2001, Jeffes et al. [42] published the results of a multicenter, phase II study of ALA-PDT using blue light (417 nm). A 14- to 18-hours incubation was used on AK lesions of the face and scalp in 36 patients. A total of 70 lesions were treated. Light exposure duration was 16 minutes and 40 seconds, now considered standard of treatment. At 8 weeks following a single treatment, 88% of lesions cleared. Due to the extended time of incubation, an increased rate of phototoxic-related side effects was observed. These adverse effects included erythema and edema. A second phase II study was conducted with the same protocol, this time in a total of 64 patients [51]. All of the patients had 75% or more clearance of AK lesions following one treatment. However, 14% of patients required reduced power density during blue light irradiation due to intolerable side effects including stinging and burning. A final phase II study was a dose-ranging study of ALA solution from concentrations of 2.5–30% ALA. Clearance of AKs occurred in a dose-dependent manner, and a 20% concentration was selected as the most ideal concentration for use in ALA-PDT with blue light [51].

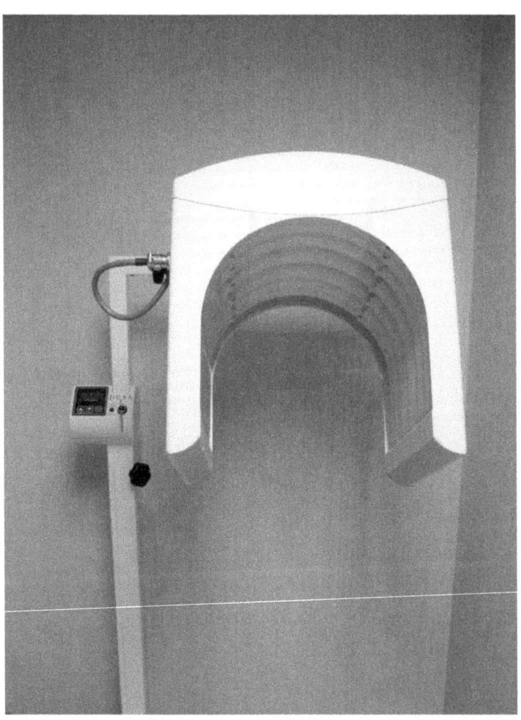

Fig. 2.3 Noncoherent blue lamp is a common choice for photoactivating aminolevulinic acid (ALA) in the United States. The Blu-U (DUSA Pharmaceuticals, Inc., Wilmington, MA) emits light at a bandwidth of approximately 417 ± 5 nm (Courtesy of DUSA Pharmaceuticals, Inc., Wilmington, MA)

Piacquadio et al. [52] followed in 2004, publishing the results of a phase III clinical trial. The same long incubation and illumination times were used as in the phase II trial. A total of 243 patients with nonhyperkeratotic AKs were treated. Complete clearance at 12 weeks following one PDT session was 70%. A second treatment resulted in a complete clearance rate of 88%. Facial lesions responded more favorably than scalp lesions, with complete response rates of 78 and 50%, respectively, at week 12 following treatment. In terms of patient feedback, 94% of patients rated their cosmetic outcome following PDT as good or excellent. A recurrence rate analysis for this treatment cohort between 8 and 12 weeks post-treatment was 5% [51].

Several other studies examining the use of blue light in ALA-PDT for the treatment of nonhyperkeratotic AKs followed. In 2002, Gold [53] reported on facial AKs treated with blue light PDT. The response rate was favorable with 83% clearance. A separate study by Goldman and Atkin [46] demonstrated similar results. In both studies, photorejunative effects on the treated areas of the skin were noted.

In 2004, Touma et al. [6] reported on the efficacy of short-contact ALA-PDT. Not only did this allow for PDT to be conducted in a single clinic visit rather than over 2 days, but side effects related to the longer 14–18 h incubations were reduced. In this study, 17 patients with AKs of the face and scalp were treated with ALA using incubation times of 1, 2, or 3 h. A clearance rate of 93, 84, and 90% were achieved in the 1-, 2-, and 3-hour incubation groups, respectively. Clearance rates were maintained through 5 months of follow-up. In addition, this was the second study with blue light to demonstrate a modest but significant improvement in photoaging.

Work by Tschen et al. [41] confirmed earlier findings. This phase IV study of 101 patients with 6–12 AKs used a 14–18 hour ALA incubation time. After the first PDT, a complete clearance of 72–76% was observed, which increased to 86% with a second treatment.

Green Light. One study by Fritsch et al. [54] used a green light source for the treatment of AKs with ALA-PDT. The focus of this study was on patient discomfort. Compared to a red light source, light irradiation with a green light source (543–548 nm) was less painful in the treatment of facial AKs during PDT.

Yellow-Orange Light: PDL. Long-PDL (585–595 nm) (Fig. 2.4) target the chromophore oxyhemoglobin, allowing selective destruction of blood vessels. As actinic keratoses often appear as erythematous scaly plaques, the inflammatory nature of these lesions can be targeted with this vascular laser. Alexiades-Amenakas and Geronemus [47] were the first to report on its use in ALA-PDT. Thirty-six patients and a total of 3,622 lesions were treated. Location of lesions included the face and scalp (2,620 lesions), extremities (949), and trunk (53). ALA was applied with either a 3 hour, unoccluded incubation versus a 14–18 hour incubation. No difference in clearance was observed between the two incubation time groups. Clearance rates were highest for head lesions at 100%. According to this large cohort study, it appeared that PDL at subpurpuric doses allows an efficient and less painful means of accomplishing PDT.

In 2003, Smith et al. [55] published a three-arm study on 36 patients with AKs. One arm received treatment with low concentration 5-FU, the other two arms received ALA-PDT – using either a PDL or blue light for photoactivation. A short, 1 hour unoccluded incubation was used. Clearance rates at 4 weeks follow-up were similar for 5-FU and ALA-PDL (79% vs. 80%). Clearance rates of PDT using a blue light source were lower (60%). Additionally, improvements in global photodamage, hyperpigmentation, and tactile roughness were observed [55].

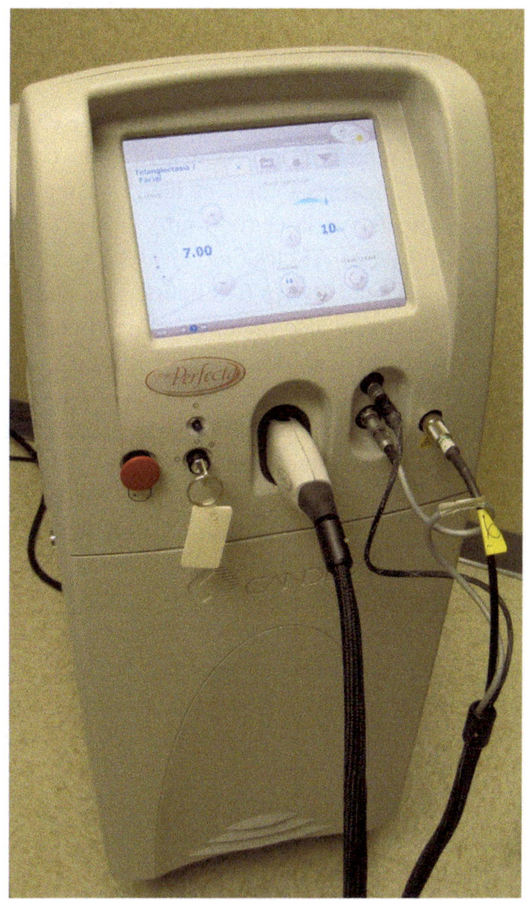

Fig. 2.4 Pulsed dye lasers (PDL) may be used as a light source for ALA-PDT to target individual lesions including AKs, sebaceous hyperplasia, and solar lentigines (Vbeam Perfecta [595 nm] laser image printed courtesy of Candela Corporation, Wayland, MA)

Red Light Sources. The longer wavelength of red light allows deeper tissue penetration. Red light is used frequently during PDT with MAL. Red light may also be used for photoactivation of PpIX during ALA-PDT. Several laser and light sources emit wavelengths in the red light spectrum, usually targeted around 630 nm. These include the argon pumped dye laser, excimer laser, metal halide lamps, and red LED lamps.

Red Light from Laser Sources. One of the earliest studies reporting on ALA-PDT was completed by Calzavara-Pinton et al. [1] using an argon pumped dye laser (630 nm). In the treatment of 50 facial AK lesions, 20% ALA cream was applied topically for 6–8 hours. The study's patient population also included a mixed pool of 85 total patients with diagnoses of Bowen's disease, SCCs, BCCs, and AKs. In terms of AK outcomes, a clearance rate of 100% was achieved at 24–36 months posttreatment.

The initial phase I clinical study for FDA-approval of ALA in PDT also utilized an argon pumped dye laser. Thirty-nine of the forty enrolled patients completed the dose-ranging study. Jeffes et al. [56] used 0–30% ALA topically with an extended incubation time of 14–18 hours. Ninety-one percent clearance was obtained in thin to well-developed AKs on the face and scalp that were treated with 30% ALA. Extremity treatment was not as successful with only 45% clearance of AKs on the limbs. Hyperkeratotic AKs did not respond well to therapy, and the small number of treated hyperkeratotic lesions precluded statistical analysis.

Recently, Nakano et al. [17] reported on the use of an excimer laser (630 nm) in patients of darker skin types. Thirty Japanese patients with AKs were divided into two groups based on lesion appearance. The first group included subjects with AK lesions 10 mm or less in diameter with the second group including larger lesions greater than 10 mm in diameter. Patients received three ALA-PDT sessions weekly for 3 weeks. A clinical and histological clearance of 100% was obtained in the small AK lesions group during the 1-year follow-up period. In the cohort with larger AK lesions, 6 of the 20 patients experienced residual lesions or recurrence. These findings are consistent with the poor penetration of ALA through thicker, hyperkeratotic lesions and resulting lower AK clearance rates.

Incoherent Red Light Sources. Metal halide lamps emitting a spectrum of light from 580 to 740 nm have been used in numerous ALA-PDT studies. Using the Waldmann/PDT 1200 lamp, 36 lesions in 10 patients were treated topically with ALA for 6 hours under occlusion followed by red light irradiation. On 28th day following treatment, the clearance of face and scalp lesions was 71%. Patient experienced pain and burning and mild postprocedure erythema.

Several studies followed shortly thereafter reporting clearance rates of facial AKs between 77 and 99%. Karrer et al. [57] treated 24 patients and 200 scalp and facial lesions with a clearance rate of 84% at 1 month following PDT. Kurwa et al. [44] used a metal halide lamp for ALA-PDT to treat the dorsal hands, resulting in a 79.5% decrease in AKs lesions. Itoh et al. [58] treated Japanese patients with AKs on the face, neck, and extremities. With two or more treatments, clearance rates at 12 months were higher for lesions on the head and neck (81.8%) compared with the extremities (55.6%). No serious adverse effects were reported in these patients with darker skin types. Markham and Collins [21] treated four patients with topical ALA under occlusion for 4 hours for scalp AKs. Three patients cleared following treatment, and the remaining patient had significant improvement at 6 months. Varma et al. [59] treated 88 patients with ALA-PDT using a red lamp for a variety of diagnoses including AKs (127 lesions), Bowen's disease (50), and superficial BCC (62). Complete clearance rate for AKs after one and two treatments were 77 and 99%, respectively. However, the recurrence rate at 12 months was 28%. Mild stinging, tingling, or burning was reported by most patients. Another study also treated patients of mixed diagnoses. AKs, BCC, and SCC-in situ in 762 patients were treated by Moseley et al. [60]. Ninety-two percent of AKs cleared after two treatments, with 100% clearance after three PDT sessions. Finally, Clark et al. [19], using a topical 20% ointment, treated 207 patients with 483 lesions. An impressive 91% clearance was observed clinically at a median of 48 weeks following treatment.

Broad Band/Visible Light Sources. The earliest light sources used for the treatment of AKs during the modern PDT era produced unfiltered, noncollimated light for photoactivation. Following the work by Kennedy et al. [48], Wolf et al. [5] in 1993 reported on the complete clearance of nine AKs after one round of treatment using a slide projector for a light source. Fink-Puches et al. [61] used a modified halogen slide projector with four filter cutoffs at 515, 530, 570, and 610 nm. AK lesions of the head, neck, forearms, and dorsal hand lesions were treated with 20% ALA for 4 hours under occlusion prior to light irradiation. Overall complete response after one treatment was 64%, increasing to 85% with a second treatment. Head and neck lesions responded better than extremity lesions. Head and neck complete response rates varied from 93 to 100% depending on the spectrum of light used for treatment. Forearms and hands had a lower response rate ranging from 33 to 53%. Overall complete response rate at 36 months was 23% for filtered light and 71% for full spectrum light.

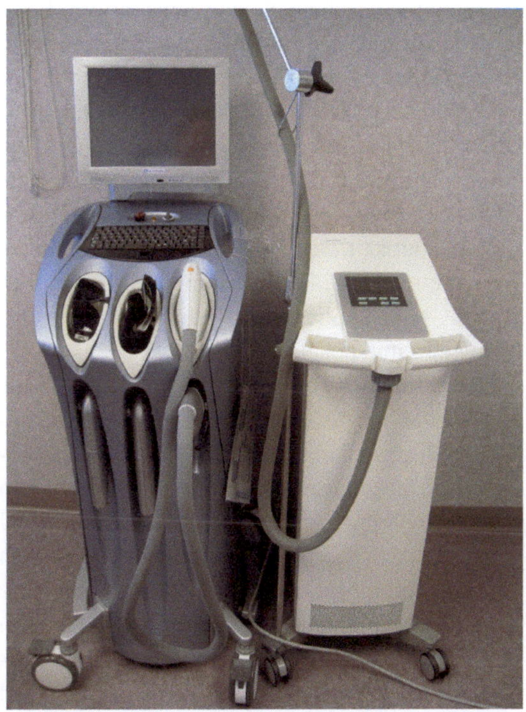

Fig. 2.5 Intense pulsed light (IPL) devices are particularly effective in ALA-PDT for photorejuvenation. Cooled conductive gel and forced air cooling units minimize discomfort during treatment (Lumenis One IPL device courtesy of Lumenis, Inc., Santa Clara, CA)

IPL devices (Fig. 2.5) are powerful tools for treating the signs of photoaging. Their use in photorejuventation with ALA-PDT is discussed in a separate section of this chapter. However, a small study by Kim et al. [62] documented the use of ALA-IPL for the treatment of AKs exclusively. Twelve facial AK lesions in seven patients were treated with one session of ALA-PDT. At 12 weeks follow-up, 50% of lesions cleared. This clearance rate is markedly lower than reported averages, but it is difficult to formulate sound conclusions based on the small sample size.

Combination Therapy for AK Treatment

Several small case studies have demonstrated a possible synergistic effect of ALA-PDT with other treatment options for AKs. Combination 5-FU cream with PDT was tested in a study by Gilbert [63]. Fifteen patients with multiple AKs completed a 5-day course of nightly 5-FU cream to the face followed by short-contact PDT activated by an IPL light source. A clearance rate of 90% was observed at 1 year follow-up. Shaffelburg [64] conducted a split-face study of 24 patients with multiple AKs, in which ALA-PDT was performed on the entire face. One-half of the face was also randomized to receive additional subsequent treatment with a 12-week regimen of imiquimod. Clearance rates at 12 months were superior on the combination treatment side, with 89.9% complete lesion clearance compared with 74.5% on the ALA-PDT treatment side alone.

Photorejuvenation

Definition of Photoaging

Photodamage is a marker of cumulative ultraviolet exposure and senescent changes to the skin. Not only can the appearance be of concern to the patient, but it can also lead to pre-cancerous conditions with the development of actinic keratoses [65]. The characteristic appearance of photodamaged skin includes sallow discoloration, inelasticity, rhytid formation, pigmentary alteration, ecstatic vessels/telangiectasias, and textural alterations [18]. Global photodamage scales have been developed for scoring the severity of skin involvement. Dover used a

5-point scale in evaluating several categories of photodamage including fine surface lines, mottled pigmentation, sallowness, tactile roughness, coarse wrinkling, and global photodamage [66]. Working from this initial scale, others have added facial erythema, telangiectasias, sebaceous gland hyperplasia, and facial AKs as separate categories in the evaluation of photodamage [67, 68].

Light Sources in ALA-PDT Photorejuvenation

Many of the same lasers and light sources effective in ALA-PDT for the treatment of AKs have the added benefit of inducing photorejunative effects on the skin. Chromophores targeted during PDT treatment may include vessels, melanin, and even collagen [67]. Blue light only allows for a photochemical effect in PDT with less tissue penetration than other light sources such as IPL and PDL. The latter sources penetrate deeply enough to target vessels, pigment, and collagen [69]. The choice of which light source to use for ALA-PDT ultimately depends on such factors as the condition being treated, efficacy, cost of use, and availability of equipment.

Treatment Results of ALA-PDT in Photorejuvenation

Studies relating to the treatment of photodamage with ALA-PDT are organized in the section below according to the light source employed. A summary of these studies is provided in Table 2.2.

PDT with Blue Light. Despite the shallow penetration of blue light, it still appears to improve the signs of photoaging following ALA-PDT. The first indication that blue light had photorejuvenative effects in PDT was with the phase II/III clinical trials for FDA-approval of Levulan for nonhyperkeratotic AKs. In these studies, significant improvement in the signs of photoaging was noted after treatment [42, 52, 70].

Photorejuvenation studies using the blue light source have also been conducted by Goldman and Atkin [46], where a blue light source was used to illuminate the face after the topical application of ALA. Thirty-two patients with photodamage and AKs were treated with one session of ALA-PDT using a 1-h ALA incubation followed by Blu-U activation. AKs showed a 90% improvement in terms of photorejuvenation parameters, a 72% improvement in skin texture, and a 59% improvement in skin pigmentation. Gold [53] reported on the dual use of blue light ALA-PDT for AKs and photoaging. The treatment of nonhyperkeratotic facial AKs also resulted in an improvement of skin elasticity and texture in patients with photodamaged skin.

Touma et al. [6] studied the effectiveness of ALA and blue light illumination in the treatment of AKs and diffuse photodamage. Eighteen patients with facial non-hypertrophic AKs and mild to moderate facial photodamage were evaluated. Short-contact ALA was applied from 1 to 3 hours with subsequent exposure to blue light. At 1 and 5 month follow-up intervals, there was a significant reduction in AKs. In addition, marked improvement in photodamage parameters such as skin quality, fine wrinkling, and sallowness were observed. Other markers of photodamage, such as pigmentary changes and coarse wrinkling showed little to no improvement. Patients were also satisfied with the procedure, with 80% of patients rating their results as good to excellent. Other findings make this an intriguing study. This clinical study was pivotal in shifting treatment of AKs from long, 14–18 hour incubation times to shorter contact times. In addition, study patients were pretreated with microdermabrasion prior to topical ALA application, leading to more uniform and rapid penetration of ALA.

A final study by Smith et al. [55] examined the use of blue light ALA-PDT in diffuse photodamage. As discussed in the section "Actinic Keratoses (AK)" of this chapter, this study was a three-arm study comparing topical, low concentration 5-FU to two forms of short-contact ALA-PDT – one arm with activation from a blue light source, the other with a PDL. While one patient in the 5-FU group discontinued due to a confluent erythematous reaction, all patients in the ALA-PDT group completed the study. In both ALA-PDT groups, patients experienced improvement in global photodamage, hyperpigmentation, and tactile roughness. The ALA-PDL was more successful in treating pigmentation, while blue light had lower response

Table 2.2 Published clinical studies on ALA-PDT for photorejuvenation

References	ALA preparation	Location of photodamage/study design	Incubation period (hours)	# Patients	Light source (emission λ, nm)	Response	Follow-up (months)
Ruiz-Rodriguez et al. [65]	20% Emulsion	Face and scalp, more than or equal to one AK and chronic photodamage; two PDT sessions	4, Occluded	17 (38 AKs)	IPL (590–1,200)	87% CR of AKs; excellent cosmesis	3
Goldman and Atkin [46]	20% Solution	Face, long-incubation PDT	15–20	32	Blue light (417)	94% CR of AKs; improved skin texture, pigmentation	3–6
Smith et al. [55]	20% Solution, two sessions	Face, scalp	1	35	Blue light (417) or PDL (595)	80% CR for AKs with blue light; 60% CR for PDL; both demonstrated improvement in global photodamage, tactile roughness, and hyperpigmentation	1
Touma et al. [6]	20% Solution	Facial AK and mild–moderate photodamage	1–3	17	Blue light (417)	Improvement in photo-damage markers, including skin quality, fine rhytides, and sallowness	1–5
Avram and Goldman [74]	20% Solution	Facial photodamage (with AKs) treated with one ALA-IPL session	1	17	IPL	69% CR of AKs; improvement in telangiectasias, dyspigmentation, skin texture	3
Alster et al. [75]	20% Solution	Split-face comparison, IPL vs. ALA-IPL	1–3	10	IPL (500–1,200)	ALA-IPL treated side showed greater improvement	6
Dover et al. [66]	20% Solution	Split-face comparison, IPL vs. ALA-IPL (five treatment sessions)	0.5–1	20	IPL (515–1,200)	Greater improvement in ALA-IPL over IPL only for global photoaging, pigmentation, and fine lines only	1

(continued)

Table 2.2 (continued)

References	ALA preparation	Location of photodamage/study design	Incubation period (hours)	# Patients	Light source (emission λ, nm)	Response	Follow-up (months)
Key [78]	20% Solution	Face, subpurpuric doses of PDL	1	12	PDL (585)	Improvement in majority of photodamage parameters with ALA-PDL; no improvement with PDL alone	1
Lowe and Lowe [72]	5–20% Cream	Forearm, periorbital	0.5–2	6	Red light (633)	Mild improvement noted in photoaging	0.25
Marmur et al. [76]	20% Solution	Split-face comparison, IPL vs. ALA-IPL (1 treatment)	1	7	IPL	Microscopic changes demonstrated greater type I collagen on ALA-IPL side	N/A
Gold et al. [68]	20% Solution	Split-face comparison, IPL vs. ALA-IPL (three treatment sessions)	0.5–1	16	IPL (550/570 cutoff filters-1,200)	ALA-IPL results superior to IPL alone	1–3
Serrano et al. [77]	1–2% Gel	Multiple application, low concentration ALA-PDT to face, neck, hands (three treatment sessions)	0.5–1	8/26 Patients with photoaging; 18/26 treated for acne, vitiligo	IPL (530–1,200) or yellow-red lamp (550–630)	90% of cases with hyperpigmentation improvement; erythema (85%), skin texture (100%)	6

rates to global photoaging. Interestingly, the blue light ALA-PDT was the only treatment arm to have photoaging completely resolve in one patient.

PDT with Red Light. Two of the three studies regarding red light PDT for the treatment of photoaging used MAL rather than ALA. These studies by Szeimies et al. [43] and Pariser et al. [71] demonstrated excellent cosmetic results and are discussed in Chap. 16.

One small pilot study conducted by Lowe and Lowe [72] investigated the use of ALA-PDT for the treatment of photoaging on the forearm and periorbital region. Escalating concentrations of ALA (5–20%) and increasing incubation times (30–120 min) were used prior to light irradiation with a red light source (633 nm). Mild improvement in signs of photoaging was noted at 7 days following treatment.

PDT with IPL. IPL is a light source that emits noncollimated, noncoherent light with wavelengths in the range of 515–1,200 nm, which corresponds to the visible light and near-infrared spectrum [20]. Various filters can be used to block certain wavelengths below the cut-off point of the desired filter. IPL treatments improve many of the signs of photoaging, including pigmentation in the form of solar lentigines, erythema, and telangiectasias due to vascular ectasia/damage, as well as fine wrinkling [20]. Like the PDL, IPL treatments also promotes neocollagenesis [73]. Although IPL alone has been proven effective in the treatment of photodamage, the addition of ALA to IPL treatment (ALA-IPL) appears to be more effective in treating photodamaged skin. Clinical examples of ALA-IPL treatment for photorejuvenation are illustrated in Figs. 2.6 and 2.7.

In 2002, Ruiz-Rodriguez et al. [65] investigated the treatment of photodamage and AKs using ALA-PDT with IPL as the light source for photorejuvenation. Seventeen patients with various degrees of photodamage and AKs (38 AKs total) underwent therapy with ALA-IPL. A total of two treatments were performed 1 month apart. Treatments were well-tolerated. At 3 months follow-up, 87% of AKs disappeared and marked cosmetic improvement was noted in wrinkling, coarse skin texture, pigmentary changes, and telangiectasias.

Multiple studies followed the initial results of Ruiz-Rodriguez and coworkers. Avram and Goldman [74] evaluated the combined use of ALA-IPL for the treatment of photorejuvenation with

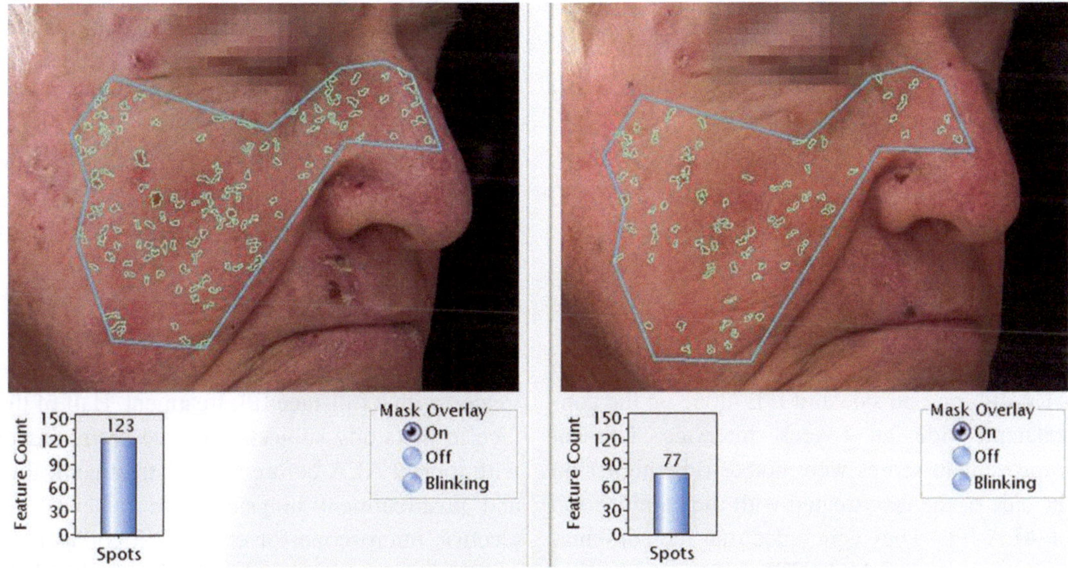

Fig. 2.6 Complexion analysis of the right cheek of a white male before and after one ALA-PDT session for photorejuvenation. A 47% decrease in *brown spots* (solar lentigines) was quantified using the computer software system

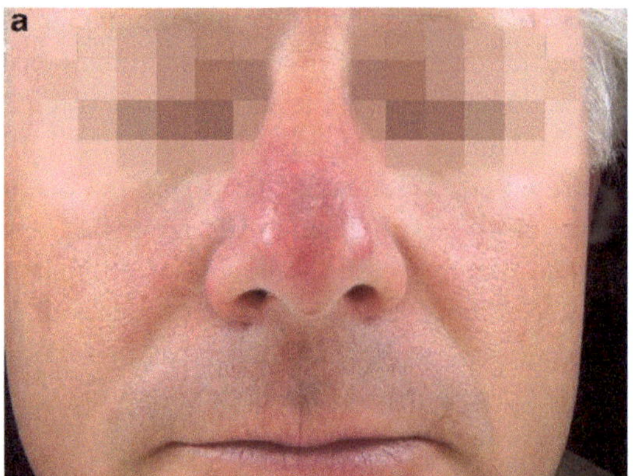

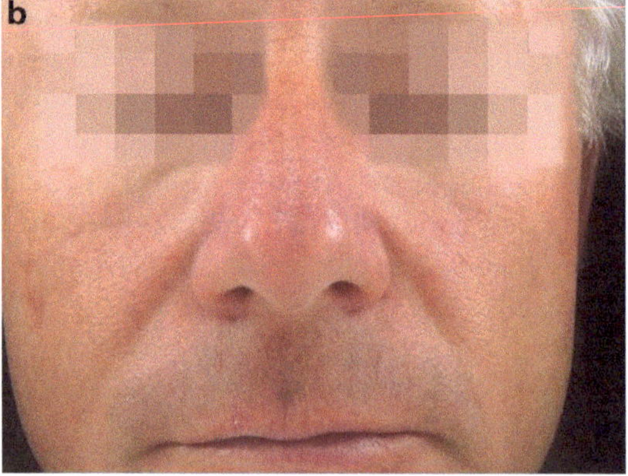

Fig. 2.7 (**a**) White male with moderate erythema and telangiectasias concentrated over the nose on a background of mild/moderate photodamage. The patient had received a single treatment of IPL without significant clearance. (**b**) Significant improvement after one treatment of ALA-PDT

one treatment session. Sixty-nine percent of the AKs responded to the use of ALA-IPL. Additionally, a 55% improvement in telangiectasias, 48% improvement in pigment irregularities, and 25% improvement in skin texture were observed.

Alster et al. [75] also examined the use of IPL in ALA-PDT. Ten patients with mild to moderate photodamage underwent two sessions of split-face treatment. Patients received treatment with ALA-IPL on one side and IPL alone on the contralateral side at 4-week intervals. Clinical improvement scores were noted to be higher on the side of the face treated with the combination of ALA-IPL. They concluded that the combination of topical 5-ALA+IPL is safe and more effective than IPL alone for the treatment of facial rejuvenation.

Another split face study on ALA-IPL versus IPL alone was performed by Dover et al. [66]. In this study, 20 subjects had 3 split-face treatments 3 weeks apart. Half of the face was treated with ALA followed by IPL treatment and the other half was treated with IPL alone. A blinded investigator was used to evaluate global photodamage, fine lines, mottled pigmentation, tactile roughness, and sallowness during the study. They concluded that pretreatment with ALA followed by IPL resulted in greater improvement in global photoaging (80% vs. 50%) and mottled pigmentation (95% vs. 65%). Successful results were also noted for fine lines for the ALA-IPL side compared with the IPL side alone (55% vs. 20%). Although tactile roughness and sallowness were noticeably better, pretreatment with ALA did not enhance the results of using IPL alone. It was important to note that both modes of treatment were well tolerated and that no significant differences in the side effect profiles were observed. This study was important not only for its demonstration and safety of IPL in the use of ALA-PDT, but for the development of a photodamage rating scale.

A final split-face comparative study for photorejuvenation using ALA-IPL versus IPL alone was performed by Gold et al. [68]. Thirteen patients received short-contact ALA-IPL on one side of the face and IPL alone on the contralateral side. Photoaging categories including fine wrinkling (crow's feet), tactile skin roughness, mottled pigmentation, telangiectasias, and AKs were evaluated. All demonstrated a better response on the side of the face treated with ALA-PDT. This study demonstrated the enhancing effects of ALA-PDT in IPL photorejuvenation.

Marmur et al. [76] conducted a pilot study to assess the ultrastructural changes seen after ALA-IPL photorejuvenation. Seven adult subjects were treated with a full-face IPL treatment. Half of the face in the study subjects received pretreatment with topical ALA before the IPL treatment. Pre- and posttreatment biopsies were reviewed by electron microscope for changes in collagen. A greater increase in type I collagen was noted in the subjects that were pretreated with ALA-IPL as opposed to the group treated with IPL alone.

They concluded that the addition of ALA-PDT using IPL could be superior to IPL alone.

A more recent study by Serrano et al. [77] in 2009 examined the use of ALA-IPL for the treatment of acne, vitiligo, and photoaging. Twenty-six patients in total completed the study, eight of which were in the photoaging treatment arm. Low concentration ALA (1–2%) was used for incubation prior to light exposure. Improvement in several photoaging parameters were noted in the majority of patients. One hundred percent of cases had skin texture improvement; erythema/telangiectasia, and hyperpigmentation were improved in 85 and 90% of cases, respectively. Eighty-eight percent of patients were satisfied with the results after three sessions of ALA-PDT.

PDT with PDL. PDL have also been studied as a light source for photorejuvenation in ALA-PDT. PDL targets oxyhemoglobin as a chromophore according to the theory of selective photothermolysis. But thermal energy generated in the surrounding areas adjacent to targeted blood vessels may also result in photorejuvenative effects. Subpurpuric doses from the PDL alter dermal collagen and may improve skin texture [20].

Alexiades-Amenakas and Geronemus [47] found ALA-PDT with the 595 nm PDL was successful in treating face and scalp AKs. Additionally, in this large study of 2,561 lesions, areas treated showed signs of photorejuvenation.

Key [78] treated 14 patients with long-incubation ALA (12 h) followed by photoactivation using a PDL. Improvement was noted following ALA-PDL in terms of skin texture, tactile quality, and brown spots, although the degree of vascularity and seborrheic keratoses were unaffected by treatment. The lack of improvement in blood vessel lesions is curious given that PDL targets the vasculature.

Summary of Findings for ALA-PDT in AK Treatment and Photorejuvenation. These results show the potential usefulness of a variety of lasers and light sources in the treatment of actinic keratoses and in the improvement of photodamage and photorejuvenation utilizing 5-ALA based PDT treatments. Beyond the treatment of AKs, ALA-PDT offers beneficial cosmetic outcomes in photorejuvenation.

Patient Selection for ALA-PDT

Thoughtful selection of eligible patients for ALA-PDT benefits both physician and patient. Patients should be carefully screened at an initial clinical consultation for inclusion and exclusion criteria for PDT. Physicians should gauge whether a patient has an accurate understanding and realistic expectations of the procedure. This will maximize patient's results, reduce patient's anxiety, and ensure the PDT is conducted smoothly on the day of the procedure. A comprehensive consent that explains the risks, benefits, and complications of therapy as well as treatment alternatives should be reviewed with patients carefully prior to treatment.

Exclusion Criteria

Patients should be screened for important exclusion criteria prior to undergoing PDT. A history of photosensitivity including porphyria, photodermatoses, and photosensitizing medication use should preclude treatment [46, 56, 67]. Many studies have excluded patients from treatment if they have undergone treatment with systemic retinoids, chemotherapeutic agents, or immunotherapy in the past 6 months [42, 56, 72]. Pregnant or nursing women and individuals with an active infection should not undergo treatment [41, 42]. Patients should refrain from topical retinoids, alpha hydroxy acids, and chemical peels approximately 1 month prior to treatment [56].

Unique Patient Populations

Solid organ transplant recipients (OTR) suffer from a 10 to 250-fold increase in AKs due to their ongoing immunosuppressive therapy [79]. In addition, the precancerous and cancerous lesions developing in the OTR population are often more aggressive [79], requiring frequent and ongoing cancer surveillance. PDT, a safe and effective treatment option for precancerous and malignant lesions, offered a new treatment modality for controlling AKs and nonmelanoma skin cancers in the OTR population. Although initial response rates of AKs following PDT were comparable in the OTR patient population compared with normal controls [80], longer-term follow-up demonstrated statistically significant decreases in clearance rates in the OTR population. In addition, SCC of the dorsal hands and forearms were not prevented in OTRs in a 2-year follow-up study, although there was a trend toward decreased keratotic regions in the areas treated [81]. PDT may still be a viable treatment option in this population, but it may require adjustments to typical treatment protocols including increased frequency of PDT sessions [80] and use of longer wavelengths (red light) for deeper skin penetration [81].

Treatment Protocol

Skin Preparation

Optimal results following ALA-PDT can be achieved with proper preparation prior to the procedure itself. The stratum corneum is a major barrier to the penetration of 5-ALA [22, 51]. Hyperkeratotic lesions must be treated with light curettage prior to 5-ALA application. Otherwise, ALA is preferentially absorbed by the hyperkeratotic scale rather than the lesion intended for treatment [21]. Some physicians use occlusion to improve delivery of 5-ALA through thicker lesions. Tegaderm™, opaque Mepore®, or Glad Press-N-Seal® may be used for these purposes.

Methods of proper skin preparation to reduce stratum corneum thickness also include light chemical peels, tape stripping, microdermabrasion, and degreasing of the skin with acetone [16, 69, 82, 83]. All the above measures can improve the absorption of ALA by the skin [22]. We routinely use a vibrating microdermabrasion system (Vibraderm, Great Plains, TX) (Fig. 2.8) with subsequent acetone degreasing to prepare the skin for 5-ALA application (Fig. 2.9).

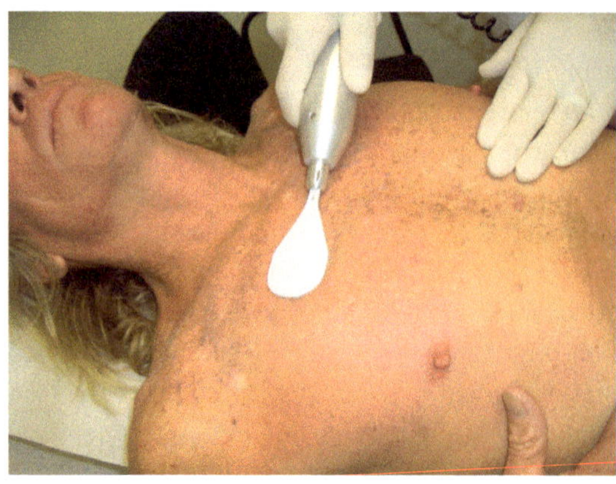

Fig. 2.8 Proper skin preparation prior to ALA application removes excess layers of the stratum corneum and improves ALA penetration. We use a vibrating microdermabrasion device for 5 min prior to acetone degreasing

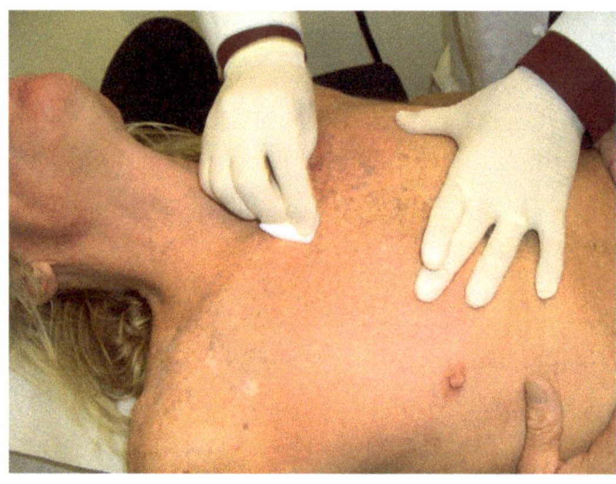

Fig. 2.9 Acetone-soaked gauze following microdermabrasion enhances ALA delivery. Firm pressure should be used during scrubbing to remove excess skin lipids and keratinocytes

Incubation Time

5-ALA is FDA-approved for use with a 14–18 hour incubation and subsequent photoactivation with blue light [10]. However, longer incubation times often results in an increased severity of adverse effects following ALA-PDT (Fig. 2.10) [42], and furthermore, shorter incubation times (1–3 h) have demonstrated similar efficacy in AK clearance [6, 55]. We routinely use a 60-minute incubation time in the treatment of AKs or for photorejuvenation. When treating thicker, larger, or more invasive lesions, we extend the incubation time to 3 hours and occlude the treated area with Glad Press 'N Seal®.

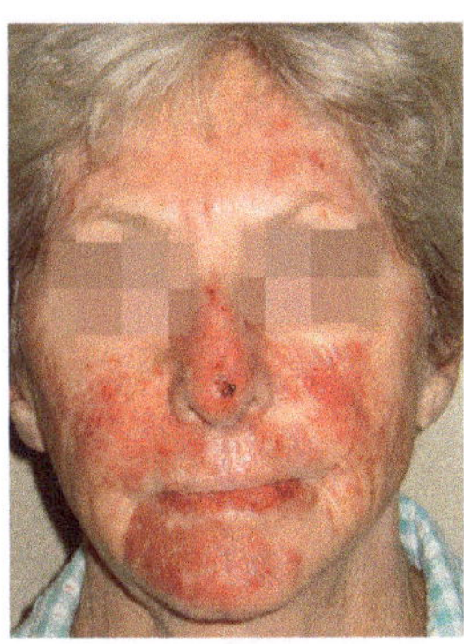

Fig. 2.10 Moderate/severe phototoxic reaction due to extended ALA incubation period. This woman had ALA-PDT with a 3-hour, unoccluded incubation. The patient denied UV exposure for the 36 h following photodynamic therapy (PDT)

Light Sources

Blue, red, green, and broad-band light sources may be used to activate PpIX during ALA-PDT for AKs or photorejuvenation. There is some evidence that blue light may be more effective for superficial AKs due to the shorter wavelength and increased potency during PDT of blue light [69]. Green light was found to cause less pain than red light in the treatment of AKs [54]. Red light has a deeper depth of penetration, but is often used with MAL rather than ALA. Broad band light sources including IPL have the advantage of improving signs of photodamage. It is our practice, both in the treatment of AKs and photorejuvenation, to use multiple light sources during ALA-PDT. With a typical treatment, we treat individual lesions first with subpurpuric doses of a PDL, followed by full-face treatment by an IPL, and lastly illumination with a blue and/or red light source. It should be noted that the IPL also results in hair reduction, so judicious use should be exercised in hair-bearing areas such as the scalp and beard area.

Patient Comfort and Photoprotection and Follow-Up

We do not routinely use topical or intralesional anesthesia prior to ALA-PDT. With a 1-hour incubation time, our clinical experience is that the procedure is well-tolerated by the overwhelming majority of patients. We use forced air cooling (see Fig. 2.5) and refrigerated conductive gel during the IPL portion of photoactivation, and a cooling fan with aerosolized water during blue light exposure. For longer incubation periods, the use of oral analgesics, topical lidocaine preparations, and ice packs in conjunction with PDT may increase patient's comfort [46].

Immediately following treatment, we apply an aloe vera-based gel to the treated skin to calm erythema and irritation. A sunblock (physical blocker) containing zinc oxide and titanium dioxide is applied to the treated skin. To avoid phototoxicity during daylight hours, our patients are scheduled for treatment in the late afternoon, so they may depart the clinic during twilight hours. Patients are given a protective visor if the face was treated, and patients are asked to wear sunglasses and protective clothing during their ride home.

We instruct patients to avoid sunlight and bright indoor light sources for 36 hours following treatment. We request patients return to clinic at 1 week and 2 months following PDT for routine follow-up. We perform subsequent rounds of ALA-PDT at 1–2 months intervals. We counsel patients to anticipate two ALA-PDT sessions for the treatment of AKs, while photorejuvenation, especially when sebaceous hyperplasia is present, usually requires three to four sessions. These recommendations are consistent with consensus guidelines from the American Society of Photodynamic Therapy [9].

Clinical Technique

Summarized below is our treatment protocol for ALA-PDT [2]. This is supplied as an example, but is by no means the only way to successfully perform PDT. This may be used as a general guideline and practitioners must decide for themselves the most effective and efficient use of ALA-PDT in their office.

Aminolevulinic Acid-Photodynamic Therapy for Actinic Keratoses and Photorejuvenation

1. Cleanse the patient's skin with mild soap and water (Cetaphil cleanser or Neutrogena Foaming Facial Wash).
2. Peform microdermabrasion with the Vibraderm over the treated area (Fig. 2.8).

3. Scrub the skin virgorously using a 4×4 in. acetone-soaked gauze (Fig. 2.9).
4. Break the two glass ampules in the Levulan Kerastick as per the package insert [10]. Shake the stick for about 2 min.
5. Apply the ALA solution to the treatment area. This is best accomplished by painting the Levulan on using the application stick. At least two coats of the solution are recommended, and the entire contents of the Kerastick should be used. It is important to get close to the eyes, otherwise it will be apparent that the periorbital skin was not treated.
6. Allow the Levulan to incubate for 60 minutes on the skin. The patient should remain indoors during the incubation period.
7. Remove the Levulan prior to any light treatment by requesting the patient to wash his or her face with a gentle soap and water.
8. Activate the Levulan with the appropriate light source(s):
   - AKs: PDL is used to target individual lesions at subpurpuric settings, followed by 16 minutes and 40 seconds of treatment with blue light. The Blu-U should be positioned approximately 2 inches from the treatment area.
   - Photorejuvenation +/– AKs: PDL is used to target individual lesions at subpurpuric settings including AKs, sebaceous hyperplasia, solar lentigines, and telangiectasias. IPL treatment follows, using a double pulse and 560 nm cut-off filter for Fitzpatrick skin types I–III. Fluence, pulse duration, and pulse delay settings are determined according to skin type and type of photodamage. Lastly, the patient is treated with the Blu-U and/or red-light in a similar manner to the AK protocol (Fig. 2.11).
9. Wash the patient's face again to remove any residual Levulan on the skin's surface.
10. Apply soothing gel or lotion (we recommend an aloe vera-based gel) to the treated area after the illumination period.
11. Apply a physical sunblock containing zinc oxide and titanium dioxide to the treated area. Instruct the patient on strict photoprotection for the following 36 hours. The patient is to remain indoors, out of direct sunlight.
12. Patients are given Avene Thermal Spring Water spray to apply to their skin four to six times a day.
13. Repeat the treatment in 4–8 weeks. If there was little reaction, increase the incubation time or reevaluate your skin preparation technique.

Safety, Adverse Effects, and Complications

Expected side effects following ALA-PDT are related to the phototoxic nature of treatment and are usually mild in nature. Pain and burning may be experienced during light irradiation. Shorter incubation times decrease the severity of side effects. Expected phototoxic side effects include erythema, edema, stinging/burning, pruritus, and crusting. Pigmentary changes, whealing, and vesiculation may also occur [12, 41, 43]. Erythema and mild crusting occur in most patients following treatment, usually resolving in 1–2 weeks [60]. Hypopigmentation is rare, and hyperpigmentation, with an incidence as high as 27% following ALA-PDT [41], is usually mild in nature. More pronounced reactions are correlated with disease burden. Typically, repeat treatments are less painful than previous ones.

In patients with extensive phototoxic reactions (Fig. 2.12), especially in cases when patients are exposed to UV radiation in the 24–36 hours following treatment, topical therapy may be necessary to address erythema, edema, and crusting. Topical steroid creams and ice packs may be used on the treated area until the symptoms subside. All patients should be screened for a history of cold sores and appropriate HSV prophylaxis begun prior to treatment in such cases [2].

Pain management, especially with shorter incubation times (e.g., 1 hour), is usually a nonissue. Reassurance to the patient and "talk-esthesia" by a caring member of the clinical staff is usually more than adequate to comfort any patient's anxiety and pain. However, the use of cooling fans, Avene Thermal Water Spray, forced air cooling systems, Xylocaine spray, and even oral non-narcotic pain medication have been used successfully to mitigate pain during ALA-PDT [6, 41, 60].

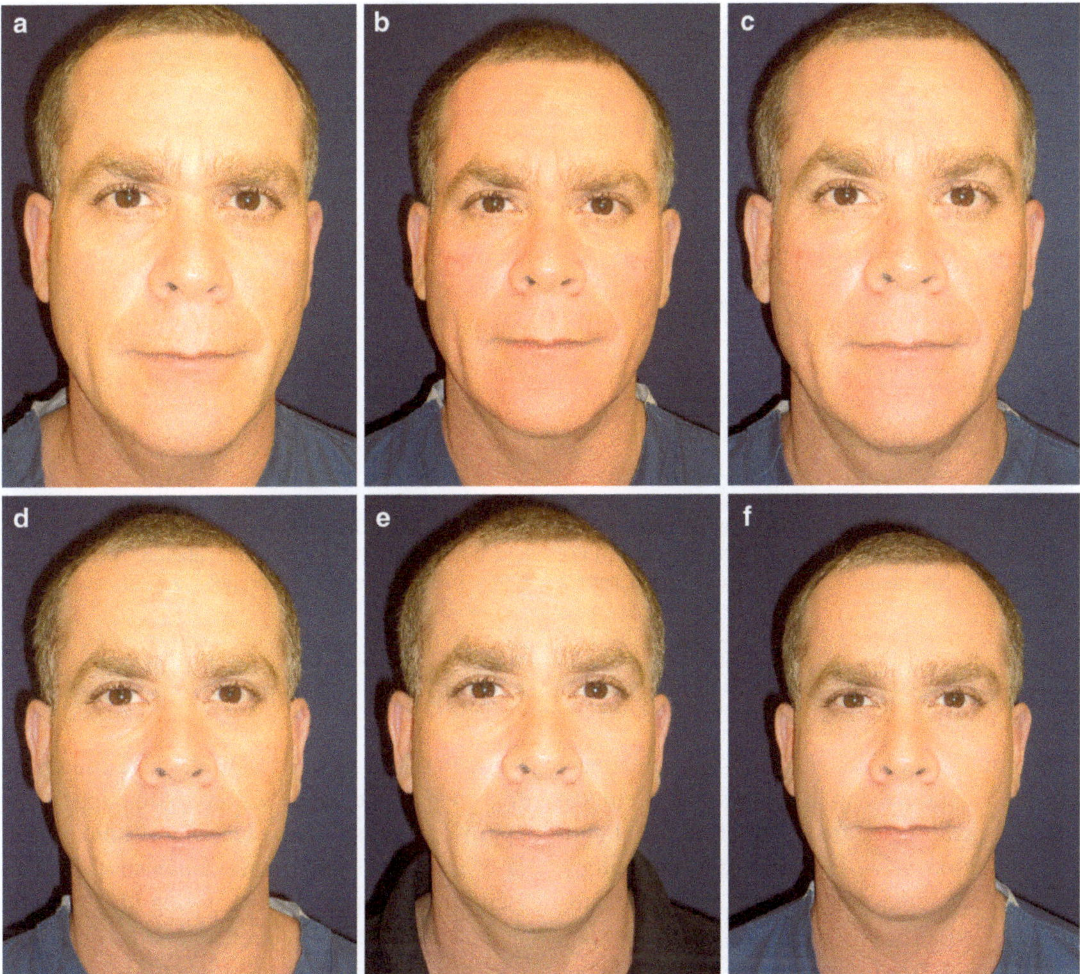

Fig. 2.11 (**a**) Frontal view of a 51-year-old male with photodamage consisting of numerous solar lentigines. (**b**) One day after ALA-PDT treatment. Levulan ALA was applied to entire treatment area for 1 h, unoccluded. IPL treatment with Lumenis One using a 560 nm cut-off filter, double pulse of 4 and 4 ms with a 10 ms delay at a fluence of 18 J/cm^2 followed by a 10-min exposure with the Blu-U. Note the erythema and crusting of all actinically damaged skin. (**c**) Two days after PDT treatment, further increase in erythema is seen in areas of actinically damaged skin. (**d**) Three days after PDT treatment, resolution of erythema begins. (**e**) Four days after PDT treatment, further resolution of erythema. (**f**) Seven days after PDT treatment, complete resolution of erythema (This figure was published in Goldman MP, Dover JS, Alam M, editors. Procedures in cosmetic surgery: photodynamic therapy. 2nd ed. Philadelphia, PA: Elsevier; 2007, Copyright Elsevier 2007 [38])

Patients should be counseled to practice strict photoprotection for 24–36 hours following treatment. Titanium dioxide and zinc oxide-containing sunblocks are preferred, in addition to protective clothing and sunglasses. Excessive UV radiation from sunlight, as well as intense spotlights, photocopy machines, photographic flashlights, and medical examining lights/lamps should be avoided during the period of photosensitivity. Indoor light is usually not a concern, but patients should avoid bright sources of light, even while indoors [12].

Not unexpectedly, if patients require a second treatment, the adverse effects as well as treatment pain are usually much less than those experienced with the initial treatment. We believe that the decrease is due to the resolution of most of the clinical and subclinical photodamage which occurs during the initial treatment.

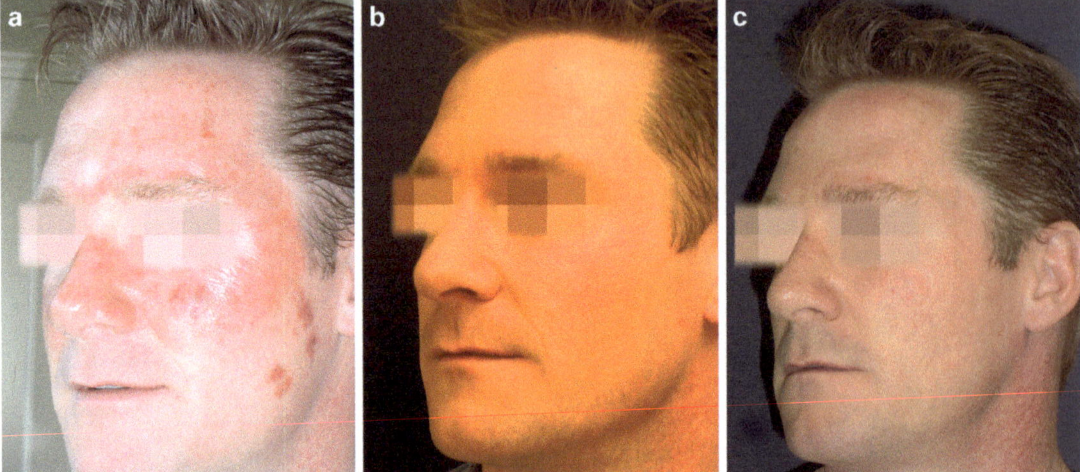

Fig. 2.12 (**a**) Mild to moderate phototoxic reaction due to sunlight exposure in the 24 hours following an ALA-PDT session. (**b**) Six months post-procedure, the patient demonstrated marked improvement in photodamage without postinflammatory hyperpigmentation. (**c**) Four year follow-up with durable photorejuvenative effects

Expected Benefits

Many of the benefits of ALA-PDT treatment have been addressed in the discussion of clinical studies regarding the treatment of AKs and photorejuvenation. ALA-PDT is a safe, efficacious, and well-tolerated treatment for AKs, with the added benefit of addressing photoaging. Clearance of AK lesions with PDT is superior from a cosmetic standpoint compared to conventional treatments such as liquid nitrogen [46]. A few studies have evaluated patient satisfaction with PDT. A study by Tierney et al. [45] followed patient satisfaction in 39 patients following ALA-PDT. In this study, patients reported statistically significant better recovery compared with other treatments including cryotherapy or surgical excision. A borderline statistically significant improvement was achieved with PDT for overall cosmetic outcome patient satisfaction compared with other therapies. Morton et al. [84] also found that patients preferred the overall treatment procedure and cosmetic outcome of ALA-PDT compared with cryotherapy. Patient satisfaction was high in the stage III clinical trial by Piacquadio et al. [52]. Ninety-four percent of patients through the cosmetic results following PDT were good to excellent.

Conclusion

ALA-PDT is a safe and effective treatment for nonhyperkeratotic lesions. Although FDA-approved for use with a blue light source, other laser and light sources have demonstrated promise in the treatment of AKs during PDT. Shorter incubation times maintain AK clearance rates but decrease the occurrence of phototoxic adverse events. With careful patient selection, ALA-PDT allows selective field treatment of precancerous skin lesions with improvement in overall photodamage. Patient satisfaction is high and cosmetic results can be excellent.

References

1. Calzavara-Pinton PG, Venturini M, Sala R. Photodynamic therapy: update 2006. Part 1: photochemistry and photobiology. J Eur Acad Dermatol Venereol. 2007;21:293–302.
2. Nootheti PK, Goldman MP. Aminolevulinic acid-photodynamic therapy for photorejuvenation. Dermatol Clin. 2007;25:35–45.
3. Ericson MB, Sandberg C, Stenquist B, Gudmundson F, et al. Photodynamic therapy of actinic keratosis at varying fluence rates: assessment of photobleaching, pain and primary clinical outcome. Br J Dermatol. 2004;151:1204–12.

4. Nakaseko H, Kobayashi M, Akita Y, Tamada Y, et al. Histological changes and involvement of apoptosis after photodynamic therapy for actinic keratoses. Br J Dermatol. 2003;148:122–7.
5. Wolf P, Rieger E, Kerl H. Topical photodynamic therapy with endogenous porphyrins after application of 5-aminolevulinic acid. J Am Acad Dermatol. 1993;28:17–21.
6. Touma D, Yaar M, Whitehead S, Konnikov N, et al. A trial of short incubation, broad-area photodynamic therapy for facial actinic keratoses and diffuse photodamage. Arch Dermatol. 2004;140:33–40.
7. Tsai T, Ji HT, Chiang PC, Chou RH, Chang WSW, Chen CT. ALA-PDT results in phenotypic changes and decreased cellular invasion in surviving cancer cells. Lasers Surg Med. 2009;41:305–15.
8. MacCormack MA. Photodynamic therapy in dermatology: an update on applications and outcomes. Semin Cutan Med Surg. 2008;27:52–62.
9. Nestor MS, Gold MH, Kauvar ANB, Taub AF, et al. The use of photodynamic therapy in dermatology: results of a consensus conference. J Drugs Dermatol. 2006;5:140–54.
10. Product information (package insert): Levulan (R) Kerastick (TM) (aminolevulinic acid HCl) for topical solution, 20%. DUSA Pharmaceuticals, Inc., Wilmington, MA, USA; 2009.
11. Fotinos N, Campo MA, Popowycz F, Gurny R, et al. 5-Aminolevulinic acid derivatives in photomedicine: characteristics, application and perspectives. Photochem Photobiol. 2006;82:994–1015.
12. Kalka K, Merk H, Mukhtar H. Photodynamic therapy in dermatology. J Am Acad Dermatol. 2000;42:389–413.
13. Gaullier JM, Berg K, Peng Q, Anholt H, et al. Use of 5-aminolevulinic acid esters to improve photodynamic therapy on cells in culture. Cancer Res. 1997;57:1481–6.
14. Peng Q, Warloe T, Berg K, Moan J, et al. 5-Aminolevulinic acid-based photodynamic therapy. Cancer. 1997;79:2282–308.
15. Kasche A, Luderschmidt S, Ring J, Hein R. Photodynamic therapy induces less pain in patients treated with methyl aminolevulinate compared to aminolevulinic acid. J Drugs Dermatol. 2006;5:353–6.
16. Goldberg DJ. Photodynamic therapy in skin rejuvenation. Clin Dermatol. 2008;26:608–13.
17. Nakano A, Tamada Y, Watanabe D, Ishida N, et al. A pilot study to assess the efficacy of photodynamic therapy for Japanese patients with actinic keratosis in relation to lesion size and histological severity. Photodermatol Photoimmunol Photomed. 2009;25:37–40.
18. Zakhary K, Ellis DAF. Applications of aminolevulinic acid-based photodynamic therapy in cosmetic facial plastic practices. Facial Plast Surg. 2005;21:110–6.
19. Clark C, Bryden A, Dawe R, Moseley H, et al. Topical 5-aminolevulinic acid photodynamic therapy for cutaneous lesions: outcome and comparison of light sources. Photodermatol Photoimmunol Photomed. 2003;19:134–41.
20. DeHoratius DM, Dover JS. Nonablative tissue remodeling and photorejuvenation. Clin Dermatol. 2007;25:474–9.
21. Markham T, Collins P. Topical 5-aminolaevulinic acid photodynamic therapy for extensive scalp actinic keratoses. Br J Dermatol. 2001;145:502–4.
22. Kalisiak MS, Rao J. Photodynamic therapy for actinic keratoses. Dermatol Clin. 2007;25:15–23.
23. Gold MH. Pharmacoeconomic analysis of the treatment of multiple actinic keratoses. J Drugs Dermatol. 2008;7:23–5.
24. Drake LA, Ceilley RI, Cornelison RL, et al. Guidelines of care for AKs. J Am Acad Dermatol. 1995; 32:95–8.
25. Stockfleth E, Kerl H. Guidelines for the management of actinic keratoses. Eur J Dermatol. 2006;16: 599–606.
26. Lehmann P. Methyl aminolaevulinate-photodynamic therapy: a review of clinical trials in the treatment of actinic keratoses and nonmelanoma skin cancer. Br J Dermatol. 2007;156:793–801.
27. Berking C, Herzinger T, Flaig MJ, Brenner M, Borelli C, Degitz K. The efficacy of photodynamic therapy in actinic cheilitis of the lower lip: a prospective study of 15 patients. Dermatol Surg. 2007;33:825–30.
28. Marks R. Epidemiology of nonmelanoma skin cancer and solar keratoses in Australia: a tale of self-immolation in Elysian fields. Australas J Dermatol. 1997;38:S26–9.
29. Diepgen TL, Mahler V. The epidemiology of skin cancer. Br J Dermatol. 2002;146:1–6.
30. Osborne JE. Skin cancer screening and surveillance. Br J Dermatol. 2002;146:745–54.
31. Marks R, Rennie G, Selwood TS. Malignant transformation of solar keratoses to squamous cell carcinoma. Lancet. 1988;1:795–7.
32. Glogau RG. The risk of progression to invasive disease. J Am Acad Dermatol. 2000;42(1 Pt 2):23–4.
33. Czarnecki D, Meehan CJ, Bruce F, Culjak G. The majority of cutaneous squamous cell carcinomas arise in actinic keratoses. J Cutan Med Surg. 2002;6:207–9.
34. Cockerell CJ, Wharton JR. New histopathological classification of actinic keratosis (incipient intraepithelial squamous cell carcinoma). J Drugs Dermatol. 2005;4:462–7.
35. Ortonne JP. From actinic keratoses to squamous cell carcinoma. Br J Dermatol. 2002;146:S20–3.
36. Hurwitz RM, Monger LE. Solar keratosis: an evolving squamous cell carcinoma. Benign or malignant? Dermatol Surg. 1995;21:184.
37. Moy RL. Clinical presentation of actinic keratoses and squamous cell carcinoma. J Am Acad Dermatol. 2000;42:8–10.
38. Bäumler W, Wetzig T. Clinical application of fluorescence diagnosis. In: Goldman MP, Dover JS, Alam M, editors. Procedures in cosmetic dermatology: photodynamic therapy. 2nd ed. Philadelphia, PA: Elsevier; 2008. p. 149–60.
39. Salasche SJ. Epidemiology of actinic keratoses and squamous cell carcinoma. J Am Acad Dermatol. 2000;42:4–7.

40. Cockerell CJ. Histopathology of incipient intraepidermal squamous cell carcinoma ("actinic keratosis"). J Am Acad Dermatol. 2000;42:11–7.
41. Tschen EH, Wong DS, Pariser DM, Dunlap FE, Houlihan A, Ferdon MB. Photodynamic therapy using aminolaevulinic acid for patients with nonhyperkeratotic actinic keratoses of the face and scalp: phase IV mulicentre clinical trial with 12-month follow up. Br J Dermatol. 2006;155:1262–9.
42. Jeffes EW, McCullough JL, Weinstein GD, Kaplan R, Glazer SD, Taylor JR. Photodynamic therapy of actinic keratoses with topical aminolevulinic acid hydrochloride and fluorescent blue light. J Am Acad Dermatol. 2001;45:96–104.
43. Szeimies RM, Karrer S, Radakovic-Fijan S, Tanew A, Galzavara-Pinton PG, Zane C, et al. Photodynamic therapy using topical methyl 5-aminolevulinate compared with cryotherapy for actinic keratosis: a prospective, randomized study. J Am Acad Dermatol. 2002;47:258–62.
44. Kurwa HA, Yong-Gee SA, Seed PT, et al. A randomized paired comparison of photodynamic therapy and topical 5-fluorouracil in the treatment of actinic keratoses. J Am Acad Dermatol. 1999;41:414–8.
45. Tierney EP, Eide MJ, Jacobsen G, Ozog D. Photodynamic therapy for actinic keratoses: survey of patient perceptions of treatment satisfaction and outcomes. J Cosmet Laser Ther. 2008;10:81–6.
46. Goldman MP, Atkin DH. ALA/PDT in the treatment of actinic keratosis: spot versus confluent therapy. J Cosmet Laser Ther. 2003;5:107–10.
47. Alexiades-Amenakas MR, Geronemus RG. Laser-mediated photodynamic therapy of actinic keratoses. Arch Dermatol. 2003;139:1313–20.
48. Kennedy JC, Pottier RH, Pross DC. Photodynamic therapy with endogenous protoporphyrin IX: basic principles and present clinical experience. J Photochem Photobiol B. 1990;6:143–8.
49. Dijkstra AT, Majoie IML, van Dongen JWF, van Weelden H, et al. Photodynamic therapy with violet light and topical δ-aminolaevulinic acid in the treatment of actinic keratosis, Bowen's disease and basal cell carcinoma. J Eur Acad Dermatol Venereol. 2001;15:550–4.
50. Ross EV, Anderson RR. Laser-tissue interactions. In: Goldman MP, editor. Cutaneous and cosmetic laser surgery. Philadelphia, PA: Elsevier; 2006. p. 1–26.
51. Ormrod D, Jarvis B. Topical aminolevulinic acid HCl photodynamic therapy. Am J Clin Dermatol. 2000;2:133–9.
52. Piacquadio DJ, Chen DM, Farber HF, et al. Photodynamic therapy with aminolevulinic acid topical solution and visible blue light in the treatment of multiple actinic keratoses of the face and scalp: investigator-blinded, phase 3, multicenter trials. Arch Dermatol. 2004;140:41–6.
53. Gold MH. The evolving role of aminolevulinic acid hydrochloride with photodynamic therapy in photoaging. Cutis. 2002;69:8–13.
54. Fritsch C, Stege H, Saalmann G, Goerz G, et al. Green light is effective and less painful than red light in photodynamic therapy of facial solar keratoses. Photodermatol Photoimmunol Photomed. 1997;13:181–5.
55. Smith S, Piacquadio D, Morhenn V, Atkin D. Short incubation PDT versus 5-FU in treating actinic keratoses. J Drugs Dermatol. 2003;2:629–35.
56. Jeffes WJ, McCullagh JL, Weinstein GD, Fergin PE, et al. Photodynamic therapy of actinic keratosis with topical 5-aminolaevulinic acid. Arch Dermatol. 1997;133:727–32.
57. Karrer S, Bäumler W, Abels C, Hohenleutner U, et al. Long-pulse dye laser for photodynamic therapy: investigations in vitro and in vivo. Lasers Surg Med. 1999;25:51–9.
58. Itoh Y, Nineomiya Y, Henta T, Tajima S, et al. Topical delta-aminolevulinic acid-based photodynamic therapy for Japanese actinic keratoses. J Dermatol. 2000;27:513–8.
59. Varma S, Wilson H, Kurwa HA, Gambles B, et al. Bowen's disease, solar keratoses and superficial basal cell carcinomas treated by photodynamic therapy using a large-field incoherent light source. Br J Dermatol. 2001;144:56–574.
60. Moseley H, Ibbotson S, Woods J, Brancaleon L, Lesar A, Goodman C, et al. Clinical and research applications of photodynamic therapy in dermatology: experience of the Scottish PDT centre. Lasers Surg Med. 2006;38:403–16.
61. Fink-Puches R, Hofer A, Smolle J, Kerl H, et al. Primary clinical response and long-term follow-up of solar keratoses treated with topically applied 5-aminolevulinic acid and irradiation by different wave bands of light. J Photochem Photobiol B. 1997;41:145–51.
62. Kim HS, Yoo JY, Cho KH, Kwon OS, et al. Topical photodynamic therapy using intense pulsed light for treatment of actinic keratosis: clinical and histopathologic evaluation. Dermatol Surg. 2005;31:33–7.
63. Gilbert D. Treatment of actinic keratoses with sequential combination of 5-fluorouracil and photodynamic therapy. J Drugs Dermatol. 2005;4:161–3.
64. Shaffelburg M. Treatment of actinic keratoses with sequential use of photodynamic therapy and imiquimod 5% cream. J Drugs Dermatol. 2009;8:35–9.
65. Ruiz-Rodriguez R, Sanz-Sánchez T, Córdoba S. Photodynamic photorejuvenation. Dermatol Surg. 2002;28:742–4.
66. Dover JS, Bhatia AC, Stewart B, Arndt KA. Topical 5-aminolevulinic acid combined with intense pulsed light in the treatment of photoaging. Arch Dermatol. 2005;141:1247–52.
67. Zane C, Capezzera R, Sala R, Venturini M, Calzavara-Pinton P. Clinical and echographic analysis of photodynamic therapy using methylaminolevulinate as sensitizer in the treatment of photodamaged facial skin. Lasers Surg Med. 2007;39:203–9.

68. Gold MH, Bradshaw VL, Boring MM, Bridges TM, et al. Split-face comparison of photodynamic therapy with 5-aminolevulinic acid and intense pulsed light versus intense pulsed light alone for photodamage. Dermatol Surg. 2006;32:795–803.
69. Uebelhoer NS, Dover J. Photodynamic therapy for cosmetic applications. Dermatol Ther. 2005;18: 242–52.
70. Jeffes EWB. Levulan: the first approved topical photosensitizer for the treatment of actinic keratosis. J Dermatol Treat. 2002;13:S19–23.
71. Pariser DM, Lowe NJ, Stewart DM, Jarratt MT, et al. Photodynamic therapy with topical methyl aminolevulinate for actinic keratosis: results of a prospective randomized multicenter trial. J Am Acad Dermatol. 2003;48:227–32.
72. Lowe NJ, Lowe P. Pilot study to determine the efficacy of ALA-PDT photorejuvenation for the treatment of facial ageing. J Cosmet Laser Ther. 2005;7: 159–62.
73. Goldberg DJ. New collagen formation after dermal remodeling with intense pulsed light sources. J Cutan Laser Ther. 2000;2:59–61.
74. Avram DK, Goldman MP. Effectiveness and safety of ALA-IPL in treating actinic keratoses and photodamage. J Drugs Dermatol. 2004;3:S36–9.
75. Alster TS, Tanzi EL, Welch EC. Photorejuvenation of facial skin with topical 20% 5-aminolevulinic acid and intense pulsed light treatment: a split-face comparison study. J Drugs Dermatol. 2005;4:35–8.
76. Marmur ES, Phelps R, Goldberg DJ. Ultrastructural changes seen after ALA-IPL photorejuvenation: a pilot study. J Cosmet Laser Ther. 2005;7:21–4.
77. Serrano G, Lorente M, Reyes M, Millán F, et al. Photodynamic therapy with low-strength ALA, repeated applications and short contact periods (40-60 minutes) in acne, photoaging, and vitiligo. J Drugs Dermatol. 2009;8:562–8.
78. Key DJ. Aminolevulinic acid-pulsed dye laser photodynamic therapy for the treatment of photoaging. Cosmet Dermatol. 2005;18:31–6.
79. Oseroff A. PDT as a cytotoxic agent and biological response modifier: implications for cancer prevention and treatment in immunosuppressed and immunocompetent patients. J Invest Dermatol. 2006;126:542–4.
80. Dragieva G, Hafner J, Dummer R, Schmid-Grendelmeier P, et al. Topical photodynamic therapy in the treatment of actinic keratoses and Bowen's disease in transplant recipients. Transplantation. 2004;17:115–21.
81. de Graaf YGL, Kennedy C, Wolterbeek R, Collen AFS, et al. Photodynamic therapy does not prevent cutaneous squamous-cell carcinoma in organ-transplant recipients: results of a randomized-controlled trial. J Invest Dermatol. 2006;126:569–74.
82. Lee WR, Tsai RY, Fang CL, Liu CJ, Hu CH, Fang JY. Microdermabrasion as a novel tool to enhance drug delivery via the skin: an animal study. Dermatol Surg. 2006;32:1013–22.
83. Katz BE, Truong S, Maiwald DC, Frew KE, George BA. Efficacy of microdermabrasion preceding ALA application in reducing the incubation time of ALA in laser PDT. J Drugs Dermatol. 2007;6:140–2.
84. Morton S, Campbell S, Gupta G, Keohane S, Lear J, Zaki I, et al. Intraindividual, right-left comparison of topical methyl aminolaevulinate photodynamic therapy and cryotherapy in subjects with actinic keratoseis: a multicentre, randomized controlled study. Br J Dermatol. 2006;155:1029–36.
85. Morton CA, Whitehurst C, Moseley H, et al. Development of an alternative light source to lasers for photodynamic therapy: clinical evaluation in the treatment of pre-malignant non-melanoma skin cancer. Lasers Med Sci. 1995;10:165–71.
86. Fijan S, Honigsmann H, Ortel B. Photodynamic therapy of epithelial skin tumors with delta-aminolaevulinic acid and desferrioxamine. Br J Dermatol. 1995;133:282–8.
87. Szeimies RM, Karrer S, Sauerwald A, Landthaler M. Photodynamic therapy with topical application of 5-aminolevulinic acid in the treatment of actinic keratoses: an initial clinical study. Dermatology. 1996;192: 246–51.

3 5-Aminolevulinic Acid: Acne Vulgaris

Amy Forman Taub

Abstract

Photodynamic therapy (PDT) with 5-aminolevulinic acid (ALA) is a widely used, although off-label, treatment for moderate to severe acne in the USA. Still in its infancy, this treatment has confounded our better wisdom for best practices as studies have been limited and largely carried out in small, investigator-initiated clinical trials. Still, some consensus does emerge on the best light sources, incubation times, expected outcomes and long-term course. The most common light sources for this treatment are intense pulsed light (IPL), pulsed dye laser (PDL), blue light, and red light. Most studies in the USA, although not controlled, randomized or blinded, indicate that IPL and PDL are more effective than blue light for acne, whereas red light with ALA has been little evaluated. This makes sense as the sebaceous gland (SG) is approximately 1 mm below the surface of the skin and the majority of blue light does not penetrate to that depth. Studies have supported that very short ALA incubation periods ranging from 15 to 30 min are effective for the treatment of acne. The author postulates that there is a follicular penetration that precedes transepidermal transit that accounts for the efficacy of short contact PDT. PDT for acne with 5-ALA for the treatment of moderate to severe acne is a very efficacious and safe procedure that is significantly underutilized in the USA due to lack of FDA approval and insurance reimbursement as well as some convenience factors.

Introduction

Photodynamic therapy (PDT) with either 5-aminolevulinic acid (ALA) or methyl aminolevulinate (MAL) applied topically has shown efficacy in the treatment of acne vulgaris in small, investigator-initiated clinical trials. Although neither photosensitizing agent is FDA-cleared for the treatment of acne by PDT, both – ALA as Levulan® Kerastick® (Dusa Pharmaceuticals, Wilmington, Mass) and MAL cream as Metvix™ (PhotoCure ASA, Norway) – are cleared for the photodynamic treatment of nonhyperkeratotic actinic keratosis (AK) of the face and scalp. Indocyanine green (ICG) and methylene blue are two other noncommercially available photosensitizers that have been studied for acne treatment

A.F. Taub (✉)
Department of Dermatology, Northwestern University Medical School, Chicago, IL, USA
and
Advanced Dermatology, Lincolnshire, IL, USA
e-mail: drtaub@advdermatology.com

M.H. Gold (ed.), *Photodynamic Therapy in Dermatology*,
DOI 10.1007/978-1-4419-1298-5_3,

with PDT. MAL-PDT is being covered elsewhere in this book and is not included in this discussion.

Literature Review

The topical use of ALA in PDT was introduced and evaluated by Kennedy et al. [1]. As ALA penetrates epidermal cells, it enters the heme biosynthetic (Fig. 3.1) pathway and is converted to protoporphyrin IX (PpIX), a photosensitive compound [2]. ALA-induced PpIX is selective such that it only occurs in certain cells and tissues, and it has been found that strong PpIX fluorescence occurs in tumors or abnormalities that exist in the epidermis [2]. As ALA-induced PpIX accumulates in the epidermal cells, the ALA-treated area is irradiated with light which, in the presence of molecular oxygen, activates PpIX to form singlet oxygen, an unstable intermediate that destroys the cells in which it is produced [3]. For photoactivation to occur, the light used in the treatment must include wavelengths absorbed by PpIX (Fig. 3.2).

PpIX also accumulates in pilosebaceous units [4]. In their 2000 landmark study, Hongcharu et al. [5] confirmed this finding (Fig. 3.3). They took advantage of this property by applying ALA-PDT to 23 patients in the treatment of mild to moderate acne of the back. In this randomized, single-blinded and controlled study, 20% topical ALA was applied with 3 h occlusion, and 150 J/cm^2 broadband light (550–700 nm) was given. One arm of patients had clearance of acne for 10 weeks after a single treatment with another arm reporting 20 weeks of clearance after four treatments. This study laid the foundation for the use of ALA-PDT in the treatment of acne as it was the first study to present clinical, microbiological, and histologic evidence that ALA-PDT with

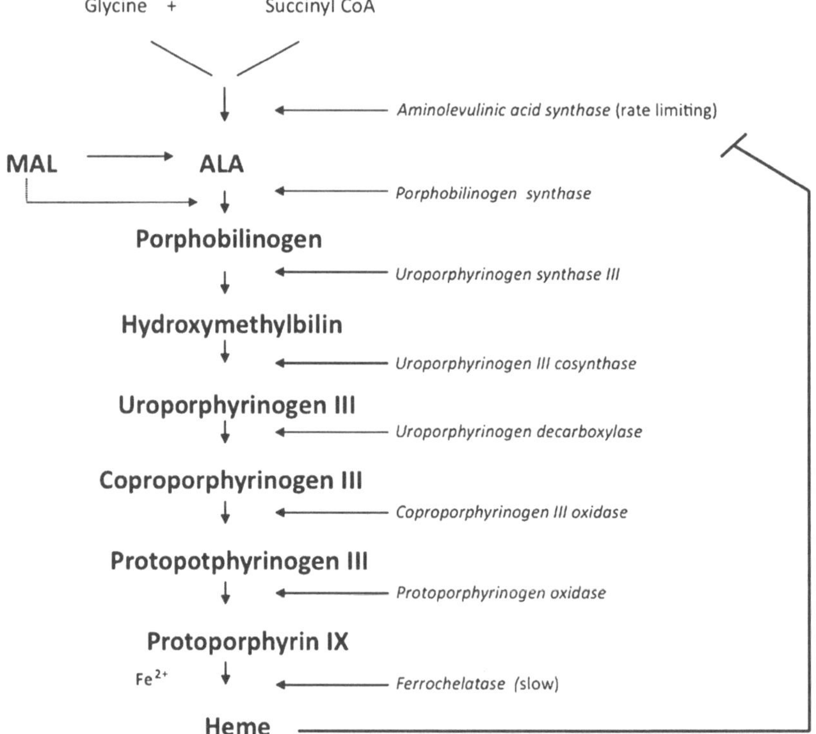

Fig. 3.1 Metabolic pathway of ALA. ALA is in the biochemical pathway of the manufacture of heme from glycine and succinyl CoA, present in every human cell. The conversion from Gly/CoA to ALA is the rate limiting step. By supplying exogenous ALA, one can bypass the rate limiting step, resulting in a net increase of Protoporphyrin IX, due to the fact that Ferrochetalase, the enzyme that converts PpIX to Heme, is relatively slow

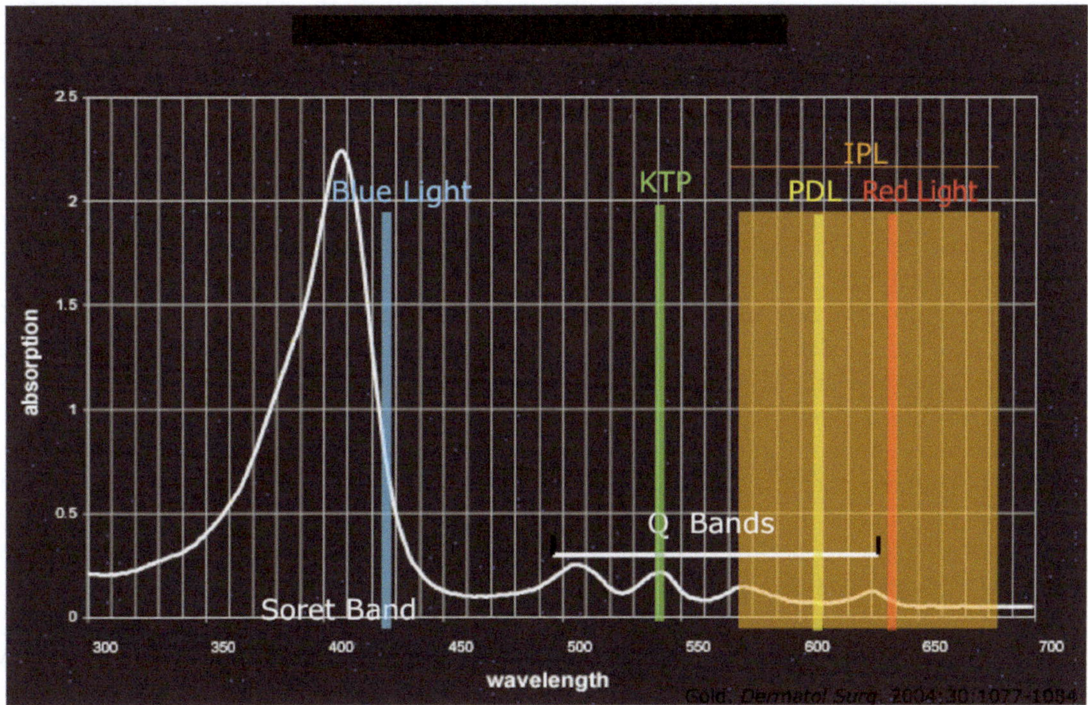

Fig. 3.2 PpIX absorption peaks. The maximum absorption peak of ALA is around 390–400 nm, referred to as the Soret Band. The so-called Q bands are lower peaks that span from 510 to 630 nm (from Gold and Goldman [36], with permission of Wiley)

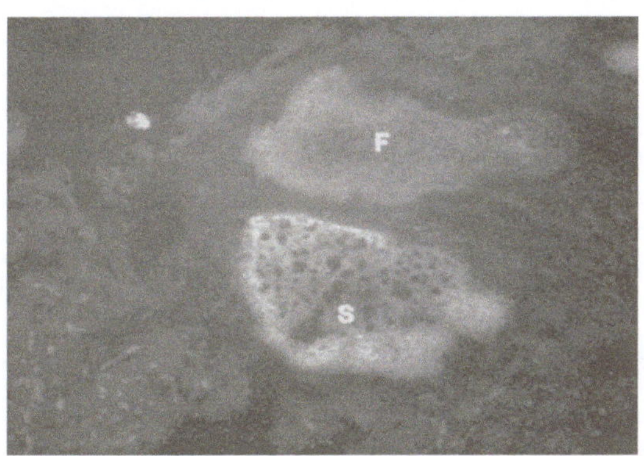

Fig. 3.3 PpIX production in Sebaceous Gland. Fluorescence microscopy shows PpIX production greater in sebaceous gland(s) than in hair follicle (reprinted by permission from Macmillan Publishers Ltd., from Hongcharu et al. [5])

broadband visible light activation was effective. The authors also suggested a mechanism of action by demonstrating decreased sebum excretion and bacterial fluorescence, as well as damaged sebaceous glands (SGs). Although the treatment was effective, the reported adverse effects were quite severe and included transient hyperpigmentation, superficial exfoliation, and crusting. In another early study, Itoh et al. [6] used ALA-PDT to treat a single facial lesion of a patient with intractable acne. They allowed ALA to remain in contact with the lesion for 4 h before irradiation with a 630-nm PDL. The treated lesion was resolved with a single treatment and did not recur for at least 8 months. This study showed that a single treatment with polychromatic visible light activation was effective against intractable facial acne.

These encouraging early results stimulated other investigators to further explore the use of ALA-PDT for acne of the face and other locations. The mechanism of ALA-PDT was examined by Pollock et al. in their randomized, blinded and controlled study of 15 patients treated with ALA-PDT on back acne with activation by laser-generated red light at 635 nm after 3 h of incubation of ALA [7]. The authors found a reduction in lesion count, uniquely to the ALA-PDT site, after the second of three weekly treatments. Although, there was reported reduction neither in the population of skin surface *P. acnes* nor in sebum excretion after ALA-PDT Pollack et al. attributed their contrasting mechanism of action-related results to the broadband wavelengths used by Hongcharu et al. as possibly responsible for the reduced sebum excretion and reduced bacterial fluorescence observed in their study.

In a controlled study, Goldman and Boyce [8] showed that ALA-PDT with blue light was more effective against acne than blue light alone and showed that short-contact ALA of only 15 min provided efficacy and minimal adverse effects. This was the first study to limit ALA incubation time to ≤1 h for the photodynamic treatment of acne.

Gold et al. [9] were the first to use IPL for ALA-PDT for acne and demonstrated its effectiveness. Twenty patients were treated for moderate to severe facial acne weekly for 4 weeks with a 1-h incubation of 20% ALA topical solution. The device used was a novel intense pulsed light (IPL) and heat source that emitted 430–1,100-nm radiation at 3–9 J/cm^2 fluences. Twelve weeks after final treatment, there was a 72% clearance in the 12/15 patients that responded to the treatment. Taub [10] confirmed the efficacy of short-contact (15–30 min incubation) ALA for patients with moderate to severe refractory acne. Eleven out of the eighteen treated patients had failed treatment with isotretinoin. The results showed that electrical optical energy (ELOS) (IPL [580–980 nm] with bipolar radiofrequency) technology was effective as an activator of ALA, as well as confirming that blue light was effective (Fig. 3.4).

In a subsequent randomized study of patients with moderate to severe acne, this author compared IPL, blue light, and ELOS devices as activators in ALA-PDT [11]. Acne grade and lesion count data showed 70, 50, and 30% improvement associated with activation by IPL, ELOS, and blue light, respectively, 3 months after 3 monthly treatments. The conclusion was that IPL was the superior light source for acne. (Fig. 3.4). Alexiades-Armenakas showed that ALA-PDT with long-pulsed, PDL activation was effective against a variety of acne lesion types with minimal adverse effects [12] (Fig. 3.5).

The results of these studies culminated in a consensus recommendation for the treatment of acne [13]: "Consensus panel members agreed that ALA PDT provides (1) the best results when used to treat inflammatory and cystic acne and (2) modest clearance when used to treat comedonal acne, although recent data shows that ALA PDT is effective against comedonal acne when the long-pulsed PDL is used [12]. They also agreed that (1) acneiform flares may occur after any treatment, including ALA PDT, and (2) although not supported by extensive documentation, PDL activation provides the best results in ALA PDT for acne. One member (Dr. Nestor) stated that only PDL with ALA PDT has maintained clearance of acne lesions for up to 2 years, even in patients resistant to other treatments." (To the author's knowledge, Dr. Nestor's data has not been published.)

The pioneers of ALA-PDT for acne had formed an overall impression that IPL and PDL are superior light activators over blue light. This has been

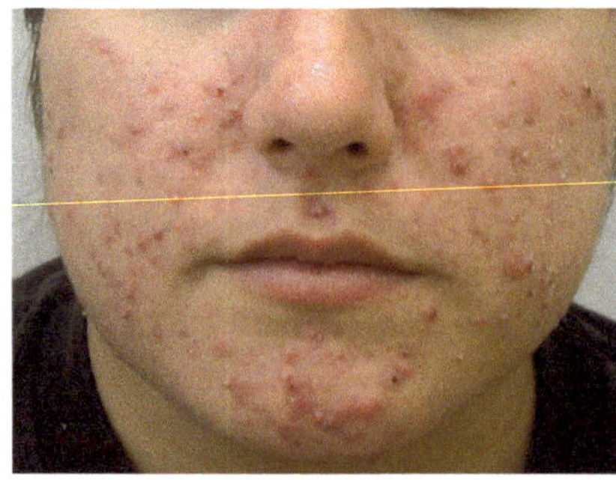

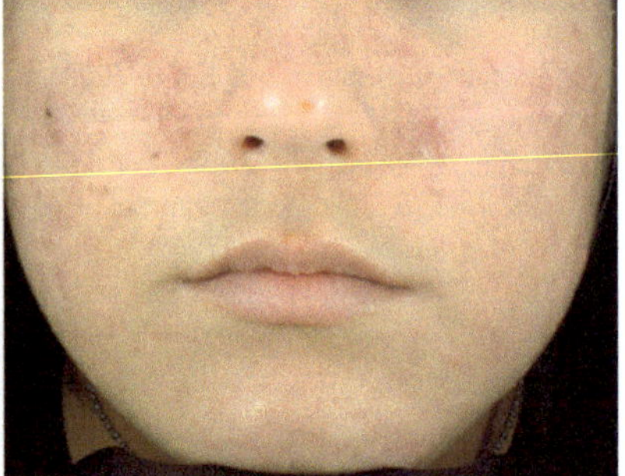

Fig. 3.4 Blue Light and ALA before and after 1 month after 3 treatments with a 15-min incubation time and blue light (photo courtesy of Amy Forman Taub, MD)

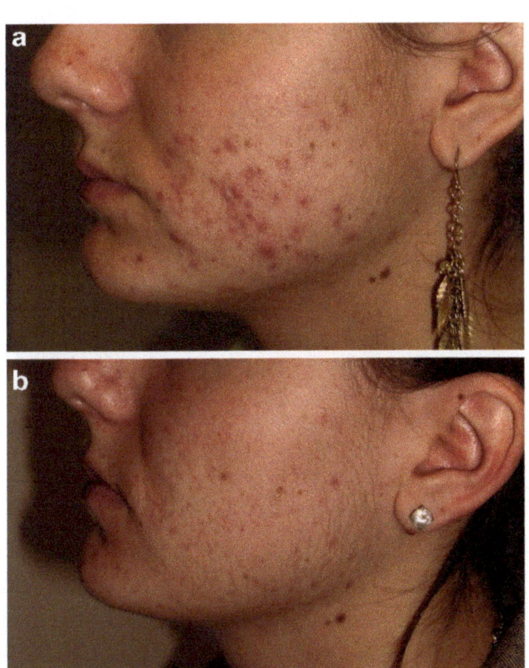

Fig. 3.5 (**a**) Before and (**b**)7 months after ALA-PDT with pulsed dye laser (photo courtesy of Macrene Alexiades-Armenakas, MD)

confirmed by two subsequent studies. Twenty patients with a split face treatment of blue light alone vs. 10% ALA with blue light found that there was no statistical difference in the clearance of lesions between the two sides [14]. These findings are consistent with a much larger scale study (unpublished Phase II trial sponsored by DUSA pharmaceuticals), utilizing 20% ALA and blue light for acne patients. In this study, 266 patients with acne severity of grades 3 or 4 participated. There were four arms split evenly: with ALA and exposure of 5 J/cm^2, without ALA and exposure of 5 J/cm^2, with ALA with a 10-J/cm^2 dosage or without ALA and a 10-J/cm^2 dosage. All patients had a 45-min incubation ± 15 min. There was no significant difference between dosage arms or between ALA with blue light vs. blue light alone. All patients did have some improvement and it ranged from 13 to 64% with patients with grade 4 acne showing more improvement than grade 3 acne patients in all arms.

More recently, a study utilizing 10% ALA and red light demonstrated that PDT does effectively reduce the area and density of macrocomedones utilizing a cyanoacrylate follicular biopsy [15]. Thirty-two patients suffering from acne participated in another randomized, prospective, single blind study [16]. All patients were treated with liposomal 0.5% 5-ALA, IPL and keratolytic peeling agents for an average of 5.7 treatments and over an average of 7.8 months achieved a mean improvement of 68.2%. Side effects were minimal.

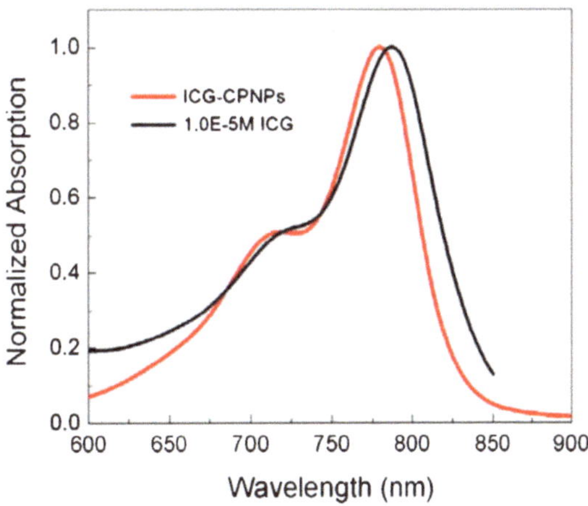

Fig. 3.6 ICG absorption spectrum (from Mills et al. [37], with permission)

Ten patients with recalcitrant localized acne and 22 patients with diffuse acne were treated in another study with either intralesional PDT and 30 min of incubation with PDL (powder from the Levulan Kerastick mixed with normal saline) or conventional PDT with PDL and 90 min under occlusion (treated prior to the application of 20% 5-ALA with a 23% glycolic acid peel), respectively [17]. All groups had a significant reduction in inflammatory acne, but the intralesional PDT resulted in quicker response times and fewer side effects. One has to question whether the use of a peeling agent immediately prior to PDT as well as the long incubation time resulted in more complications than would be expected from PDT alone.

The use of ICG in combination with a 803–810-nm diode laser has been reported by three groups. ICG is a photosensitizing dye used to evaluate hepatic function, blood volume, and cardiac output (Fig. 3.6). In a complex, multifaceted study, Tuchin et al. reported that multiple treatments yielded more favorable results than a single treatment and attributed to the efficacy to bacterial suppression [18].

Lloyd and Mirkov [19] evaluated the effect of long pulse, 810-nm diode laser (Cynosure, Inc.) energy on enlarged SGs of a single patient pre-loaded with ICG. After confirming penetration of ICG into the enlarged gland, the authors performed a laser-tissue interaction analysis to determine the appropriate treatment parameters to selectively damage the enlarged ICG-loaded glands. After finding that the laser energy of 810-nm with 50 ms pulse duration, 40 J/cm^2, and 4-mm spot size are required for optimal, selective destruction of enlarged SGs (>200 μm), they applied an ICG microemulsion to 10 sites on the backs of patients with active acne, covered the areas with occlusive dressing for 24 h, cleansed the areas, and treated them with the laser. Fluorescence microscopy and histologic studies of the treated areas revealed selective necrosis of the targeted glands, whereas clinical observations and serial photographs showed an improvement in acne at the treated area at 3, 6, and 10 months after the treatment. The authors concluded that the diode laser had selectively and safely damaged enlarged SGs.

In a similar study conducted by Genina et al., [20] it was reported that the ICG-diode laser protocol provided the best results in patients with moderate to severe acne. In a more recent study, 0.6% topical ICG, with a 30-min incubation period, was utilized for the treatment of acne and also yielded beneficial results [21]. Both of these studies utilize a diode laser in this near infrared range (Lightsheer, Lumenis,). In the latter study, both single and multiple treatment groups were performed and it was a split face control, with one side receiving laser only. Both sides noted improvement without statistical difference, although there was a statistical difference in patient satisfaction with the ICG applied side.

Methylene blue was utilized as a photosensitizer in a recent study for acne therapy with PDT [22]. This photosensitizer was manufactured in a liposomal form and utilized for acne with a 15-min incubation period under occlusion and irradiated with a red light diode laser for two treatments. There was an improvement of 2 grades of acne 12 weeks after the treatment with over 90% of the patients improving. This article meticulously outlines the manufacture of the product, the testing of same, the proof that only the liposomal variant was taken up by the SG, as well as the demonstration that it was NOT taken up by other chromophores. Thus, this increases the specificity of this liposomal preparation and thereby decreases the potential for complications. There were no reported complications in their clinical study. The peaks of absorption of methylene blue's peaks of absorption are 610 and 660 nm, which are in the optical window (600–1,300 nm) (Fig. 3.7). This is a range of wavelengths that do not target other endogenous chromophores, making posttreatment exposure to visible light less likely to cause continued activation of the photosensitizer and therefore less downtime.

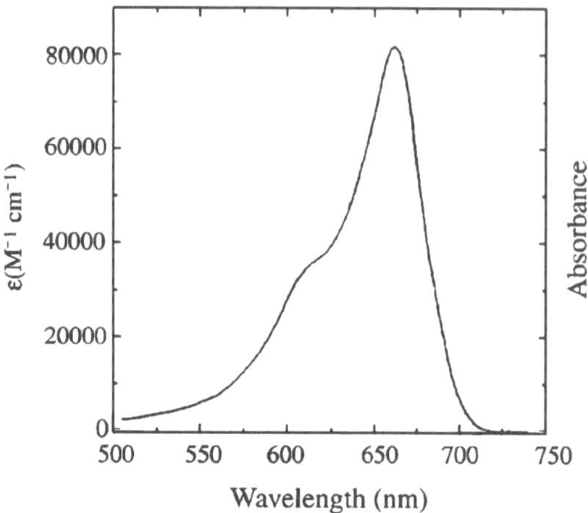

Fig. 3.7 Absorption spectrum of methylene blue

Although the efficacy of PDT in the treatment of acne has been established in these small clinical trials, the mechanism is not completely understood. Clinical data has been correlated with changes in sebum excretion [4] damage to SGs, [4, 5] *P. acnes* levels [4] and PpIX fluorescence [23].

Hongcharu et al. suggested that topical ALA-PDT may (1) inhibit sebum secretion by injuring SGs, (2) sterilize sebaceous follicles by killing *P. acnes*, and (3) reduce follicular obstruction by altering keratinocyte shedding and hyperkeratosis. Although many authors believe that there is a correlation with destruction or alteration of SGs, precisely how the SGs are affected and whether the effect can be measured by sebum secretion rates are controversial, making the true mechanism of action of ALA-PDT treatment for acne still speculative.

There is a continuing need for randomized, blinded, placebo-controlled studies of 5-ALA, ICG or methylene blue in the photodynamic treatment of acne. Consistent beneficial results can potentially lead to an FDA approval of such treatments and increase the acceptance of PDT as a mainstream viable alternative for acne therapy. Understanding the mode of action of ALA-PDT in the treatment of acne may shed light on the relative roles of sebum excretion, *P. acnes*, hair follicles, and other factors in the pathogenesis of acne itself.

Light Sources

The proper light source is critical for success and minimization of side effects in PDT for acne. The light needs to be able to reach the level of the SG, which is estimated to be about 1 mm below the epidermal surface. Unquestionably, some portion of blue light does reach the level of the SG as evidenced by the treatment of acne with blue light alone. However, the energy that is focused on the center of the SG may not be of sufficient magnitude to create the photochemical response needed to affect the gland cells themselves, as opposed to the bacteria around and within them. Red light, on the other hand, appears to penetrate quite well. It is used to treat basal cell carcinomas with PDT, and is estimated to penetrate the surface of the skin to approximately 1.5 mm. Unfortunately, side effects from the red light appear to be limiting the practical application of the treatment as this has been associated with severe crusting, pustulation, and downtimes ranging up to weeks [23]. It is unclear if this is due to the red light dosimetry, the MAL, the incubation period or the fact that it is continuous as opposed to pulsed light.

In reviewing the literature, the best results from light sources for PDT acne with ALA occur with the use of PDL and IPL. Both PDL and IPL employ wavelengths with the requisite depth to reach the SG. It is possible that pulsing the light at its high peak power at short pulse duration leads to the pronounced effect with fewer side effects. The off time between pulses may spare the epidermis; alternatively, the intensity of continuous light may explode the gland as opposed to inducing apoptosis, causing additional inflammation. Additional inflammatory material in the dermis might induce pustulation, crusting, acne flares, etc. Although still effective as it could eradicate the SG, the secondary side effects of continuous wave light may make its use intolerable. The target of PDL and IPL devices is melanin and hemoglobin, both found mainly in the deepest layer of the epidermis and the superficial dermis. The aim is to heat these targets preferentially without overheating of the epidermis. PDL and IPL are designed to have dynamic cooling or surface cooling to reduce the overheating of the epidermis. The cooling that accompanies them may also be a large factor in keeping down the reaction at the level of the epidermis as well as deeper in the gland. There are studies confirming that heat increased the amount of photodynamic reaction that occurs and cool inhibits it [24].

Another possible light source for PDT is ambient light. There has always been a faction of scientists who believe that light sources are superfluous in PDT and the real energy source causing the photosensitizing chemical reaction is ambient light. It is possible, but unlikely, that ambient light could produce enough energy at the level of the SG to be of use for acne treatment. It would be very difficult to control for dosimetry, leading one to expect suboptimal clinical responses and a potentially higher rate of complications, but this is speculative at best.

In conclusion, only light sources that can reach the SG (at least 1 mm below the epidermis) with high peak powers can induce SG demise. For ALA-PDT, those light sources include red light, IPL, and PDL. Pulsed lasers may be better than continuous wave light due to their being able to achieve high peak power while avoiding the threshold that allows gland contents to leak into the dermis, that may lead to excessive inflammation and side effects [25]. It is possible that lower doses and/or shorter incubation times might be able to achieve a better balance for red light with ALA-PDT.

Photosensitizers

Since the title of the chapter is ALA-PDT for acne, this precludes much discussion of methyl aminolevulinic acid photosensitizers. Because there is another chapter on MAL for PDT, we briefly review other photosensitizers for PDT for acne.

The chemistry of the reaction, the absorption spectrum for aminolevulinic acid and the types of chemical reactions leading to cell death has been covered earlier in this chapter. Of main interest in acne therapy is the localization of photosensitizer into the SG.

Data on two photosensitizers other than ALA and MAL has been published as effective agents in the reduction of acne. One is idocyanine green (ICG), a dye used primarily as a diagnostic aid for blood volume determination, cardiac output, or hepatic function. In 2002, ICG was first evaluated as a potential photosensitizer for acne when a study documented that it was absorbed preferentially in the SG, which could lead to a necrosis of the SGs and a reduction of acne [19]. As mentioned earlier, a recent study demonstrated the use of 0.6% topical of ICG utilized with a 30-min incubation period for the treatment of acne yielding beneficial results [21]. In both studies, a diode laser in the near infrared range of 800 nm was utilized as this is recognized as the peak absorption of ICG. (Lightsheer, Lumenis,). Although ICG is readily available in an injectable form, there is no established formula or commercial preparation in usage. As a result of this, Dr. Lloyd's group has ceased using this therapy for acne (personal communication). One important advantage that ICG would have over ALA is lack of absorption in the visible or UV range, making it unlikely that exposure to outside light would extend the period of photosensitivity, thus diminishing potential complications and making it easier to get people to comply with therapy.

Another photosensitizer shown to be capable of killing different types of bacteria and viruses is methylene blue [26, 27]. This substance is utilized in human beings for a variety of things, including the treatment of methemoglobinemia, urolithiasis, and cyanide poisoning. Methlyene blue has been shown to be nontoxic to human tissues for over 100 years [28]. As discussed previously, this photosensitizer was manufactured in a liposomal form and utilized for acne. Investigators implemented a 15-min incubation period under occlusion and irradiated the treatment area with a red light diode laser for a total of two treatments. The data illustrated significant improvement of 2 grades of acne after 12 weeks. Over 90% of the patients in the study showed improvement. This article serves as an excellent reference in regards to how the product was manufactured, the testing of its efficacy, and provides evidence that only the liposomal variant was exclusively taken up by the SG and not by other chromophores. This increases specificity and decreases the potential for complication. There is also less downtime associated with the use of methlyene blue as the photosensitizer's peaks of absorption are 610 and 660 nm. These fall within the range of wavelengths that do not affect most other endogenous chromophores, ceasing the concern of continued activation posttreatment as visible light is unlikely to activate the photosensitizer.

The specificity of the liposomes for SGs would lead one to suspect that uptake in the epidermis is minimal. It would be interesting to see if a red light LED would be capable of similar results and complications as this is more ubiquitous, less expensive light source, and does not require as highly skilled an operator as a laser would.

In the USA, 20% 5-ALA (referred to as ALA) is available in only one commercialized form, the Levulan Kerastick, a single use system that contains the powder and the proprietary vehicle developed by DUSA Corporation for maximal absorption into the epidermis. The original study for the approval of Levulan for the treatment of actinic keratoses showed that maximal epidermal penetration takes place at 14–18 h. Thus, the package insert and FDA approval for the use of Levulan is for a 14–18-h incubation (i.e., overnight), use

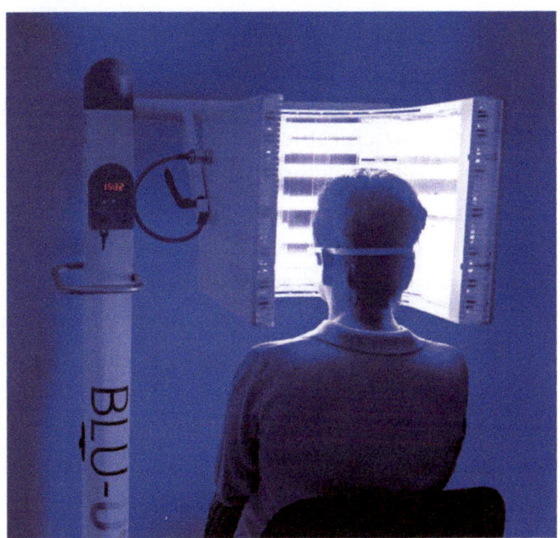

Fig. 3.8 BLU-U® Blue Light Photodynamic Therapy Illuminator Model 4170 (courtesy of DUSA Pharmaceuticals, Inc., Wilmington, MA)

with the Blu-U device (415 nm) (Fig. 3.8) and usage for actinic keratoses only. Use of a Kerastick with the BLU-U device for acne is strictly an off-label usage. The BLU-U is approved for the treatment of acne by the FDA by itself. An unpublished and very disappointing study using Levulan and BLU-U device for the treatment of acne showed that the control side (Kerastick with vehicle only) vs. the active arm Kerastick with ALA performed well for acne at two different doses, 5 and 10 J/cm^2. In fact, both arms irradiated with blue light showed a better improvement on the vehicle only side than the ALA side. The arms irradiated with blue light also showed better improvement in grade 4 acne vs. grade 3 acne, in inflammatory acne vs. noninflammatory acne, and at 6 weeks of follow-up than at 3 weeks of follow-up. The incubation time was 45 min ± 15 min. How can one interpret these findings? The baffling conclusion was that there was more of an improvement seen when utilizing the vehicle over utilizing active solution. The only way to explain this would be to say that somehow the ALA actually inhibited the blue light's effect on the bacteria. As matter of pure speculation, one could pick any of the following wildly counterintuitive possibilities: (1) ALA partially damaged the bacteria not enough to kill them but to render them less susceptible to the endogenous photosensitization from the light, (2) The vehicle acts as a photo-clearing agent for the light to be more greatly absorbed and adding levulan to it reduced this ability, (3) The vehicle is better absorbed by SGs without ALA than with it, (4) the killed P. acnes due to the levulan bolus caused more inflammation than the live bacteria. Since we did not have an arm with blue light alone (without kerastick vehicle), we cannot judge if any of the above even matter, as there are plenty of published studies showing that blue light alone (in various different protocols) causes destruction of the acne bacteria and clinically up to a 70% improvement in inflammatory acne by itself.

Why did not this become standard therapy when it first came out? The results did not seem to last and people required treatment twice per week for 8 weeks, which was impractical for many. There also seemed to be a large variability in response. A patient's success with the treatment was likely based on killing P. acnes, which regrows within a few months if not weeks, necessitating frequent treatments. In addition, the treatment was not covered by insurance. Many patients got discouraged by the need for frequent maintenance. Currently, there are many handheld devices which can deliver both blue and red light [29]. The combination of red and blue light has proven successful in the treatment of acne. Red light is capable of penetrating to the level of the SG to kill the P.acnes that cannot be reached by the blue light. The red light could also heat the SG enough to cause remodeling, shrinkage, or apoptosos of cells. The blue light is efficient in killing P. acnes that is more superficial. The main problem with the handheld devices is the compliance factor. People often do the treatments only when they need them, so they often wind up on a roller coaster, chasing their eruptions with treatments instead of using their devices routinely to prevent breakouts. A major component of the mechanism that has yet to be understood is how the photosensitizer enters the SG. Identifying the factors that increase the ability of ALA to penetrate the SG and the kinetics of both its arrival in the SG and its manufacture of PpIX would be absolutely critical to our improving the results of

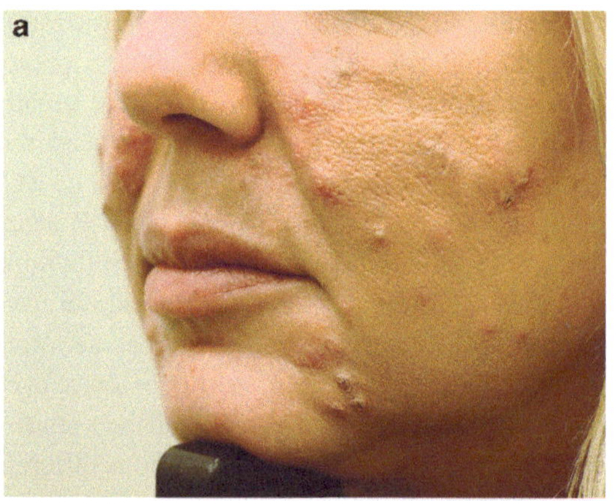

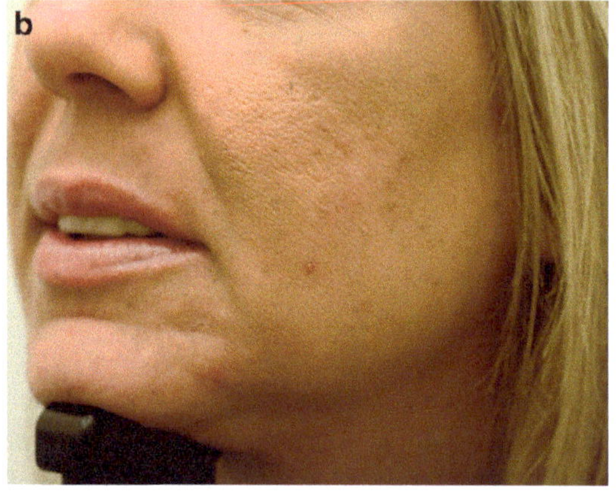

Fig. 3.9 Short contact ALA for acne. (**a**) Before and (**b**) 2 weeks after two treatments with ALA incubated for 30 min and the BLU-U illuminator (blue light) for 4 min (photo courtesy of Amy Forman Taub, MD)

PDT for acne. The author has long believed that there is a much quicker absorption into the SG than into the epidermis due to her positive clinical experience with very short incubation periods of 15 min with ALA-PDT [10] (Fig. 3.9). There is, in fact, transfollicular absorption pathway that is completely separate from transepidermal diffusion [30, 31]. The penetration of hair follicles by substances also has different kinetics than that of a transepidermal pathway. Hair follicle absorption can take place in as little as 5–15 min, whereas transcutaneous absorption usually takes at least 1 h. Of course, there are a huge number of factors influencing this: the size of the penetrating molecules, the lipophilicity of the substance, the temperature of the skin, the thickness of the stratum corneum, ad infinitum. Another method of attempting to localize material into the SG is to encapsulate it into a liposome. These are structures that present a lipophilic face and hence penetrate more quickly into a lipophilic area such as that of sebum-rich follicular orifice.

It remains to be determined which photosensitizers are optimal for acne. ALA has an advantage in that it is commercially available and has a propensity to be absorbed by SG cells. Methylene blue and ICG could be viable alternatives that might result in less posttreatment toxicity. There is reason to also consider MAL, although its use has been fraught with severe side effects in acne. However, as stated above, this could easily be due either to the long incubation periods, the continuous wave length that is usually employed with it, or the combination of the two.

In order to optimize ALA as a photosensitizer for acne, it would be ideal to either perform a rapid treatment to avoid epidermal uptake and "PDT effect," or to find something that could be applied topically or used systemically that could inactivate the remaining PpIX and thus the ensuing 48 h of light sensitivity.

Incubation Time

Incubation times have been alluded to in the sections on photosensitizers and light sources. The ideal incubation time would leave enough time for the photosensitizing agent to reach the SG and synthesize enough PpIX to effect a good photochemical reaction while minimizing nonspecific epidermal uptake.

Almost all of the work on incubation times has been done with respect to the treatment of AK. The work of getting an essentially hydrophilic solution across the stratum corneum barrier and through the epidermis and down to the basal layer of the epidermis where most cytologically atypical epidermal cells are found is difficult. The original research indicated that this was accomplished only after a 14–18 h incubation period; this is still on the FDA label of ALA. Clinical studies thereafter demonstrated that a very good clinical response could be achieved by 3 h incubations with ALA. This was subsequently whittled down to a 1-h incubation [32], which is currently the standard of care in the USA for facial AK and blue light PDT. Through trial and error, most practitioners have come to the conclusion that 2 h create more "PDT effect" (i.e., redness, peeling, and burning discomfort) for some efficacy gains, but not substantial enough to warrant the increased severity of side effects. Areas of the face and scalp (arms, legs, back, and chest) typically do need the 2 h incubation with occlusion as the epidermis is thicker and has fewer appendages.

Practically, none of this significantly matters for acne. In fact, this author believes that the briefer the incubation for acne the better, as having a good absorption of ALA into the epidermis would only lead to side effects since the penetration target is the SG. If you believe the author's hypothesis that the first absorption of ALA takes place via the hair follicle, then a short incubation time would be ideal: it would reach the target successfully without time to be absorbed substantially in the epidermis. For that reason, preparation of the epidermis with keratolytics, retinoids, or microdermabrasion for PDT for acne only makes sense in that it removes the keratolytic plug in the acne lesion, not because it strips the stratum corneum.

Protocols

There are no clearly established protocols for PDT for acne. Using commercially available ALA in the USA, most practitioners have used 15–60 min incubations with or without pretreatment of the skin. Pretreatment can be as simple as conventional acetone degreasing of the skin or as complex as acetone followed by microdermabrasion. Microdermabrasion definitely decreases the time for PDT effect to be seen in the epidermis, in fact increasing the erythema that ensues from a 10-min exposure to ALA vs. a 1-h exposure without microdermabrasion [33]. Common topical pretreatment consists of salicylic acid preparations or retinoids, although some practitioners avoid these for fear of exacerbated side effects. Most commonly used protocols are listed in Table 3.1.

Protocols for PDT for Acne

Postoperative Care

Postoperative care involves meticulous avoidance of UV light for 48 h. It is most convenient for the patients to schedule their PDT late in the afternoon or evening, which makes it mainly one full daytime to avoid the sun. Use of sunscreen is not sufficient protection. It is very important to utilize a physical blocker preferably one containing more than 5% zinc oxide, as PDT is activated by both UVA and visible light. A hat and sunglasses are also recommended. It needs to be explained and reiterated multiple times to patients that car travel is not protected as UVA and visible light penetrate window glass. It is difficult for teenagers to avoid sun especially in the summer, and they sometimes do get affected by a significant PDT effect, which can lead to the loss of school days.

If a patient calls with a burning sensation, after treatment it is highly effective to prescribe oral steroids for a few days (e.g., 40 mg Prednisone or 4 mg Dexamethasone for 3–4 days). This ameliorates the pain within a few hours. In addition, the author prefers Avene Cooling Gel, which is nothing more than spring water that has been made into a gel, but it is highly soothing. A similar product, a low mineral water spray, was investigated and found to significantly improve discomfort for

Table 3.1 Protocols for PDT with ALA for acne

PDT with ALA for Acne	Preferred	Alternative
Incubation time (min)	15–30	60
Light source	IPL, PDL	Blue/red light
Skin Prep	Acetone + Clarisonic	Microdermabrasion
Interval/# Treatments	Q 3–4 weeks X 3–4	Q 2 weeks X 4
Maintenance	Q 2–3 months	Q 6 months

up to 1 week after PDT [34]. Biafine is another current product which appears to assist in rapid healing [35].

At the author's practice, it is standard to schedule a follow-up visit at 1, 3, and 6 months after the final PDT. Maintenance planning is decided at that time and depend on the degree of long-term clearance.

Economic Factors

Unfortunately, economic factors are of paramount importance in the treatment of acne with PDT. Because this is an off-label indication, no major insurance companies cover the treatment. Due to the fact that the therapy is more effective with PDL and IPL than blue light, it is more expensive to provide and less available as fewer practitioners have these light sources. However, if one were to consider the relative overall costs of each therapy regardless of insurance coverage, PDT would be favorable relative to isotretinoin therapy and longer-term therapies with oral and topical acne modalities for moderate to severe acne.

If isotretinoin is ever taken off the market, PDT will quickly become the treatment of choice for severe or nonresponsive acne. In one clinical trial, eleven out of eighteen patients had failed isotretinoin, but were successfully treated with PDT [10]. Although we do not have good data on the long-term efficacy or how much maintenance therapy would be necessary to keep these patients clear, anecdotal evidence suggests that reasonable maintenance therapy (e.g., no more than 4 times per year) can maintain results. Some patients experience long-term clearance after one treatment course of PDT (Fig. 3.10).

Reflections of Clinical Experience

PDT for moderate to severe acne is a very reliable treatment method. It is in alignment with patient's desire to be free of internal medications and their attendant side effects. It gives a cosmetic improvement to the skin that is beyond what would be expected from clearance of acne lesions and postinflammatory marks with time alone, such as improved skin integrity and skin brightening. It appears to have a preventative effect on nascent scarring.

There is nothing clinical in the author's view that should keep PDT from being considered first-line therapy for moderate to severe acne. The factors holding it back include economic

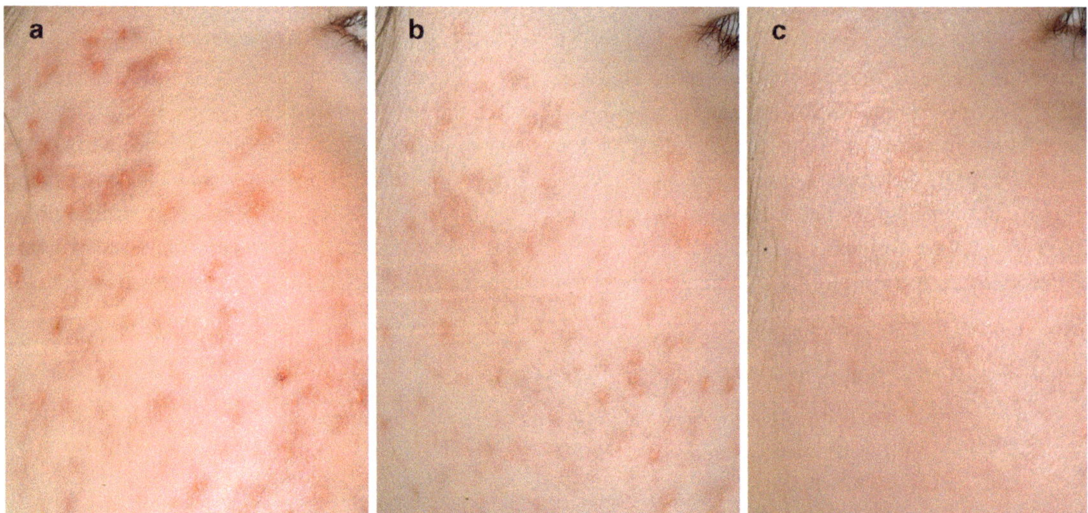

Fig. 3.10 Long-term skin improvement after PDT for acne. (**a**) Patient before and (**b**) 3 months and (**c**) 1 year after PDT for acne (photo courtesy of Mark Nestor, MD, PhD, Center for Cosmetic Enhancement, Avantura, FL)

and postoperative constraints. Patients and their families seem to want to exhaust all options that are reimbursed by insurance before turning to PDT. Many cannot afford it, although one wonders if many of these same adolescents are getting braces which are far more expensive. Only very motivated families seem to want to pursue it: families with elite athletes (Fig. 3.11), performers, etc. Another major factor is that adolescents find it difficult to spend 48 h in relative darkness. It is very possible that with very short incubation PDT there would be fewer PDT effects. Some practitioners use blue light after IPL or PDL to "photobleach" their patients, i.e., to activate the remaining PpIX so that it is not available to incubate for longer periods of time which can reduce the potential for severe PDT effect. If very severe, the PDT effect in a teenager is rather devastating often the patient refuses to go to school until they are healed and the parents worry severely. These practical factors need to be addressed if PDT for acne is ever to become a mainstream therapy.

PDT for Acne: Future Outlook

The future is still bright for PDT for acne. There are many people with moderate to severe refractory acne who cannot be treated with traditional therapies or for whom those therapies have proven to be ineffective or ephemeral. In addition, the further potential restriction of isotretinoin or an increase in bacterial resistance of the acne bacteria as well as the call by many to avoid antibiotics as much as possible (doxycycline and minocycline both being effective alternatives for methicillin-resistant *staph aureus*) leads to the conclusion that alternative treatments for acne are still very much needed. Hopefully in the next decade, we can elucidate best practices for PDT and culminate that in FDA approval for this process. Without this, although a very important alternative, PDT will not be a mainstream therapy for acne. If we can achieve this step, PDT will become standard therapy due to its excellent efficacy, cosmesis, and lack of systemic side effects.

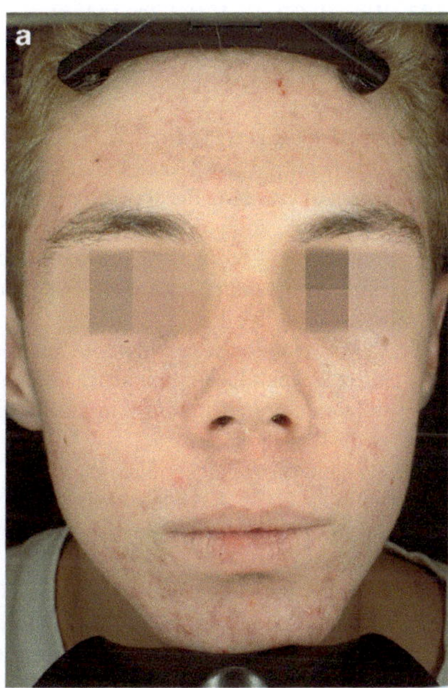

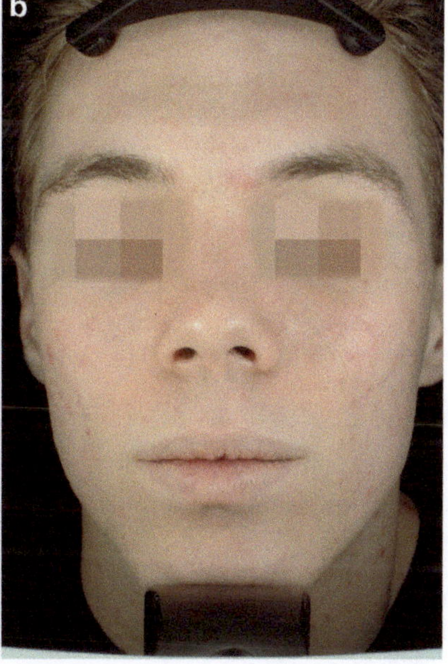

Fig. 3.11 Long term treatment with PDT. Elite high school athlete who failed all traditional acne medications and whose parents refused to allow him to take isotretinoin. (**a** and **b**) He was maintained on PDT with IPL for over 2 years (photo courtesy of Amy Forman Taub, MD)

References

1. Kennedy J, Pottier R, Pross D. Photodynamic therapy with endogenous protoporphyrin IX: basic principles and present clinical experience. J Photochem Photobiol B. 1990;6:143–8.
2. Kennedy J, Pottier R. Endogenous protoporphyrin IX, a clinically useful photosensitizer for photodynamic therapy. J Photochem Photobiol B: Biol. 1992;14: 275–92.
3. Weishaupt K, Gomer C, Dougherty T. Identification of singlet oxygen as the cytotoxic agent in photoinactivation of a murine tumor. Cancer Res. 1976;36:2326–9.
4. Divaris D, Kennedy J, Pottier R. Phototoxic damage to sebaceous glands and hair follicles of mice after systemic administration of 5-aminolevulinic acid correlates with localized protoporphyrin IX fluorescence. Am J Pathol. 1990;136:891–7.
5. Hongcharu W, Taylor C, Chang Y, Aghassi D, Suthajariya K, Anderson RR. Topical ALA-photodynamic therapy for the treatment of acne vulgaris. J Invest Dermatol. 2000;115:183–92.
6. Itoh Y, Ninomiya Y, Tajima S, Ishibashi A. Photodynamic therapy of acne vulgaris with topical delta-aminolaevulinic acid and incoherent light in Japanese patients. Br J Dermatol. 2001;144:575–9.
7. Pollock B, Turner D, Stringer M, Bojar RA, Goulden V, Stables GI, Cunliffe WJ. Topical aminolaevulinic acid-photodynamic therapy for the treatment of acne vulgaris: a study of clinical efficacy and mechanism of action. Br J Dermatol. 2004;151:616–22.
8. Goldman M, Boyce S. A single-center study of aminolevulinic acid and 417 NM photodynamic therapy in the treatment of moderate to severe acne vulgaris. J Drugs Dermatol. 2003;2:393–6.
9. Gold M, Bradshaw V, Boring M, Bridges TM, Biron JA, Carter LN. The use of a novel intense pulsed light and heat source and ALA-PDT in the treatment of moderate to severe inflammatory acne vulgaris. J Drugs Dermatol. 2004;3(6 suppl):S15–9.
10. Taub AF. Photodynamic therapy for the treatment of acne: a pilot study. J Drugs Dermatol. 2004;3(6 suppl): S10–4.
11. Taub AF. A comparison of intense pulsed light, combination radiofrequency and intense pulsed light, and blue light in photodynamic therapy for acne vulgaris. J Drugs Dermatol. 2007;10:1010–6.
12. Alexiades-Armenakas M. Long-pulsed dye laser-mediated photodynamic therapy combined with topical therapy for mild to severe comedonal, inflammatory, or cystic acne. J Drugs Dermatol. 2006;5:45–55.
13. Nestor M, Gold M, Kauvar A, Taub A, Geronemus RG, Ritvo EC. The use of photodynamic therapy in dermatology: results of a consensus conference. J Drugs Dermatol. 2006;5:140–54.
14. Akaraphanth R, Kanjanawanitchkul W, Gritiyarangsan P. Efficacy of ALA-PDT vs blue light in the treatment of acne. Photodermatol Photoimmunol Photomed. 2007;23(5):186–90.
15. Fabbrocini G, Cacciapuoti S, De Vita V, Fardella N, Pastore F, Monfrecola G. The effect of aminolevulinic acid photodynamic therapy on microcomedones and macrocomedones. Dermatology. 2009;219(4):322–8.
16. de Leeuw J, van der Beek N, Bjerring P, Martino Neumann HA. Photodynamic therapy of acne vulgaris using 5-aminolevulinic acid 0.5% liposomal spray and intense pulsed light in combination with topical keratolytic agents. J Eur Acad Dermatol Venereol. 2010;24:460–9.
17. Ryou JH, Lee SJ, Park YM, Kim HO, Kim HS. Acne-photodynamic therapy with intra-lesional injection of 5-aminolevulinic acid. Photodermatol Photoimmunol Photomed. 2009;25(1):57–8.
18. Tuchin V, Genina E, Bashkatov A, Simonenko GV, Odoevskaya OD, Altschuler GB. A pilot study of ICG laser therapy of acne vulgaris: photodynamic and photothermolysis treatment. Lasers Surg Med. 2003;33:296–310.
19. Lloyd J, Mirkov M. Selective photothermolysis of the sebaceous glands for acne treatment. Lasers Surg Med. 2002;31:115–20.
20. Genina E, Bashkatov A, Simonenko G, Odoevskay OD, Tuchin VV, Altschuler GB. Low-intensity indocyanine-green laser phototherapy of acne vulgaris: pilot study. J Biomed Opt. 2004;9:828–34.
21. Kim BJ, Lee HG, Woo SM, Youn JI, Suh DH. Pilot study on photodynamic therapy for acne using indocyanine green and diode laser. J Dermatol. 2009;36:17–21.
22. Fadel M, Salah M, Samy N, Mona S. Liposomal methylene blue hydrogel for selective photodynamic therapy of acne vulgaris. J Drugs Dermatol. 2009;8(11):983–90.
23. Wiegell SR, Wulf HC. Photodynamic therapy of acne vulgaris using methyl aminolaevulinate: a blinded, randomized, controlled trial. Br J Dermatol. 2006;154: 969–76.
24. van den Akker JT, Boot K, Vernon DI, Brown SB, Groenendijk L, van Rhoon GC, Sterenborg HJ. Links Effect of elevating the skin temperature during topical ALA application on in vitro ALA penetration through mouse skin and in vivo PpIX production in human skin. Photochem Photobiol Sci. 2004;3(3):263–7. Epub 2004 Feb 13.
25. Lyte P, Sur R, Nigam A, Southall MD. Links heat-killed Propionibacterium acnes is capable of inducing inflammatory responses in skin. Exp Dermatol. 2009;18:1070–2.
26. Zolfaghari PS, Packer S, Singer M, Nair SP, Bennett J, Street C, et al. In vivo killing of *Staphylococcus aureus* using a light-activated antimicrobial agent. BMC Microbiol. 2009;9:27.
27. Schagen FH, Moor AC, Cheong SC, Cramer SJ, van Ormondt H, van der Eb AJ, et al. Photodynamic treatment of adenoviral vectors with visible light: an easy and convenient method for viral inactivation. Gene Ther. 1999;6(5):873–81.
28. Salah M, Samy N, Fadel M. Methylene blue mediated photodynamic therapy for resistant plaque psoriasis. J Drugs Dermatol. 2009;8(1):42–9.

29. Sadick NS. Handheld LED array device in the treatment of acne vulgaris. Drugs Dermatol. 2008;7(4):347–50.
30. Scheuplein RJ. Mechanism of percutaneous absorption. II. Transient diffusion and the relative importance of various routes of skin penetration. J Invest Dermatol. 1967;48(1):79–88.
31. Kao J, Hall J, Helman G. In vitro percutaneous absorption in mouse skin: influence of skin appendages. Toxicol Appl Pharmacol. 1988;94(1):93–103.
32. Touma D, Yaar M, Whitehead S, Konnikov N, Gilchrest BA. A trial of short incubation, broad-area photodynamic therapy for facial actinic keratoses and diffuse photodamage. Arch Dermatol. 2004;140(1):33–40.
33. Katz BE, Truong S, Maiwald DC, Frew KE, George D. Efficacy of microdermabrasion preceding ALA application in reducing the incubation time of ALA in laser PDT. J Drugs Dermatol. 2007;6(2):140–2.
34. Goldman MP, Merial-Kieny C, Nocera T, Mery S. Comparative benefit of two thermal spring waters after photodynamic therapy procedure. J Cosmet Dermatol. 2007;6(1):31–5.
35. Garcia BD, Goldman MP, Gold MH. Comparison of pre- and/or post photodynamic therapy and intense pulsed light treatment protocols for the reduction of post procedure-associated symptoms and enhancement of therapeutic efficacy. J Drugs Dermatol. 2007;6(9):924–8.
36. Gold MH, Goldman MP. 5-aminolevulinic acid photodynamic therapy: where we have been and where we are going. Dermatol Surg. 2004;30(8):1077–84.
37. W. Mills, J. Adair, and E. Altinoglu, Novel approach to safe and highly efficient cancer imaging, SPIE Newsroom, 9 Feb 2009, http://dx.doi.org/10.1117/2.1200901.1459.

4 Photodynamic Therapy for the Treatment of Sebaceous Gland Hyperplasia

Michael H. Gold

Abstract

Sebaceous gland hyperplasia (SGH) is seen routinely in both traditional medical and in surgical or esthetic-based dermatologic practices. Treatment options vary and will be reviewed herein; ALA-PDT has proven efficacious in the treatment of SGH.

Sebaceous gland hyperplasia (SGH) is seen routinely in both traditional medical and in surgical or esthetic-based dermatologic practices. They arise from the sebaceous gland, which are most abundant on the face, back, chest, and the upper outer portions of the arms [1]. These glands are known to form acini, aggregates of different sized glands that arise from the hair follicles. The acini empty into networks of continuous ducts, which empty into the pilary canal. As these cells mature as sebocytes, they move from the periphery of the gland into the central excretory sebaceous ducts. Lipids then accumulate with the sebocytes and when they rupture, they release their lipid-rich cytoplasm, and then die [2, 3]. This material, along with the desquamating cells of the associated hair follicle, then travels to the skin surface as sebum [1].

Sebaceous gland size and degree of activity vary according to both age and circulating levels of androgens. These glands are large at birth, and then become small until one reaches puberty; with increasing androgen activity at puberty, the glands tend to grow once again. The peak activity of the glands usually is seen in those between 20 and 30 years of age. Then one usually notes shrinkage of these glands, as ones androgen levels decrease with increasing age.

Lesions may grow over time and hence the name SGH. It occurs when cellular turnover is reduced, and undifferentiated cells crowd the glandular lobules, causing an increase in the size of the glands themselves. They usually are most apparent about the face, and although larger than normal sebaceous glands, only secrete small amounts of sebum because their cells are small and undifferentiated [4–6].

SGH lesions are benign and occur for the most part in the adult population. They have been associated with many other conditions and can occur in earlier ages when patients are immunosuppressed. They have also been reported in those receiving immunosuppression therapies such as cyclosporine [7, 8]. SGH also has been reported in families [9] and in other genetically described syndromes, which supports a potential genetic role in the development of SGH [9–14]. SGH lesions appearing at puberty [15, 16] and what

M.H. Gold (✉)
Gold Skin Care Center, Tennessee Clinical Research Center, Nashville, TN, USA
and
Department of Dermatology, Vanderbilt University School of Medicine and Vanderbilt University School of Nursing, Nashville, TN, USA
e-mail: goldskin@goldskincare.com

M.H. Gold (ed.), *Photodynamic Therapy in Dermatology*,
DOI 10.1007/978-1-4419-1298-5_4,

are known as giant SGH lesions [17, 18] have also been described.

SGH lesions are typically round, flesh-colored papular aggregates, which arise from the proliferating sebaceous glands. There is a ductal opening or central umbilication, which occurs as a result of the dilated excretory duct. Lesions of SGH usually occur as individual lesions, although multiple lesions are not uncommonly seen. The forehead, nose, and cheek areas are the most commonly seen sites for lesions of SGH to occur [6, 19]. The etiology of SGH is not known although, as noted, genetics may play a role. The differential diagnosis, although usually not difficult to distinguish, may include other entities such as sebaceous nevus, sebaceous adenoma, sebaceous epithelioma, basal cell carcinoma, molluscum contagiosum, and xanthomas all may be confused with lesions of SGH [20].

The majority of patients coming into our offices for treatment for SGH come in for strictly cosmetic reasons [20]. When determining an optimal therapy for SGH lesions, one must consider that these are benign lesions, and thus all therapeutic modalities should treat the lesions and not result in textural changes to the skin or scarring.

Treatment Modalities for SGH

A variety of treatment options have been reported to be successful in treating the lesions of SGH. These have included the use of a variety of topical therapies, oral isotretinoin, cryotherapy with liquid nitrogen, various acid preparations including trichloroacetic acid, electrodessication and curettage, intralesional desiccation, and a variety of laser systems [21–31]. Details for most of these therapies will not be covered here; previous reports have reviewed them in detail.

Oral isotretinoin has shown promise in clearing lesions of SGH, usually within 2–6 weeks of therapy [21–23]. Recurrences routinely have been reported once therapy with oral isotretinoin has been discontinued. Because of the I Pledge program and similar restrictive programs regarding the use of oral isotretinoin except for its main indication, recalcitrant cystic acne and the use of it in lesions of SGH are limited in today's world.

A variety of destructive modalities have been reported for treating SGH. With all modalities described above, the principal limiting factor associated with all of the treatments is scarring. Also, posttreatment hypopigmentation and postinflammatory hyperpigmentation have also been reported. Care must be taken if any of these modalities are used in treating SGH.

A variety of lasers have also been described as useful in treating SGH lesions. These have included the argon, the CO_2, as well as the pulsed dye laser (PDL) and the 1,450 nm near infrared laser. The first two may also lead to scarring and so their uses are limited. In 1984, Landthaler et al. [29] noted preliminary promising results treating five patients with SGH lesions and an argon laser. Treatments were multiple and given 3 weeks apart. The authors attributed its success to the laser's nonspecific coagulative effect. Marsili et al. [30] used a focused CO_2 laser to treat several conditions noted on the skin of a patient with rhinophyma. SGH lesions associated with the rhinophyma were noted to resolve.

The 585-nm PDL has become the mainstay of laser therapy for the treatment of SGH lesions, and a variety of clinical reports have shown its usefulness in its treatment with minimal, if any adverse results. Schonermark et al. [22] reported in 1997 the successful use of the PDL in the treatment of a single SGH lesion on the forehead of one patient and multiple SGH lesions in another patient. After three laser treatments, the single lesion resolved and remained clear for a 13-month follow-up period. The second patient was followed for 9 months; recurrences were not noted in this case as well. The theory of selective photothermolysis was given as to why the lesions resolved without scarring with the target chromophore hemoglobin, which is found in the blood vessels supplying these lesions. Others have also reported their successes with the PDL [30].

The 1,450 nm near-infrared laser has also been reported to have success in treating lesions of SGH. This laser has been used to selectively destroy sebaceous glands and has had its most success in the treatment of acne vulgaris. No et al. [32]

evaluated the efficacy of the 1,450 nm laser in treating 330 lesions of SGH in 10 patients. Patients were treated 1–5 times at 5–6 week intervals. They noted that from these therapies, lesions of SGH responded with 84% of lesions reducing in size by 50% and that 70% had been reduced more than 75%. The authors reported one patient with an atrophic scar and one patient with temporary postinflammatory hyperpigmentation. Because the main target chromophore for this laser is water, the authors speculated that heat, or via a thermal effect, was the main mechanism for the SGH destruction.

ALA-PDT for SGH

The use of ALA-PDT has been referenced throughout this textbook and will not be reviewed here. Nonetheless, it is imperative to note that the use of ALA-PDT for the treatment of SGH is considered off-label in regard to the FDA indications, namely nonhyperkeratotic AK lesions of the face and scalp utilizing a 14–18-h drug incubation period and 16 min and 40 s of blue light.

What is the evidence for the use of ALA-PDT in the treatment of SGH? Five clinical studies have been published in the medical literature – and will be reviewed here. Horio et al. [20] were the first to describe the successes of ALA-PDT in the treatment of SGH. The authors, in 2003, treated facial SGH lesions of a 61-year-old Japanese man with a 10-year history of multiple SGH lesions. ALA was utilized as a photosensitizer and was occluded for 4 h prior to light therapy. The light therapy utilized was a Halogen light source, >620 nm. The larger papular lesions of SGH did not clear completely but were noted to become smaller after three treatment sessions. Smaller lesions of SGH responded with complete clearance. The patient was followed for 1 year. There were associated burning, edema, erythema, scaling, and pigmentary changes noted after the therapies, but they were tolerated and indicated a potential effect for PDT in the treatment of SGH.

Other authors have reported successes in treating SGH lesions with shorter, more tolerable incubation times and a variety of lasers and light sources. In 2003, Alster and Tanzi [33] reported their experiences with ten patients treated with ALA-PDT and a PDL as a light source. The incubation time for these ten patients was for 1 h, and the patients received either one or two treatments at 6-week intervals. For comparison, the authors used matched lesions on the same patient – some left treated with the PDL alone and others left untreated. Patients were evaluated for upward of 3 months. The combination of ALA and the PDL were noted to clear SGH lesions with one treatment in seven patients and with two treatments in three patients. Improvements in SGH lesions treated with the combination of ALA and the PDL were noted by the authors to be superior to that of the PDL alone. The untreated lesions did not change during the treatment sessions. The treatments were found to be well tolerated by the study participants with no severe adverse events being reported. Thus they found that short-contact ALA was well tolerated and sufficient for SGH to be treated, that the PDL was a good choice for ALA drug activation, and that the combination of ALA and a PDL may clear SGH lesions faster than PDL alone.

Goldman [34], in 2003, reported his results with ALA-PDT and full-face, short-contact ALA drug incubation with either the intense pulsed light source (IPL) or a high intensity blue light source. His patients were mainly being treated for acne vulgaris; lesions of SGH were also noted to be present. Lesions were noted to be relatively clear after 2–4 treatments. The treatments were noted to be pain-free and without adverse effects.

In 2004, Richey and Hopson [35] reported on the use of ALA-PDT and a short-contact drug incubation time (1 h) and a 410-nm blue light source (BluU, Dusa Pharmaceuticals, Wilmington MA). They treated ten patients with 3-6 ALA-PDT treatments spaced 1 week apart and followed the patients for 6 months following the last treatment. All of the patients had at least partial responses to the therapy – and no scarring or other serious adverse events were noted by the authors. Some burning was noted during the therapy in several of the patients and two patients were noted to have transient hyperpigmentation. By the last treatment, 70% of the treated lesions on average were noted to be clear and did not recur during the 6-month follow-up period. Recurrence rates of up to 20% were noted, most seen within 3–4 months following the last treatment.

Gold et al. [36], in 2004, reported on their experiences with ALA-PDT and SGH lesions treating with either an IPL or a blue light source. Eleven patients were enrolled into the clinical trial. Patients received treatments once per month for four consecutive months and follow-ups were for at 4 and 12 weeks following the last treatment. The ALA drug incubation period was from 30 to 60 min. The six patients who received blue light therapy showed an average lesion reduction of 50.6% at the end of the treatment phase, which increased to 55.3% at week 4 of the follow-up and remained at 55.3% at the 12-week follow-up. Lesion recurrences were not observed during the follow-up. The five patients who received IPL therapy showed an average reduction in SGH lesions of 48.4% after the four IPL treatments, which increased to 53.4% at 4-week follow-up and 55.3% at the 12-week follow-up. There were no lesion recurrences noted in the follow-up period. Adverse events were minimal in the entire series – two patients experienced erythema persisting longer than 48 h after the therapy, and one small blister was noted in one patient which resolved quickly without sequelae.

In a subsequent ALA-PDT consensus paper, Nestor et al. [37] summarized the findings of a panel of physicians by noting that SGH lesions do respond to therapy with ALA-PDT. The feeling of the panel was that a 1-h drug incubation was necessary for the treatment to be successful and that light sources to be utilized were (from most efficacious to least) the PDL, especially when using multiple stacked pulses; followed by blue light or the IPL; then yellow, followed by red light. Double or triple pulsing with the IPL will be more beneficial than single pulsed therapy. One to two treatments at 2–5-week intervals were also noted to be best.

On a final note, as far as this author is aware, there are no clinical evaluations of MAL-PDT in the treatment of SGH. Although theoretically this will work, more clinical data is required to see if the effects with MAL-PDT can be useful. Perhaps with a deeper penetration depth with its red light treatment, lesion clearance will be seen.

Conclusions

ALA-PDT has been shown to be a safe and effective modality for the treatment of SGH lesions. These treatments can shrink existing lesions and eradicate many of them with a variety of lasers and light sources.

References

1. Habif TP. Clinical dermatology: a color guide to diagnosis and therapy. 4th ed. New York: Mosby; 2004.
2. Hogan D, Jones RW, Mason SH. Sebaceous hyperplasia. Available at: http://www.emedicine.com/derm/topic395.htm. Accessed 14 April 2006.
3. Montagna W. An introduction to sebaceous glands. J Invest Dermatol. 1974;62(3):120–3.
4. Braun-Falco O, Thianprasit M. On circumscribed senile sebaceous gland hyperplasia. Arch Klin Exp Dermatol. 1965;221:207–31.
5. Plewig G, Kligman AM. Proliferative activity of the sebaceous glands of the aged. J Invest Dermatol. 1978;70(6):314–7.
6. Luderschmidt C, Plewig G. Circumscribed sebaceous gland hyperplasia: autoradiographic and histoplanimetric studies. J Invest Dermatol. 1978;70(4):207–9.
7. Bencini PL, Montagnino G, Sala F, De Vecchi A, Crosti C, Tarantino A. Cutaneous lesions in 67 cyclosporin-treated renal transplant recipients. Dermatologica. 1986;172(1):24–30.
8. Walther T, Hohenleutner U, Landthaler M. Sebaceous gland hyperplasia as a side effect of cyclosporin A. Treatment with the CO_2 laser. Dtsch Med Wochenschr. 1998;123(25–26):798–800.
9. Grimalt R, Ferrando J, Mascaro JM. Premature familial sebaceous hyperplasia: successful response to oral isotretinoin in three patients. J Am Acad Dermatol. 1997;37(6):996–8.
10. Lynch HT, Fusaro RM, Roberts L, Voorhees GJ, Lynch JF. Muir-Torre syndrome in several members of a family with a variant of the Cancer Family Syndrome. Br J Dermatol. 1985;113(3):295–301.
11. Schwartz RA, Goldberg DJ, Mahmood F, DeJager RL, Lambert WC, Najem AZ, et al. The Muir-Torre syndrome: a disease of sebaceous and colonic neoplasms. Dermatologica. 1989;178(1):23–8.
12. Matsui Y, Nishii Y, Maeda M, Okada N, Yoshikawa K. Pachydermoperiostosis–report of a case and review of 121 Japanese cases. Nippon Hifuka Gakkai Zasshi. 1991;101(4):461–7.

13. Jansen T, Brandl G, Bandmann M, Meurer M. Pachydermoperiostosis. Hautarzt. 1995;46(6):429–35.
14. Orge C, Bonsmann G, Hamm H. Multiple sebaceous gland hyperplasias in X chromosome hypohidrotic ectodermal dysplasia. Hautarzt. 1991;42(10):645–7.
15. Dupre A, Bonafé JL, Lamon R. Functional familial sebaceous hyperplasia of the face. Reverse of the Cunliffe acne-free naevus? Its inclusion among naevoid sebaceous receptor diseases. Clin Exp Dermatol. 1980;5(2):203–7.
16. De Villez RL, Roberts LC. Premature sebaceous gland hyperplasia. J Am Acad Dermatol. 1982;6(5): 933–5.
17. Czarnecki DB, Dorevitch AP. Giant senile sebaceous hyperplasia. Arch Dermatol. 1986;122(10):1101.
18. Uchiyama N, Yamaji K, Shindo Y. Giant solitary sebaceous gland hyperplasia on the frontal region. Dermatologica. 1990;181(1):60–1.
19. Aghassi D, Anderson RR, González S. Time-sequence histologic imaging of laser-treated cherry angiomas with in vivo confocal microscopy. J Am Acad Dermatol. 2000;43(1 Pt 1):37–41.
20. Horio T, Horio O, Miyauchi-Hashimoto H, Ohnuki M, Isei T. Photodynamic therapy of sebaceous hyperplasia with topical 5-aminolaevulinic acid and slide projector. Br J Dermatol. 2003;148(6):1274–6.
21. Liu HN, Perry HO. Identifying a common–and benign–geriatric skin lesion. Geriatrics 1986;41(7):71–3, 76.
22. Schönermark MP, Schmidt C, Raulin C. Treatment of sebaceous gland hyperplasia with the pulsed dye laser. Lasers Surg Med. 1997;21(4):313–6.
23. Blanchet-Bardon C, Servant JM, Le Tuan B, Puissant A. Acquired sebaceous hyperplasia of cutis verticis gyrata type sensitive to 13-cis-retinoid. Ann Dermatol Venereol. 1982;109(9):749–50.
24. Grekin RC, Ellis CN. Isotretinoin for the treatment of sebaceous hyperplasia. Cutis. 1984;34(1):90–2.
25. Burton CS, Sawchuk WS. Premature sebaceous gland hyperplasia: successful treatment with isotretinoin. J Am Acad Dermatol. 1985;12(1 Pt 2):182–4.
26. Wheeland RG, Wiley MD. Q-tip cryosurgery for the treatment of senile sebaceous hyperplasia. J Dermatol Surg Oncol. 1987;13(7):729–30.
27. Rosian R, Goslen JB, Brodell RT. The treatment of benign sebaceous hyperplasia with the topical application of bichloracetic acid. J Dermatol Surg Oncol. 1991;17(11):876–9.
28. Bader RS, Scarborough DA. Surgical pearl: intralesional electrodesiccation of sebaceous hyperplasia. J Am Acad Dermatol. 2000;42(1 Pt 1):127–8.
29. Landthaler M, Haina D, Waidelich W, Braun-Falco O. A three-year experience with the argon laser in dermatotherapy. J Dermatol Surg Oncol. 1984;10(6): 456–61.
30. Marsili M, Cockerell CJ, Lyde CB. Hemangioma-associated rhinophyma. Report of a case with successful treatment using carbon dioxide laser surgery. J Dermatol Surg Oncol. 1993;19(3):206–12.
31. González S, White WM, Rajadhyaksha M, Anderson RR, González E. Confocal imaging of sebaceous gland hyperplasia in vivo to assess efficacy and mechanism of pulsed dye laser treatment. Lasers Surg Med. 1999;25(1):8–12.
32. No D, McClaren M, Chotzen V, Kilmer SL. Sebaceous hyperplasia treated with a 1450-nm diode laser. Dermatol Surg. 2004;30(3):382–4.
33. Alster TS, Tanzi EL. Photodynamic therapy with topical aminolevulinic acid and pulsed dye laser irradiation for sebaceous hyperplasia. J Drugs Dermatol. 2003;2(5):501–4.
34. Goldman MP. Using 5-aminolevulinic acid to treat acne and sebaceous hyperplasia. Cosmetic Dermatol. 2003;16:57–8.
35. Richey DF, Hopson B. Treatment of sebaceous hyperplasia by photodynamic therapy. Cosmetic Dermatol. 2004;17:525–9.
36. Gold MH, Bradshaw VL, Boring MM, Bridges TM, Biron JA, Lewis TL. Treatment of sebaceous gland hyperplasia by photodynamic therapy with 5-aminolevulinic acid and a blue light source or intense pulsed light source. J Drugs Dermatol. 2004;3(6):S5–8.
37. Nestor MS, Gold MH, Kauvar AN, Taub AF, Geronemus RG, Ritvo EC. The use of photodynamic therapy in dermatology: results of a consensus conference. J Drugs Dermatol. 2006;5(2):140–54.

Photodynamic Therapy for Hidradenitis Suppurativa

5

Michael H. Gold

Abstract

Hidradenitis suppurativa is a chronic, often suppurative dermatologic disorder that has been shown to principally affect apocrine gland-bearing skin. Hidradenitis suppurativa is a disease that has often been misdiagnosed, not adequately studied by clinical researchers, and often not appropriately treated by clinicians. Hidradenitis suppurativa is a difficult to treat dermatologic disorder. ALA-PDT and MAL-PDT can be used to improve the lives of those affected with hidradenitis suppurativa.

Hidradenitis suppurativa (HS) is a chronic, often suppurative dermatologic disorder that has been shown to principally affect apocrine gland-bearing skin. HS is a disease that has often been misdiagnosed, not adequately studied by clinical researchers, and often not appropriately treated by clinicians. A consensus definition of HS, adopted by the second Congress of the HS Foundation in 2009 states: "HS is a chronic, inflammatory, recurrent, debilitating, skin follicular disease that usually presents after puberty with painful deep seated, inflamed lesions in the apocrine gland-bearing area of the body, most commonly, the axillary, inguinal, and anogenital regions."

M.H. Gold (✉)
Gold Skin Care Center, Tennessee Clinical Research Center, Nashville, TN, USA
and
Department of Dermatology, Vanderbilt University School of Medicine and Vanderbilt University School of Nursing, Nashville, TN, USA
e-mail: goldskin@goldskincare.com

Historical Perspective

Human sweat glands and their functions in the body were first described in the medical literature by Purkinje in 1833 [1]. The first description of HS in the medical literature was by Velpeau in 1839 [2]. Several years later, in 1845, Robin [3] described the structure, function, and location of apocrine glands in human skin. HS was first related to apocrine gland structure and function by Verneuil in 1854 [4], when he described "hydrosadenite phlegmoneuse" as an apocrine gland disorder, later to be known simply as HS. Some have credited Verneuil with describing HS, although it appears to have been described several years earlier.

The next major clinical investigation relating to HS occurred in 1955 when Shelley and Cahn [5] reported that the etiology of HS includes keratinous plugging of the apocrine duct, dilatation of the apocrine duct, and severe inflammation of the apocrine duct. Published reports in the 1990s showed that HS is, in fact, an acne vulgaris-like

M.H. Gold (ed.), *Photodynamic Therapy in Dermatology*,
DOI 10.1007/978-1-4419-1298-5_5, © Springer Science+Business Media, LLC 2011

disorder with predominant follicular occlusion where the apocrine glands play a role predominantly in the associated perifollicular inflammatory response [6–9]. Yu and Cook showed that follicular occlusion was the primary event in HS. Kligman and Plewig [6] described what has become known as the "follicular tetrad," referring to the following clinical entities: HS, acne conglobata, dissecting folliculitis of the scalp, and pilonidal cysts. Yu and Cook [7] showed that follicular occlusion was the primary event in HS.

Epidemiology

The exact etiology for HS and the exact prevalence of HS remains unknown. This has been attributed to numerous factors, including the fact that many patients suffering from HS just do not present to physicians for treatment and that physicians often misdiagnose or have a delay in the diagnosis of HS. Prevalence rates for HS are estimated to be from 1:100 to 1:600 individuals, based on several studies [10, 11]. This translates into approximately 100,000 HS patients in the United Kingdom and over 400,000 in the United States. Further estimates state that 1% of the population is at risk for the development of HS [12], meaning that upward of two million US adults may suffer from HS. HS is considered by many to be an "orphan" disease, due to the lack of easy diagnosis, the delay in diagnosis, and relative poor therapeutic responses to therapy.

HS appears to have a genetic predisposition; clinical studies have shown from 13 to 38% of patients report a family history of HS. Both autosomal dominant and autosomal recessive type of inheritance pattern have been described. HS is more predominant in females, with a female to male predominance reported to be as high as 4:1. Female HS patients note increased disease symptoms associated with menses. Over 50% of females report a flare of the disease with their menstrual cycle [13]. Dermatologic Life Quality Index (DLQI) studies have demonstrated that HS patients have a higher impairment rating than other skin disorders studied, including acne vulgaris, eczema, or psoriasis [14–18]. Nongenetic or other environmental factors have also been described [12]. In this study of 302 HS patients, smoking and obesity have been positively associated with an increase incidence of HS. Smoking may have some role in triggering flares of HS as smoking has been found to occur in over 70% of HS sufferers, a higher rate than would be expected in the general population [19]. Other factors, such as the use of antiperspirants, the use of talcum powder, the use of deodorants, and the use of razors for hair removal, have been ruled out as risk factors for HS [20].

HS has been most commonly described as a primary skin condition. On occasion, HS has been associated with other skin disorders. These are shown in Table 5.1. The clinical presentation of HS has been well described. Inflammatory cystic lesions appear in the predominant apocrine gland-bearing skin, especially the skin of the axillae and the inguinal region. Other apocrine gland areas of the skin also can show signs and symptoms of HS; these areas are shown in Table 5.2 [21].

The typical lesions of HS are described as painful inflammatory papules, nodules, or abscesses. These lesions remain tender from several days up to 1 week or so at a time. Lesions

Table 5.1 Diseases with an association with HS

Crohn's disease
Irritable bowel syndrome
Down's syndrome
Arthritis
Graves' disease
Hashimoto thyroiditis
Sjogren's syndrome
Hyperandrogenism
Herpes simplex
Acanthosis nigricans

Table 5.2 Apocrine gland areas of the body prone to HS

Axillae
Inguinal folds
Inframammary areas
Perineal areas
Buttocks
Scrotum
Mons pubis
Abdominal folds

may be found in different stages at different times on the same individual, and on occasion, lesions become chronic and persist for a long time. This then leads to the formation of abscesses, which then lead to the development of intradermal or subcutaneous epithelial-lined sinus tracts, continuing a source of intense inflammatory activity. A recent clinical trial showed, that on average, individuals suffering from HS have 4.8 inflammatory lesions each month and that disease activity lasted upward of 20 years in this cohort of HS individuals [22].

Three phases of HS are typically described [15]:

- Primary Stage: boils appear in separate places and where nodular noninflamed precursor lesions appear as well.
- Secondary Stage: sinus tracts appear with scarring linking individual lesions.
- Tertiary Stage: coalescing, scarring, and sinus tracts predominate although inflammation and chronic discharge also appear.

These are shown clinically in Fig. 5.1 [15]. Histologic findings seen in patients are shown in Figs. 5.2 and 5.3 [23].

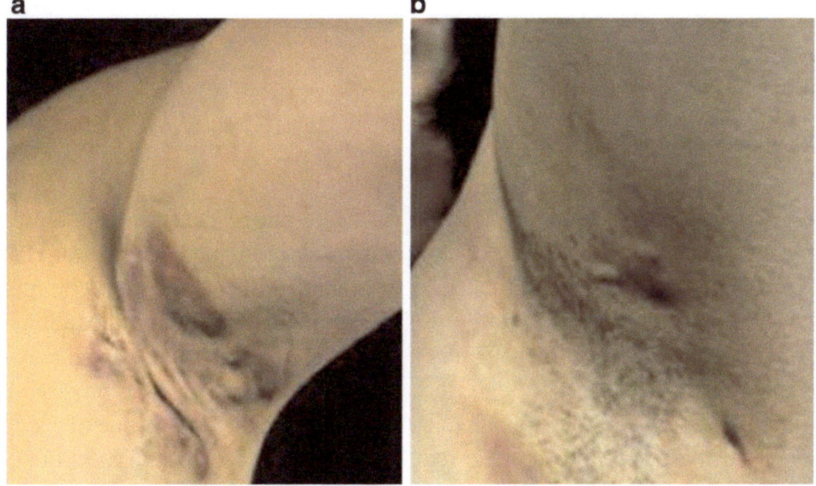

Fig. 5.1 Clinical examples of HS in secondary and tertiary stages in the axillae

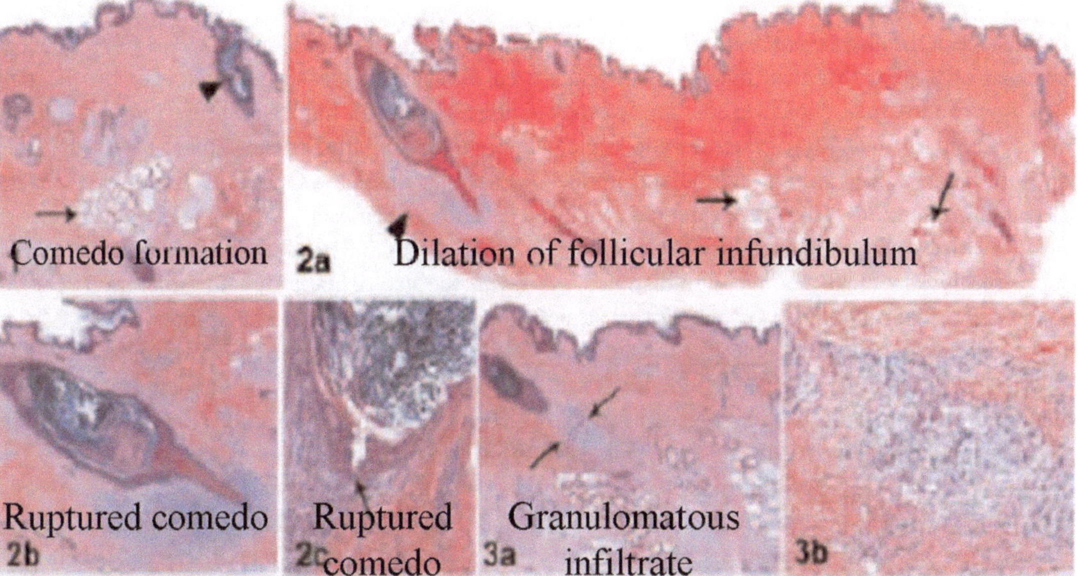

Fig. 5.2 Histological findings in an HS patient

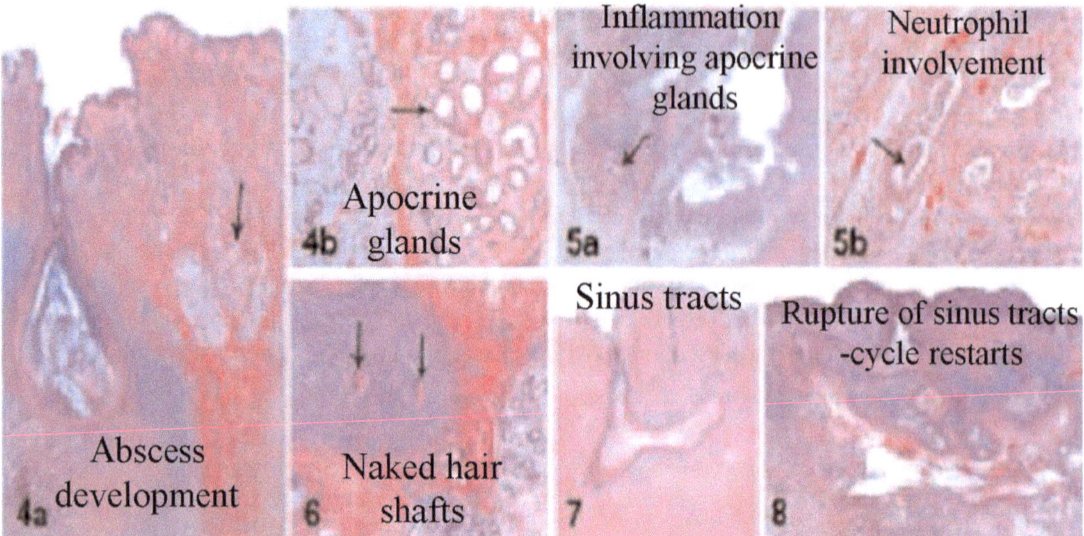

Fig. 5.3 Histological findings in an HS patient

The treatment of HS remains difficult and frustrating both for the patient and for the physician. Most physicians approach therapy of HS focusing on treating the acute disease phase and flare-ups and then considering the long-term management of the chronic phase of the disease. It is not the intent to review all of the different therapeutic options for the HS; these have been reviewed elsewhere [24]. The treatment of the acute disease phase and flare-ups vary, from medical to surgical intervention to a combination of both, all dependent on the physician treating the patient and their knowledge of the disease process and their aggressiveness of therapy. Medical management is the first line of treatment choice in the dermatology arena would include both systemic and topical antibiotics, as well as both systemic and intralesional corticosteroids. Hormonal intervention has also been used, with mixed results. The efficacies of all of these medical therapies are disputed by many authorities, although most would still argue that their use is still the first line of therapy. Systemic isotretinoin has also been used with mixed results in patients with HS. Newer medical therapies include the use of the psoriasis biologic medications, including infliximab, etanercept, and efalizumab. Clinical studies are ongoing to see if these anti-TNF medications play a role in suppressing the disease process [21].

Many suggest surgical modalities as the major mainstay in the management of HS. Incision and drainage, probably the most common of therapies performed HS treatment modality, may make the entire area more inflamed and may end up worsening the overall disease process. However, one might argue that this is one of the more common procedures performed in cases of HS, by all fields of medicine. Excision of small areas of disease activity may be performed but most would argue that wide, radical surgical excision may be the only way to truly control the disease. Most dermatologists would argue that we have all seen cases where wide surgical excision in the past actually did not halt the disease progression and might make further therapies more difficult. Lasers, such as the CO_2 and Erbium YAG lasers, have also been used, with mixed results [21].

The remainder of this manuscript will deal with the use of photodynamic therapy (PDT) in the treatment of HS, something which has been reported for the past several years and has evolved as a potential therapy for the acute phase of the disease as well as offering potential benefits in the chronic phase of HS as well.

PDT has been the focus of this text book and has been described in detail many times throughout the book. It will be reviewed only briefly here. PDT, in its simplest form, utilizes a photosensitizer, and with molecular oxygen and an appropriate light source, it can selectively destroy certain cells in the body. From previous reports, we know that the photosensitizers currently available are able to be absorbed selectively by actinically damaged skin cells, actinic keratoses (AKs), nonmelanoma skin cancer cells, and the pilosebaceous unit. Two photosensitizers are currently available in the US, although other photosensitizers with unique delivery systems are available elsewhere and covered elsewhere in this textbook.

In the US, the available photosensitizers are known as Levulan® Kerastick™ (Dusa Pharmaceuticals, Wilmington, MA) and Metvix® (Europe) or Metvixia® (PhotoCure ASA, Norway, Galderma Laboratories, Ft. Worth, TX). Levulan® is the 20% 5-aminolevulinic acid (ALA) solution while Metvix® and Metvixia® are the 16.8% methyl ester of ALA (MAL). ALA has FDA approval for the treatment of nonhyperkeratotic AKs of the face and scalp utilizing a drug incubation time of 14–18 h and treating with a blue light source (415 nm) for 16 min and 40 s. MAL has FDA approval for the treatment of nonhyperkeratotic AKs as well. Lesion preparation with a curette is recommended and the FDA label is for a 3-h drug incubation under occlusion and therapy with a red light source (630 nm). Two treatments, at a 1-week interval, are recommended as well. All other uses of ALA and MAL are considered off-label use by the FDA, and we must inform our patients of this prior to beginning therapy for other skin conditions besides its use in AKs [25].

The clinical uses of Levulan® Kerastick™ and Metvix®, Metvixia® have been reviewed in numerous drafts and have been covered in detail throughout this book. What will be reviewed, however, is that in the US, most physicians utilize ALA in a short-contact mode, which is, applying the ALA and allowing it to incubate on the skin for a shorter time period than the FDA label of 14–18 h. Clinical studies have shown its efficacy in treating skin disorders in this fashion, and short-contact ALA has become the standard of care in the US Metvix® therapy began with recommendations for a 3-h under occlusion therapy; when Metvixia® became approved in the US, the new treatment paradigm of two treatments 1 week apart and drug incubation for 1 h under occlusion became the standard; although many in the US use the medicine unoccluded with acceptable clinical results [25].

What is important and continues to be important is that in the US, many different lasers and light sources are available that have been shown to activate ALA and MAL. These are shown in Fig. 5.4, which shows the absorption spectrum of Protoporphyrin IX (PpIX). PpIX is the active form of both ALA and MAL and, as shown in Fig. 5.4, has many absorption peaks, which allows a PDT response to occur.

This author first reported the use of ALA and its successful therapy in patients with HS in 2004 [21]. Four patients with recalcitrant HS were selected for PDT therapy with ALA and a blue light source. The patients were treated with short-contact ALA and then exposed to a blue light source. The drug incubation time was between 15 and 30 min and exposure to the blue light was given for an average of 18 min. Each patient received 3–4 treatments at 1–2-week intervals and followed over time. Clearance was noted in 75–100% of the patients at the 3-month follow-up period. Clinical examples are shown in Figs. 5.5 and 5.6.

Because HS is predominantly an apocrine disorder, and not a sebaceous gland problem, it is difficult to explain how ALA-PDT works in recalcitrant HS. There is selective accumulation of PpIX in the hair follicle epithelium associated with the sebaceous glands near the disease pathology and with proper light exposure, as seen in those patients with inflammatory acne vulgaris, a PDT reaction can occur. As well, a potent anti-inflammatory response may play a major role in the resolution of these lesions. In a follow-up to the cases already presented, three of the four patients remained disease free for over 3 years, with the fourth requiring maintenance every 6 months or so.

The second report in the literature, this time utilizing MAL, did not show a positive response for PDT in the treatment of HS. Strauss et al. [26], in 2005, reported his findings with four patients

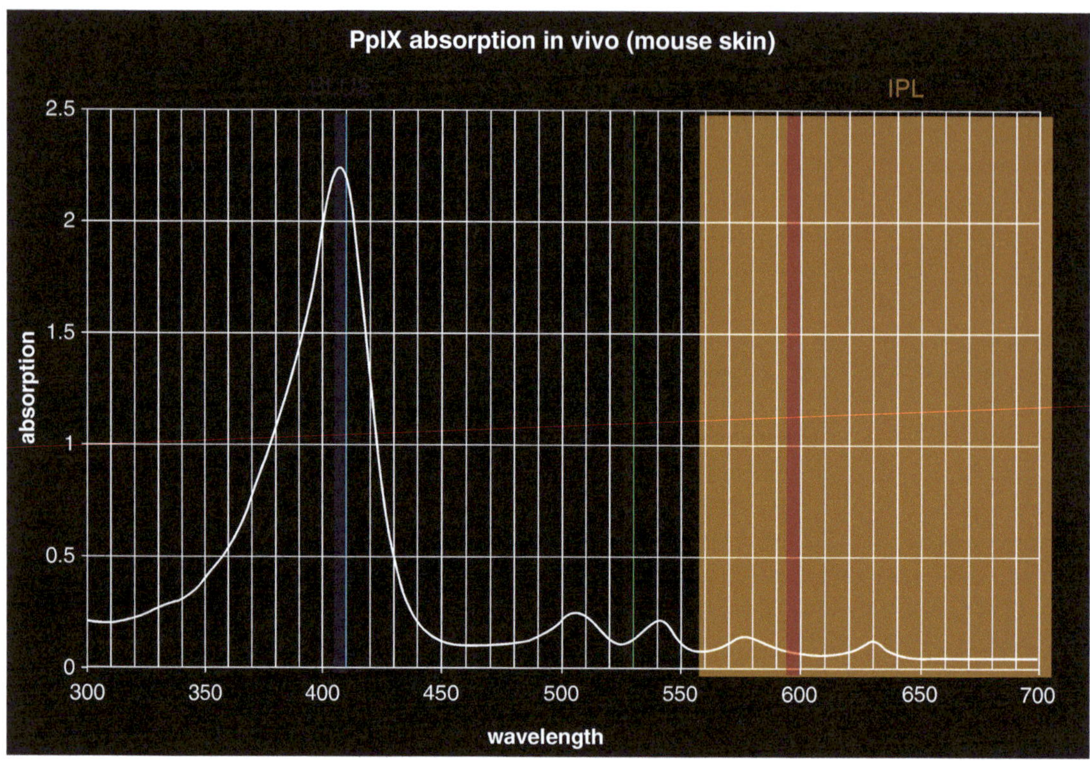

Fig. 5.4 PpIX absorption spectrum

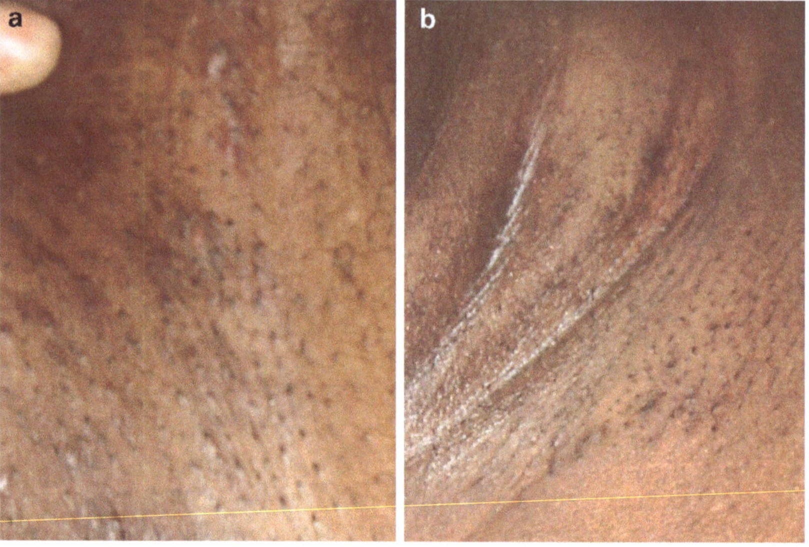

Fig. 5.5 Clinical example of HS before treatment (**a**) and after treatment (**b**) with ALA-PDT

with recalcitrant HS, utilizing Metvix®. A drug incubation of 4 h under occlusion was used in this series. Prior to each light treatment, local anesthesia was given to each site. A Ceramoptic diode laser (633 nm) was used in three patients and a broadband light source (570–640 nm) was

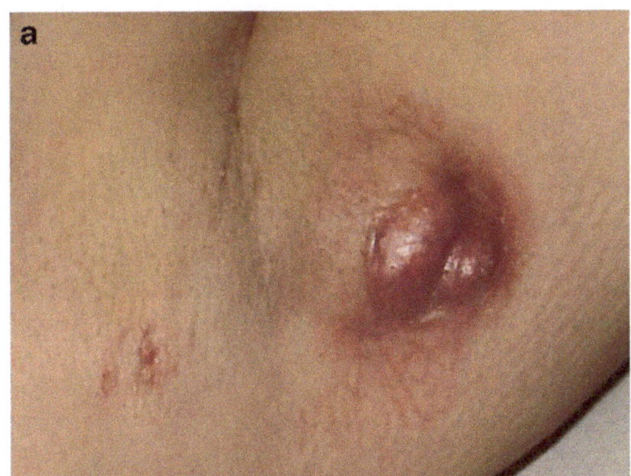

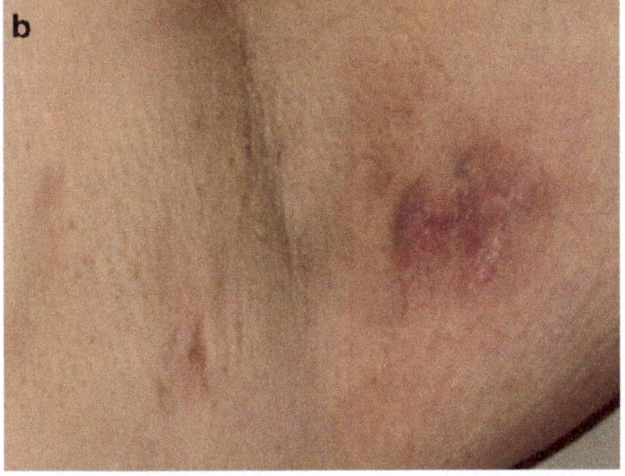

Fig. 5.6 Clinical example of HS before treatment (**a**) and after treatment (**b**) with ALA-PDT

used in one patient. Each patient was scheduled to receive 3 weekly treatments with an 8-week follow-up period. One of the patients received three treatments; one received two treatments; of these two patients, one improved and one worsened the disease activity. One of the other patients did not complete the therapy due to adverse events (severe burning and stinging) and one patient had two treatments but did not continue because of worsening of the disease process. The authors concluded that PDT was not useful in HS cases.

Since these early two reports, several other studies have been reported with ALA and various light sources. Rivard and Ozog [27] reported their experiences with ALA and HS. In their 2006 report, two patients with HS were treated with PDT. Both of the patients noted improvement following their ALA-PDT and blue light sessions, although combination therapy was used in both with either glycolic peels or vascular lasers. They noted their patients were not "cured" with PDT, although both were improved. Schweiger et al. [28] also reported their experiences with ALA and HS. Twelve patients were enrolled in their clinical trial; nine patients completed the study. Patients received once weekly ALA-PDT treatments for 4 weeks and had a 4-week follow-up visit. Treatments were performed with either the blue light source or the IPL. Three subjects noted complete clearing following the therapy; the others improved their HS symptoms. Mean lesion counts were noted to be 11.25 at baseline, 6.5 at the final treatment (50.8% reduction), and 7.5 at the week 4 follow-up visit (29.9% reduction). The IPL was found to be not as comfortable to the patients in treating their HS as compared to the blue light source.

So it appears from these case reports that ALA-PDT can be successfully utilized in the treatment of HS. Not all patients will achieve a 100% cure rate, but the disease process can definitely be minimized and brought under control. In the one MAL-PDT report, the author noted that PDT may not be useful for the treatment of HS. While his results would suggest the same, there are several issues which may explain the failures seen in that study. First, utilizing MAL with a 4-h under occlusion drug incubation will definitely increase the amount of pain and potential downtime associated with the procedure. Patients in this study also required local anesthesia, another source of pain. Pain is definitely a limiting factor for our patients undergoing PDT treatments, and we must minimize the pain component for our patients. We can do this with short-contact therapy, utilizing the medicines in an unoccluded fashion and increasing the incubation period with subsequent treatments. This is what this author proposes now and does for his patients he treats with PDT for HS. This is also the method used in a new clinical protocol that we are working on at this time.

HS is a difficult to treat dermatologic disorder. ALA-PDT and MAL-PDT can be used to improve the lives of those affected with HS.

References

1. Gordon SW. Hidradenitis Suppurativa: a closer look. J Natl Med Assoc. 1978;70:339–43.
2. Velpeau A. Dictionnaire De Médecine, Un Répertoire Général Des Sciences Médicales Sous La Rapport Théorique Et Practique. Vol. 2, 2nd ed. Paris: Bechet Jeune; 1833: 91–109; Aiselle, 1833.
3. Robin C. Note sur une espece particuliere de glandes de la peau de l'homme. Troisieme serie Zoologie Ann sc nat Paris. 1845;4:380.
4. Verneuil A. De l'hidrosadenite phlegmoneuse et des abces sudoripares. Arch Gen Med. 1854;2:537–57.
5. Shelley WB, Cahn MM. The pathogenesis of hidradenitis suppurativa. Arch Dermatol. 1955;72: 562–5.
6. Kligman AM, Plewig G. Classification of acne. Cutis. 1976;17(3):520–2.
7. Yu CC, Cook MG. Hidradenitis suppurativa: a disease of follicular epithelium, rather than apocrine glands. Br J Dermatol. 1990;122(6):763–9.
8. Attanoos RL, Appleton MA, Douglas-Jones AG. The pathogenesis of hidradenitis suppurativa: a closer look at apocrine and apoeccrine glands. Br J Dermatol. 1995;133(2):254–8.
9. Layton AM, Pace D, Cunliffe WJ, Barth J. A perspective histological study of acute hidradenitis suppurativa. Br J Dermatol. 1995;131(s44):38–9.
10. Jemec GB, Hansen U. Histology of hidradenitis suppurativa. J Am Acad Dermatol. 1996;34(6): 994–9.
11. Harrison BJ, Mudge M, Hughes LE. The prevalence of hidradenitis suppurativa in South Wales. In: Marks R, Plewig G, editors. Acne and related disorders. London: Martin Dunitz; 1991. p. 365–6.
12. Naldi L. Epidemiology. In: Jemec G, Revuz J, Leyden J, editors. Hidradenitis suppurativa. 1st ed. Heidelberg: Springer; 2006. p. 58–64.
13. Wiltz O, Schoetz Jr DJ, Murray JJ, Roberts PL, Coller JA, Veidenheimer MC. Perianal hidradenitis suppurativa. The Lahey Clinic experience. Dis Colon Rectum. 1990;33(9):731–4.
14. Fitzsimmons JS, Guilbert PR. A family study of hidradenitis suppurativa. J Med Genet. 1985;22(5): 367–73.
15. Sartorius K, Lapins J, Emtestam L, Jemec GB. Suggestions for uniform outcome variables when reporting treatment effects in hidradenitis suppurativa. Br J Dermatol. 2003;149(1):211–3.
16. Von der Werth JM, Williams HC, Raeburn JA. The clinical genetics of hidradenitis suppurativa revisited. Br J Dermatol. 2000;142:947–57.
17. Galen WK, Cohen I, Roger M, Smith H. Bacterial infections. In: Schachner LA, Hansen RC, editors. Pediatric dermatology. 2nd ed. New York: Churchill Livingstone; 1996. p. 1206–7.
18. Von der Werth JM, Jemec GB. Morbidity in patients with hidradenitis suppurativa. Br J Dermatol. 2001;144(4):809–13.
19. Breitkopf C, Bockhorst J, Lippold A. Pyodermia fistulans sinifica (akne inversa) und eauchgewohnheiten. Z Haut. 1995;70: 332–4.
20. Morgan WP, Leicester G. The role of depilation and deodorants in hidradenitis suppurativa. Arch Dermatol. 1982;118(2):101–2.
21. Gold MH, Bridges TM, Bradshaw VL, Boring M. ALA-PDT and blue light therapy for hidradenitis suppurativa. J Drugs Dermatol. 2004;3(1 suppl):32–9.
22. Von der Werth JM, Williams HC. The natural history of hidradenitis suppurativa. J Eur Acad Dermatol Venereol. 2000;14(5):389–92.
23. Sellheyer K, Krahl D. "Hidradenitis suppurativa" is acne inversa! an appeal to (finally) abandon a misnomer. Int J Dermatol. 2005;44(7):535–40.
24. Revuz J. Medical treatments of hidradenitis suppurativa: a new paradigm. Dermatology. 2007;215(2): 95–6.
25. Gold MH, Goldman MP. 5-Aminolevulinic acid photodynamic therapy: where we have been and where we are going. Dermatol Surg. 2004;30:1077–84.
26. Strauss RM, Pollock B, Stables GI, Goulden V, Cunliffe WJ. Photodynamic therapy using aminolaevulinic acid does not lead to improvement in hidradenitis suppurativa. Br J Dermatol. 2005;152:803–4.
27. Rivard J, Ozog D. Henry Ford Hospital dermatology experience with Levulan Kerastick and blue light photodynamic therapy. J Drugs Dermatol. 2006;5(6): 556–61.
28. Schwiger ES, Riddle CC, Aires DJ. 20% Aminolevulinic acid photodynamic therapy to treat hidradenitis suppurativa: description and interim results of a pilot clinical study. J Am Acad Dermatol. 2008;58(2):P428 [abstr].

6 Topical Methyl Aminolevulinate Photodynamic Therapy for the Treatment of Actinic Keratosis

Surianti Binti Md Akir and Peter Foley

Abstract

Actinic (or solar) keratosis (AK) is a common lesion in fair-skinned populations that develops as a result of solar damage to the skin. It is variously referred to as a precancerous lesion that may progress to squamous cell carcinoma (SCC) or as SCC (in situ type). Methyl aminolevulinate photodynamic therapy is still an evolving therapy for actinic keratosis that has good efficacy and provides excellent cosmetic outcomes. The objective of this chapter is to investigate the efficacy of topical methyl aminolevulinate photodynamic therapy (MAL-PDT), its cosmetic outcomes, and its side effects. Multiple electronic databases were searched for studies involving methyl aminolevulinate photodynamic therapy and actinic keratosis. Cochrane Central Register of Controlled Trials was also searched. Cited references of all trials were identified and key review articles were assessed for discussion of relevant outcomes investigated. A total of 11 studies that studied MAL-PDT to treat AK are included in this review. Four studies compared MAL-PDT and cryotherapy; three other studies compared MAL-PDT with placebo cream. Only one study compared MAL-PDT with both cryotherapy and placebo, while one report examined MAL-PDT in comparison with aminolevulic acid photodynamic therapy (ALA-PDT). The other two studies compared differences in treatment regimens, dose and treatment interval. MAL-PDT is effective as a treatment for AK lesions especially on the face and scalp. The cosmetic outcome is excellent and superior to cryotherapy in terms of minimum skin discoloration and scarring. The side effects, including skin "burning," pain, and erythema, have been reported as tolerable.

Background

Description of the Condition

Disease Definition and Clinical Features

Actinic keratosis (AK) also known as solar keratosis is a lesion induced by ultraviolet (UV) light and often seen in fair-skinned people on areas

P. Foley (✉)
Department of Dermatology, Skin and Cancer Foundation, The University of Melbourne, Carlton, Victoria, Australia
and
Department of Medicine (Dermatology), St Vincent's Hospital Melbourne, Fitzroy, Victoria, Australia
e-mail: Peter.FOLEY@svhm.org.au

M.H. Gold (ed.), *Photodynamic Therapy in Dermatology*,
DOI 10.1007/978-1-4419-1298-5_6, © Springer Science+Business Media, LLC 2011

exposed to sun including the dorsum of the hands, forearms, face, and scalp [1]. It is a very common premalignant cutaneous lesion and carries a low risk of progression to invasive squamous cell carcinoma (SCC) [2, 3]. However, as we currently do not have a means of distinguishing between AK lesions that will transform and those that will not, it would appear prudent to treat all AK lesions. AK consists of hyperkeratotic erythematous macules, papules, and patches on sun-exposed skin. They are slow-growing, small, dry, reddish-brown lesions with well-defined scales that do not flake off. They may become thick and horny and sometimes bleed. In Australia, it has been estimated that 60% of people over the age of 40 years will have at least one AK lesion [4]. AK lesions are often multiple and might be round or irregular [5].

Natural History

Any individual AK may follow one of three paths: it may regress, it may persist unchanged, or it may progress to an invasive SCC. Marks et al. reported that AK is highly associated with an increased frequency of both SCC and basal cell carcinoma (BCC) [6]. Glogau estimated that the rate at which AK lesion may progress to SCC varies from 0.025 to 16% per year [2]. The nature of its progression highlights the importance of effective therapy to eradicate the lesion as soon as possible.

Epidemiology and Causes

Evidence suggests that UV light by itself is sufficient to induce AK [3, 7]. Sensitivity to UV light is inherited, meaning that some individuals are more susceptible to develop AK. Fair-skinned, fair-haired patients, who tan poorly and burn easily, often develop the lesions. In addition, UVB-specific p53 mutations, which have been demonstrated in AK, strengthen the evidence of the role of sunlight [8]. AK lesions occur most frequently in the elderly, especially elderly men, who are also at highest risk for death or disfigurement from squamous cell cancer. There is a high prevalence in immunosuppressed individuals such as HIV patients and organ transplant recipients [9]. Other possible risk factors are cutaneous human papilloma virus (HPV), exposure to arsenic, and chronic tanning bed use. However, AK only occurs in people who are exposed to sun [8].

Treatment and Management

There are a number of treatments for AK. The appropriate treatment is generally based on the number of lesions present and the efficacy of the treatment [10]. Glogau further documented that additional variables to be considered include persistence of the lesion(s), age of the patient, history of skin cancer, tolerability of the treatment modality, and patient preference [2]. Wolf et al. suggest that the most important aspect to justify treatment is the prevention of malignancies and metastasis, followed by cosmetic reason and symptom relief [11]. Treatment options consist of destructive therapy such as cryosurgery and curettage, photodynamic therapy (PDT), and topical therapy. In patients where multiple AK lesions have developed within sun-exposed areas or fields, leading to so-called field cancerization, any therapy, such as PDT, that can be used over large areas in a single treatment session may be particularly well suited. Unfortunately, for lesions comprising large areas of the body, PDT is rarely used because of the cost involved.

Description of Intervention

Methyl Aminolevulinate Photodynamic Therapy (MAL-PDT)

Methyl aminolevulinate (MAL or Metvix™ in Australia and European countries, and Metvixia in North America) is a topical photosensitizer precursor used to treat precancerous lesions such as AK and nonmelanoma skin cancer (NMSC) such as superficial BCC and Bowen's disease [12]. In USA and Canada, 5-aminolevulinic acid (ALA or Levulan™) is widely used. Recent evidence has suggested that there is greater selectivity for neoplastic tissue with MAL in comparison to ALA [13, 14]. PDT combines the simultaneous presence of photosensitizer, in this case MAL metabolite(s), activated by an appropriate wavelength of light to damage the target cell. Braathen et al. [15] reported in the international guidelines on the use of PDT for nonmelanoma cancer that it is important to choose an appropriate light for PDT to ensure optimal photosensitizer excitation and tissue penetration.

Mechanism of MAL-PDT and Patient Preparation

Before the application of MAL cream, any crust or scales overlying the lesions are gently removed to allow for better skin penetration. After topical application of MAL, it must be left for sufficient time, usually around 3 h (under occlusion, e.g., Tegaderm), to allow for penetration of the active agent into the neoplastic cells with porphyrin production and accumulation before activation with light. During light illumination (Aktilite, 37 J/cm^2), photoactive porphyrins are excited to a higher energy state (triplet state). Upon returning to the resting state, this energy is transferred to oxygen molecules present that are transformed into cytotoxic free radicals (including hydroxyl radicals) and singlet oxygen species. The target cell is destroyed by apoptosis and necrosis action [16, 17]. Photodynamic therapy is well tolerated; it has excellent cosmetic results, and studies have documented cure rates between 69 and 93% [18, 19]. Potential adverse effects such as initial erythema, edema, a burning sensation, pain, crusting followed by hypo- or hyperpigmentation, ulceration, or scaling have been reported [18, 19].

The ideal treatment of AK must fulfill three criteria: effectiveness, good tolerance, and excellent cosmetic outcome. Areas such as the face are cosmetically sensitive areas, and patients often consider this factor when choosing a treatment. MAL-PDT may be suggested as a first-line treatment for AK lesion as it is an effective and selective targeted treatment that destroys only target cells. However, to develop treatment recommendations, it requires sufficient evidence from clinical trials and studies. This chapter examines the efficacy, cosmetic outcomes, and side effects of MAL-PDT in comparison to placebo cream, cryotherapy, and ALA-PDT. Previous studies have shown that MAL-PDT provides good clinical outcomes in the treatment of AK. MAL, the methyl ester of ALA may offer an advantage over ALA in terms of deeper skin penetration. [14] Cryotherapy, though it has almost similar efficacy as that of MAL-PDT, is reported to have poorer cosmetic outcomes.

Method

Criteria for Considering Studies for This Review

Types of Studies

Published randomized control trials (RCT) and open label trials comparing the following types of treatment were included in this review:

(a) MAL-PDT and cryotherapy
(b) MAL-PDT and placebo
(c) MAL-PDT and ALA-PDT

In addition, studies evaluating doses of PDT as well as treatment interval were also included.

Search Method for Identification of Studies

Electronic Searches

Literature search was carried out in October 2009 using MEDLINE, PubMed, and Web of Science using the search engine SuperSearch from the University of Melbourne library Web site. Another literature search was undertaken using the Cochrane Central Register of Controlled Trials (CENTRAL), with citations published between 1995 and 2009. This period was chosen because MAL-PDT is considered a new treatment and most of the studies were carried out after 2000. Articles were obtained by using the following keywords: "photodynamic therapy," "Methyl Aminolevulinate" and "actinic keratosis," "photodynamic therapy (PDT)" and "actinic keratosis." Studies were limited to the English language and adult participants. Other than that, two main journals, British Journal of Dermatology and Journal of the American Academy of Dermatology, were accessed because of their known identification for publishing the results of

MAL-PDT trials. Finally, the Cochrane database of systematic reviews was used to find other journals from the references of the studies.

Searching Other Resources

Other resources such as conference presentations and the latest guidelines on the use of photodynamic therapy for NMSC by Braathen et al. [15] were reviewed. In addition, other appropriate studies that met the inclusion and exclusion criteria were identified from the reference list of the included studies. Journals and books related to AK and PDT treatment were searched from the citation of the latest guidelines and other studies included in the review. All the references were scanned for appropriate extraction.

Inclusion and Exclusion Criteria of the Studies

The studies included in this review are those that are published in the English language. The studies included should contain the information of the primary outcome and lesion response rates in their results. Studies are excluded if the patient involved suffered from diseases other than AK, such as Bowen disease and superficial BCC. This review is specific for AK lesions only.

Types of Participants

The studies included must involve adults aged at least 18-years old who had one or more AK lesions and who were eligible for randomization to active treatment, placebo/open treatment, or other treatment. AK lesions in all participants should be diagnosed by a dermatologist by clinical assessment.

Types of Outcome Measures

Primary Outcomes

1. Lesion response to the treatment
   Lesion response is classified as either (1) complete response – defined as complete disappearance of the lesion or (2) noncomplete response – defined as incomplete disappearance of the lesion. Outcomes were measured by lesion count by inspection, photography, and palpation from baseline to follow-up, depending on the study protocol.

Secondary Outcomes

1. Cosmetic effect
   Cosmetic outcomes are defined as follows [18]:
   - Excellent: no scarring, atrophy or induration, and no or slight occurrence of redness or change in pigmentation compared with adjacent skin.
   - Good: no scarring, atrophy or induration, but moderate redness or change in pigmentation compared to adjacent skin.
   - Fair: slight to moderate occurrence of scarring, atrophy or induration.
   - Poor: extensive occurrence of scarring, atrophy or induration.

   Cosmetic outcomes were assessed by a dermatologist involved in the studies.
2. Other outcomes included side effects that are discussed here briefly. Side effects that were documented by the investigator were recorded at the end of the treatment by either interview or questionnaire.

Data Extraction

The following data were extracted from each study:

- Name of the authors and the type of study
- The primary aims of the study
- The criteria of the population of the study
- The comparator group of the study
- The results of the study

This information extracted was recorded and is presented in the results section of this review.

Assessment of Risk of Bias in Included Studies

The assessment of risk of bias (methodological quality) included an evaluation of the following components for each study:

1. Randomization procedure
2. Concealment of allocation

3. Intention to treat analysis
4. Blinding
5. Number of patients lost to follow-up

Results

Result of the Search

A total of 70 articles were obtained by using the following search strings: (MAL-PDT AND Actinic keratosis). Twenty-one articles were found in Web of Science, 23 in MEDLINE, and 26 in PubMed. All the titles and abstracts of the articles were scanned. Finally, the articles chosen were narrowed down to 20 manuscripts. After discussion with the reviewer, only 11 manuscripts that met the inclusion criteria were chosen and were then reviewed.

Description of the Studies Included

Table 6.1 illustrates the description of the studies in the review. Out of 11 studies reviewed, 3 studies compared MAL-PDT and cryotherapy; another 3 studies compared MAL-PDT with placebo cream. One study reported the outcomes of comparison with both placebo cream and cryotherapy. Only one study discussed about the difference in efficacy, cosmetic outcomes, and patient preference between MAL-PDT and ALA-PDT. The last study in Table 6.1, conducted by Tarstedt et al., compared treatment regimens using different dose and period interval between two treatments [19]. This study was included in this review because it has sufficient information on the outcomes investigated. Similarly, a study by Caekelbergh et al. was reviewed for the same reason, even though its primary aim was to investigate the cost-effectiveness between MAL-PDT and cryotherapy [20].

Methodological Quality

Table 6.2 describes the methodological quality of all studies included in this review. Six criteria were used to access methodological quality of the studies chosen. From the table, all the studies had allocation concealment and intention to treat analysis. The studies comparing MAL-PDT with placebo and ALA-PDT, as well as those comparing the treatment regimens, were considered as good-quality studies because they fulfilled at least five criteria.

The studies comparing MAL-PDT and cryotherapy were not able to fulfill three criteria because they were not double blind, and the assessment of the outcome was not blinded as well. There were minimal numbers lost to follow-up reported in the studies ranging from 0 to 17%.

Results of Included Studies

There is now a large body of evidence to support the use of MAL-PDT for the treatment of AK. Table 6.3 shows the results of the included studies. The studies might have had another primary aim, but data extracted were focused on the three outcomes reported in this review.

All the studies showed significant results in evaluating the efficacy of topical MAL-PDT compared to placebo cream. Three-month (lesion) complete response rates for MAL-PDT are consistently high at around 90% (for two treatment sessions).

Of all the studies, Szeimies et al. reported lower *patient* complete response rates after a single PDT treatment [21] (68% with MAL-PDT and 7% with placebo PDT compared with 82 and 21%, respectively, in the study conducted by Pariser et al. and 80 and 18%, respectively, from the prospective randomized study carried out by Freeman and colleagues. The latter two studies examined response after two treatment sessions 1 week apart [23, 27]). Tarstedt et al. found that a single treatment with MAL-PDT, repeated after 3 months only for non-CR lesions, was as effective as routinely using two treatments (7 days apart) [19]. MAL-PDT is now licensed for AK using a single treatment, repeated after 3 months only when necessary.

The result is slightly different in comparison with cryotherapy where the efficacy of both treatments was almost similar. The efficacy favored cryotherapy if the lesion of AK was on the

Table 6.1 Detailed descriptions of eligible studies included in the review

Author and type of study	Comparator group	Study size	Percentage of patient treated with MAL-PDT	Primary aims	Population criteria
Szeimies et al. [18] Multicenter, open, randomized, controlled study	Cryotherapy (1 session MAL-PDT vs. double freeze–thaw cryotherapy)	202 patients 732 lesions (367 treated with MAL-PDT) Follow-up: 3 months	50.5	Lesion complete response, cosmetic outcomes and patient satisfaction	Age: Older than 18 years M:F $T=66:36$ $C=58:42$ Up to 10 AK lesions
Kaufman et al. [24] Multicenter, randomized, intraindividual trial	Cryotherapy (1 session of MAL-PDT vs. single freeze-thaw cryotherapy with non-CR lesions retreated at week 12)	121 patients 1,343 lesions Follow-up: 24 weeks	100	Lesion response, cosmetic outcomes, patient preferences, safety	Age: 18 years and older Patients with nonhyper-keratotic AK 98% located on the extremities. The rest on the trunk and neck M:F=78:43 At least 4 comparable symmetrical AK of similar severity on both sides of the body
Morton et al. [26] Multicenter, randomized, intraindividual	Cryotherapy (1 session of MAL-PDT vs. double freeze–thaw cryotherapy with non-CR lesions retreated at week 12)	119 patients 1,501 lesions Follow-up: 24 weeks	100	Lesion response, cosmetic outcomes and patient satisfaction	Age: 18 years and older M:F=108:11 Diagnosed with nonhyperkeratotic AK on face and scalp AK of similar severity and number of both side of face and scalp

Author and type of study	Comparator group	Study size	Percentage of patient treated with MAL-PDT	Primary aims	Population criteria
Freeman et al. [23] Multicenter, prospective, randomized, controlled study	Cryotherapy and placebo (2 sessions of MAL-PDT or Placebo PDT (7 days apart) vs. single freeze–thaw cryotherapy)	200 patients 855 lesions (295 treated with MAL-PDT) Follow-up: 3 months	43.1	Complete response and cosmetic outcomes, patient satisfaction and tolerability	Age: 18 years and older M:F T=49:39 C=54:35 P=16:7 Mild to moderate nonpigmented AK of the face and scalp
Pariser et al. [27] Multicenter, randomized, double blind, placebo-controlled study	Placebo (2 sessions of MAL-PDT or Placebo PDT (7 days apart))	80 patients 502 lesions (260 treated with MAL-PDT) Follow-up: 3 months	52.5	Complete response rate, cosmetic outcomes, and patient satisfaction	Age: 18 years and older with 4–10 previously untreated mild to moderate nonpigmented AK on the face and scalp M:F T=36:6 P=34:4
Braathen et al. [28] Multicenter randomized, parallel-group open, study	Short (1 h) and long (3 h) incubation period and low (80 mg/g) and high (160 mg/g) concentration cream	112 patients 384 lesions Follow-up: 3 and 12 months	100	Complete response rate, lesion recurrence rate, and cosmetic outcomes	Age: 18 years and older M:F=63:49 Aged 43–91 years Most lesions located on the scalp
Pariser et al. [22] Multicenter, randomized, double blind	Placebo (2 sessions of MAL-PDT or Placebo PDT (7 days apart))	96 patients 723 lesions (363 treated with MAL-PDT) Follow-up: 3 months	51	Complete response rate, lesion recurrence rate and cosmetic outcomes	Age: 18 years and older M:F= T=42:7 P=37:10 4–10 nonpigmented, untreated AK lesions on the face and scalp
Szemies et al. [21] Multicenter, double blind randomized, placebo-controlled study	Placebo (2 sessions of MAL-PDT or Placebo PDT (7 days apart))	115 patients 832 lesions (418 treated with MAL-PDT) Follow-up: 3 months	49.6	Complete response	Age: 18 years and older M:F= T=46:11 P=45:13 4–10 nonpigmented, untreated AK lesions on the face and scalp

(continued)

Table 6.1 (continued)

Author and type of study	Comparator group	Study size	Percentage of patient treated with MAL-PDT	Primary aims	Population criteria
Caekelbergh et al. [20] Randomized, controlled, multicenter clinical trial	Cryotherapy	177 patients 781 lesions (360 treated with MAL-PDT) Follow-up: 12 months	49.7	Cost-effectiveness based on efficacy (complete response)	Patients with AK lesions
Moloney et al. [25] Single center, split scalp, comparison study	ALA-PDT (one side of scalp treated with ALA (5-h incubation) or MAL (3-h incubation) and the other side treated with other treatment 2 weeks later)	15 patients 240 lesions	100	Lesion response rate, side effects, and patient preference	Age 59–87 years with extensive scalp AK
Tarstedt et al. [19] Multicenter, randomized study	Interval between treatments (single treatment or two treatments 1 week apart)	211 patients 400 lesions Follow-up: 3 months	100	Lesion response rate, cosmetic effects, and adverse effects	Aged 18 years and older with up to 10 clinically diagnosed AK lesion on the face and scalp M:F = 82:129

M:F ratio of number of male subjects to female subjects; *T* treatment/MAL-PDT group; *P* placebo group; *C* cryotherapy group

Table 6.2 Methodological quality of included studies

Study	Allocation concealment	Participants' blinding status	Investigators' blinding status	Lesion assessment blinding status	Intention to treat analysis	Loss to follow-up (%)
Szeimies et al. [18]	Yes	Not blinded	Not blinded	Not blinded	Yes	4.45
Kaufman et al. [24]	Yes	Not blinded	Not blinded	Not blinded	Yes	3.30
Morton et al. [26]	Yes	Not blinded	Not blinded	Not blinded	Yes	5.04
Freeman et al. [23]	Yes	Blinded for placebo and not blinded for cryotherapy	Blinded for placebo and not blinded for cryotherapy	Blinded for placebo and not blinded for cryotherapy	Yes	10.78
Pariser et al. [22]	Yes	Blinded	Blinded	Blinded	Yes	0.00
Pariser et al. [27]	Yes	Blinded	Blinded	Blinded	Yes	3.75
Braathen et al. [28]	Yes	Not blinded	Not blinded	Not blinded	Yes	16.97
Caekelbergh et al. [20]	Yes	Not blinded	Not blinded	Not blinded	Yes	0.00
Szemies et al. [21]	Yes	Blinded	Blinded	Blinded	Yes	12.98
Moloney and Collins [25]	Yes	Blinded	Blinded	Blinded	Yes	6.25
Tarstedt et al. [19]	Yes	Not blinded	Not blinded	Not blinded	Yes	2.84

Table 6.3 Results of included studies

Study	Result: Lesion response	Cosmetic outcomes	Side effects
Szeimies et al. [18]	3 month lesion CR favored (non-significantly) cryotherapy 75.3% vs. 68.7%	Excellent or good cosmetic outcomes favored MAL-PDT: 96% vs. 81% (investigators) and 98% vs. 91% (patients)	43% MAL-PDT vs. 26% cryotherapy Burning sensation, skin pain
Kaufman et al. [24]	Inferior efficacy for MAL-PDT compared to cryotherapy (78% vs. 88%)	Excellent cosmetic outcomes favored MAL-PDT (79% vs. 56%) Patient preference MAL-PDT favored (59% vs. 25%)	Adverse effect: MAL-PDT (43% vs. 62%)
Morton et al. [26]	CR favored MAL-PDT (week 24 (after retreatment of non-CR lesions at week 12): 86% vs. 83%; week 12: 87% vs. 76%)	Excellent cosmetic outcomes favored MAL-PDT (77% vs. 50%)	Fewer adverse effects with MAL-PDT in comparison to cryotherapy (62.2% vs.72.3%)
Caekelbergh et al. [20]	CR favored MAL-PDT (80.7% vs. 57.3%)	Excellent cosmetic outcome for MAL-PDT over cryotherapy (83% vs.51%)	Not reported
Freeman et al. [23]	LRR favored MAL-PDT over placebo (p) and cryotherapy (c); 91% vs. 68% (c) vs. 30% (p)	Excellent cosmetic outcome: 84% vs. 51% by investigator and 76% vs. 56% by the patient	Mild to moderate local phototoxicity reaction
Pariser et al. [22]	LRR favored MAL-PDT (86.2% vs. 52.2%) CR favored MAL-PDT (59.2% vs. 14.9%)	Not investigated	In MAL-PDT group: mild to moderate severity (erythema, skin burning sensation, and pain)
Pariser et al. [27]	LRR response higher for MAL-PDT (89% vs. 38%.) CR higher in MAL-PDT with 82% vs. 21%	Excellent cosmetic outcomes in more than 90% of patients treated with MAL-PDT	Local phototoxicity reactions such as burning sensation, erythema, crusting, and pain
Braathen et al. [28]	LRR slightly higher using 3 h incubation period (85% vs. 76% with 1 h 160 mg/g, 74% with 1 h 80 mg/g and 77% with 3 h, 80 mg/g) CR: 78% for thin AK, 74% for thick after 1 h vs. 96% and 87% for 3 h	More than 75% had excellent cosmetic outcomes	Most were of mild intensity (erythema, pain of skin, pruritus, and burning sensation of the skin)
Szemies et al. [21]	LRR favor MAL-PDT: 83.3% vs. 28.7% CR favor MAL-PDT: 68.4% vs. 6.9%	Not investigated	Adverse events: pain of the skin: 55% vs. 22% Erythema: 52% vs. 5% Skin burning sensation: 36% vs. 12%
Moloney and Collins [25]	CR slightly higher in MAL-PDT than ALA-PDT (46.7% vs. 40%)	Not investigated	Pain scores higher for ALA-PDT 10/15 than MAL-PDT 2/15
Tarstedt et al. [19]	LRR was almost similar (81% for single treatment vs. 87% for double treatment) CR was almost similar (89% for single vs. 80% for double)	Cosmetic outcomes excellent for 75% of the lesions in each treatment group	Adverse effect reported in 45% patients (burning sensation of the skin, pain, erythema mostly mild to moderate intensity and of relatively short duration

CR complete response; *LRR* lesion response rate

extremities as reported by Kaufman et al. (88% vs. 78%) [24]. Other studies that involved lesions on the face and scalp were consistently showing the same result, which favored MAL-PDT over cryotherapy.

AKs often appear in cosmetically sensitive areas such as the face. Since field cancerization is a highly treatable condition, cosmetic outcome is an important consideration, and PDT may offer a significant advantage over alternative therapies in this respect (Figs. 6.1 and 6.2). As summarized in Table 6.3, a number of Phase III studies evaluating MAL-PDT in AK have provided a consistently favorable cosmetic outcome, rating outcome post MAL-PDT as "excellent" or "good" by 96, 97, and 98% of investigators [18, 23–27].

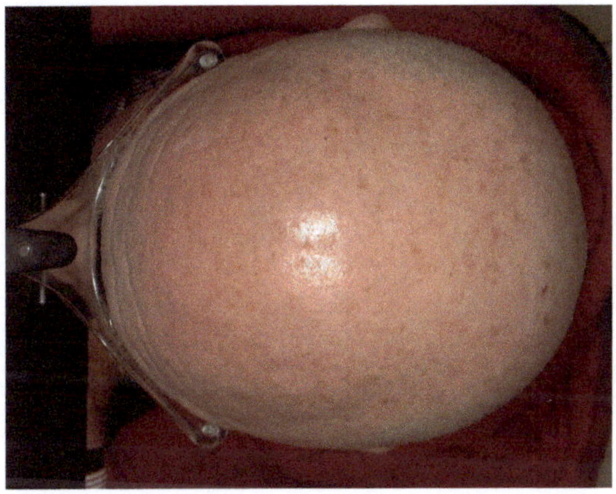

Fig. 6.1 Typical "field cancerization" changes (scalp) suitable for MAL-PDT

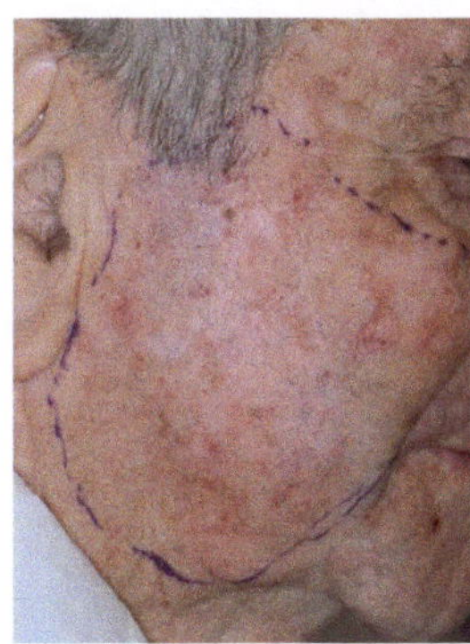

Fig. 6.2 Typical "field cancerization" changes (cheek) suitable for MAL-PDT

All the studies showed that MAL-PDT provided a consistently favorable cosmetic outcome, rated as excellent by the investigators. For example, Freeman et al. and Szemies et al. demonstrated that the cosmetic outcome with MAL-PDT was significantly superior to that achieved with cryotherapy 3 months after treatment (84% vs. 51% reporting "excellent cosmetic outcome" in the Australian multicenter study and 96% vs. 81% "excellent" or "good" in the European multicenter study, respectively) [18, 23].

The study comparing MAL-PDT with ALA-PDT showed slightly better efficacy for MAL-PDT with complete response rate of 47% in comparison to 40% in ALA-PDT [25]. However, the significance of this study was the pain intensity recorded, which was extremely high with ALA-PDT.

For comparison of treatment regimen, both single dose and double dose have almost similar efficacy. Similarly, treatment interval suggested that 1 or 3 h between cream application and illumination has minimal difference in efficacy.

In side effects evaluation, all the studies reported similar side effects of MAL-PDT, which were mostly a skin burning sensation, pain in the skin, and skin erythema. In comparison with cryotherapy, the results were inconsistent, where Szeimies et al. reported more side effects for MAL-PDT, while Morton et al. and Kaufman et al. documented fewer side effects for MAL-PDT. However, the side effects reported were well tolerated [18, 24, 26].

Discussion

Methodological Analysis

Table 6.2 shows that only one study by Pariser et al. fulfilled all the criteria for a high-quality study [22]. All studies (100%) chosen in this review performed allocation concealment. This method minimizes selection bias because subjects were randomized to be allocated to treatment or control groups. The studies that compared MAL-PDT with cryotherapy were not blinded for both investigator and subjects because of the methodological differences.

The studies that have minimal patients lost to follow-up are able to minimize attrition bias. In this review, the studies by Pariser et al. and Caekelbergh et al. documented 0% loss to follow-up [20, 22]. The highest percentage of loss to follow-up (17%) was reported by Braathen et al. [28].

The studies by Kaufman et al. and Morton et al. were of an intraindividual study design [24, 26]. This type of study is powerful as it can minimize interindividual variation that may exist if the procedure is performed in different patients. For example, in this study, the patients had a similar opinion toward the level of side effects they suffered for each of the treatments.

Placebo-Controlled Studies

The results reported in all three studies comparing MAL-PDT and placebo cream demonstrated that MAL-PDT is an appropriate treatment for multiple AK lesions based on the lesion complete response rate. There is a high observed placebo response in some studies relative to MAL-PDT. Patient complete response rates were also high in all these studies, which further strengthens the evidence of its good efficacy. The cosmetic outcomes between placebo and MAL cream have no significant differences as the procedure does not really differ in the two groups, and assessment was only performed on lesions that demonstrated a complete response. However, reported adverse effects were higher in MAL-PDT than in placebo-PDT, with frequent erythema and skin burning and pain.

Cryotherapy-Controlled Studies

There was insufficient evidence to prove that the efficacy of MAL-PDT is better than cryotherapy for all lesions from the studies chosen in this review. This is due to the fact that the location of the lesions resulted in different response rates. For example, lesions on the extremities showed almost similar efficacy with slight favoring of cryotherapy over MAL-PDT, as discussed by Kaufmann et al. [24] (Fig. 6.3). Other evidence showed that efficacy is better in AK lesions located on the face and scalp (Figs. 6.4 and 6.5). This is supported by the study conducted by Kurwa et al., suggesting that the AK lesions on the extremities might be more resistant than those on the face and scalp [29]. Kaufmann et al. also discussed that the resistance might be due to the low amount of pilosebaceous glands on the

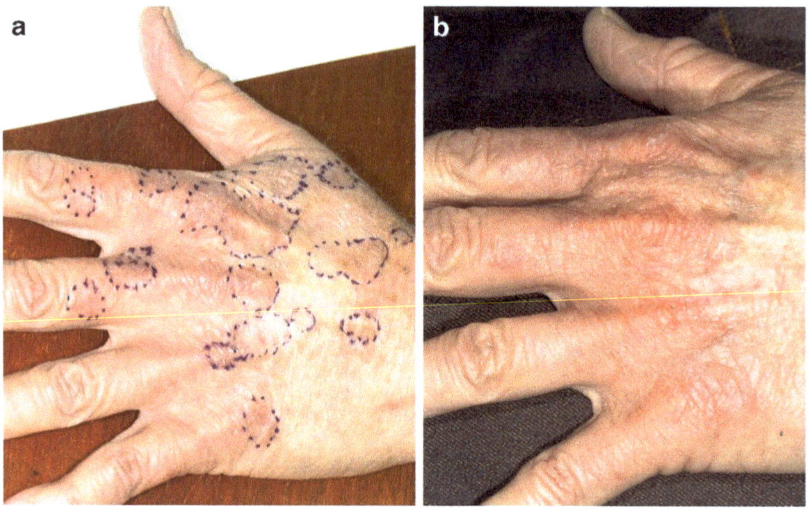

Fig. 6.3 Multiple actinic keratoses (left hand) (**a**) pre- and (**b**) 3-months post-MAL-PDT

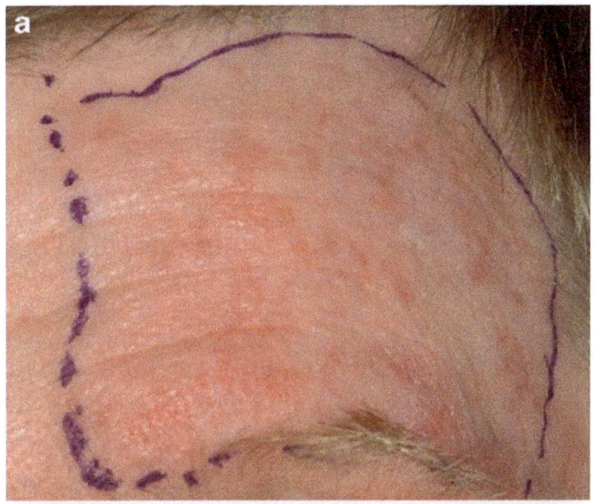

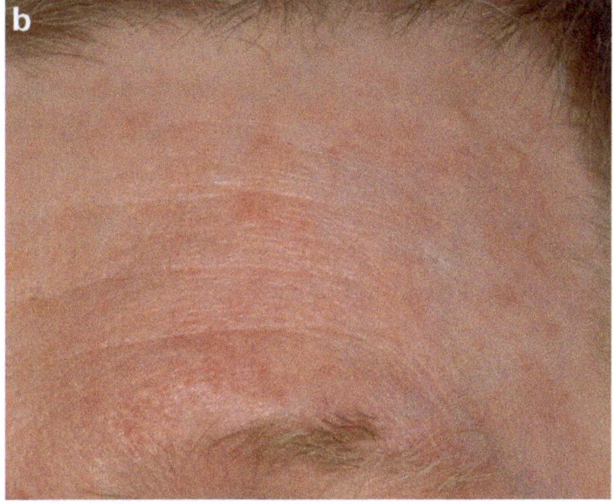

Fig. 6.4 Multiple actinic keratoses (forehead) (**a**) pre- and (**b**) 3-months post-MAL-PDT

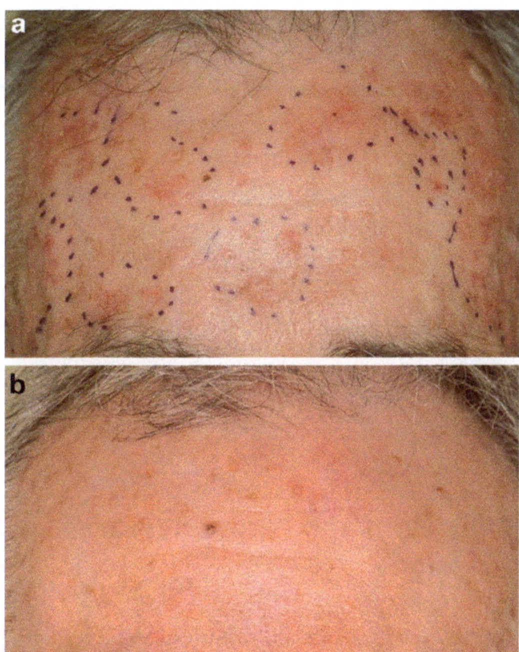

Fig. 6.5 Multiple actinic keratoses (forehead) (**a**) pre- and (**b**) 3-months post-MAL-PDT

extremities, which can reduce the absorption of MAL cream [24]. However, regarding cosmetic outcomes in terms of patient and doctor preference, MAL-PDT was superior to cryotherapy in all the studies included. Cryotherapy caused scarring and depigmentation of the skin at the treatment site and in the area surrounding the lesion. In contrast, MAL-PDT conserves the healthy skin. In terms of side effects, both treatments were safe and well tolerated. The incidence of adverse effects of MAL-PDT was consistent in all the studies with skin burning, pain, and erythema listed as frequent symptoms experienced by the patients. However, the adverse effects were reported as mild to moderate, and they were well tolerated by the subjects.

ALA-PDT Controlled Study and Regimen Comparison Study

Results showed that both ALA-PDT and MAL-PDT were effective in the treatment of AK on the face and scalp. Almost similar numbers in the lesion reduction of AK was achieved with both treatments. However, pain intensity was reported higher on ALA-PDT treated sites. There is only one study available that compared directly ALA-PDT and MAL-PDT. One theory postulates that ALA causes more pain as it is transported by γ-aminobutyric acid (GABA) receptors present in peripheral nerve endings [30]. As MAL-PDT produces slightly better efficacy and less pain intensity, most patients preferred to undergo MAL-PDT treatment rather than ALA-PDT.

The recommended regimen of MAL-PDT is 3-h incubation with 160 mg/g MAL before illumination. This review was not intended to investigate the dose and treatment interval but to investigate the efficacy of MAL-PDT. Results were consistent between previous reported studies and reaffirm the efficacy and tolerability of MAL-PDT. However, it is interesting to note that Braathen et al. pointed out an 1-h incubation time with 160 mg/g MAL to be nearly as effective as the recommended 3-h incubation (CR 76% for 1 h vs. 85% for 3 h) [28].

Tarstedt and colleagues reported that MAL-PDT was effective with either a single treatment session or two treatment sessions 1 week apart (complete response of 89% for single vs. 80% for double treatment). He suggested that single treatment is sufficient to treat AK but advised to conduct two treatments for thick AK lesions [19].

Limitations and Future Research Directions

This review has several limitations. MAL-PDT is considered a new treatment and has been approved by the United States Food and Drug administration (FDA) only in 2004. Hence, studies investigating its efficacy and cosmetic outcomes are limited. For example, there was only one published study that compared MAL-PDT and ALA-PDT. Similarly, studies involving lesions on the extremities are also limited. Most of the studies involved AK lesions on the face or scalp.

Another weakness of this review was that it did not compare the types of lesions between studies. For example, it did not compare the percentage of complete response in thin and thick lesions. It is important to consider this issue because thin lesions may give better complete response rates than thick lesions. Therefore, some studies, which reported higher complete response rates, might consist of more subjects with thin lesions. However, this was rarely reported in the studies included in the review.

Finally, this review did not compare MAL-PDT with the topical treatments, 5-fluorouracil or imiquimod. It is well known that 5-fluorouracil provides better short-term economic outcomes in comparison to MAL-PDT. However, as mentioned previously, it usually involves wide areas of AK lesion. Most of the studies available for the review compared MAL-PDT and 5-fluorouracil for BCC and Bowen's disease treatment, but not AK.

More research should be conducted for us to strengthen the existing evidence. Therefore, dermatologists can recommend MAL-PDT as a first-line treatment and provide strong evidence to the patient.

Conclusion

In conclusion, of the various treatment comparisons from the studies included in this review, MAL-PDT is particularly well suited for the treatment of AK as it offers high cure rates and minimal side effects. Moreover, it has excellent cosmetic outcomes in comparison to cryotherapy, as well as generally well-tolerated local adverse effects, and is therefore suitable for the treatment of AK lesions, particularly those on the face and scalp. Most importantly, PDT can be used over large surface areas and it therefore may be suitable for the treatment of multiple AK lesions and areas of "field cancerization"

Future research directed toward investigating MAL-PDT for the lesions on other areas of the body and comparing MAL-PDT with other topical field treatments such as 5-fluorouracil should be conducted.

References

1. Salasche SJ. Epidemiology of actinic keratoses and squamous cell carcinoma. J Am Acad Dermatol. 2000;42:4–7.
2. Glogau RG. The risk of progression to invasive disease. J Am Acad Dermatol. 2004;42:23–4.
3. Leffell DJ. The scientific basis of skin cancer. J Am Acad Dermatol. 2000;42:18–22.
4. Drake LA, Ceilley RI, Cornelison RL. Guidelines of care for actinic keratoses. J Am Acad Dermatol. 1995;32:95–8.
5. Squamous SG, Carcinoma C, Keratosis A, Keratosis S. Manual of skin disease. 5th ed. Philadelphia: JB Lippincott; 1985. 1985.
6. Marks R, Rennie G, Selwood T. The relationship of basal cell carcinomas and squamous cell carcinomas to solar keratoses. Arch Dermatol. 1998;124: 1039–42.
7. Nelson MA, Einspahr JG, Alberts DS. Analysis of the p53 gene in human precancerous actinic keratosis lesions and squamous cell cancers. Cancer Lett. 1994;85(1):23–9.

8. de Berker D, McGregor JM, Hughes BR. Guidelines for the management of actinic keratoses. Br J Dermatol. 2007;156:222–30.
9. Parrish JA. Immunosuppression, skin cancer, and ultraviolet A radiation. N Eng J Med. 2005;353(25): 2712–3.
10. Gold MH. Pharmacoeconomic analysis of the treatment of multiple actinic keratoses. J Drugs Dermatol. 2008;7(1):23–5.
11. Wolf JEJ, Talyor JR, Tschen E, Kang S. Topical 3.0% diclofenac in 2.5% hyaluronan gel in the treatment of actinic keratoses. Int J Dermatol. 2001;40:709–13.
12. Calzavara-Pinton PG, Venturini M, Sala R. Photodynamic therapy: update 2006 Part 2: clinical results. JEADV. 2007;21(4):439–51.
13. Angell-Petersen E, Sorensen R, Warloe T, Soler AM, Moan J, Peng Q, et al. Porphyrin formation in actinic keratosis and basal cell carcinoma after topical application of methyl 5-aminolevulinate. J Invest Dermatol. 2005;126(2):265–71.
14. Peng Q, Soler A, Warloe T, Nesland J, Giercksky K. Selective distribution of porphyrins in skin thick basal cell carcinoma after topical application of methyl 5-aminolevulinate. J Photochem Photobiol B. 2001; 62(3):140–5.
15. Braathen LR, Szeimies R-M, Basset-Seguin N, Bissonnette R, Foley P, Pariser D, et al. Guidelines on the use of photodynamic therapy for nonmelanoma skin cancer: an international consensus. J Am Acad Dermatol. 2007;56(1):125–43.
16. Faten G, Gilles V, Michele B, Richard B, Robert B. Photodynamic therapy with 5-aminolevulinic acid induces apoptosis and caspase activation in malignant T Cells. J Cutan Med Surg. 2001;5:8–13.
17. Noodt BB, Berg K, Stokke T, Peng Q, Nesland JM. Apoptosis and necrosis induced with light and 5-aminolaevulinic acid-derived protoporphyrin IX. Br J Cancer. 1996;74(1):22–9.
18. Szeimies RM, Karrer S, Radakovic-Fijan S, Tanew A, Calzavara-Pinton PG, Zane C, et al. Photodynamic therapy using topical methyl 5-aminolevulinate compared with cryotherapy for actinic keratosis: A prospective, randomized study. J Am Acad Dermatol. 2002;47(2):258–62.
19. Tarstedt M, Rosdahl I, Berne B, Svanberg K, Wennberg A-M. A randomized multicenter study to compare two treatment regimens of topical methyl aminolevulinate (Metvix)-PDT in actinic keratosis of the face and scalp. Acta Derm Venereol. 2005;85:1–5.
20. Caekelbergh K, Annemans L, Lambert J, Roelandts R. Economic evaluation of methyl aminolaevulinate-based photodynamic therapy in the management of actinic keratosis and basal cell carcinoma. Br J Dermatol. 2006;155:784–90.
21. Szeimies R-M, Matheson RT, Davis SA, Bhatia AC, Frambach Y, Klövekorn W, et al. Topical methyl aminolevulinate photodynamic therapy using red light-emitting diode light for multiple actinic keratoses: a randomized study. Dermatol Surg. 2009;35: 586–92.
22. Pariser D, Loss R, Jarratt M, Abramovits W, Spencer J, Geronemus R, et al. Topical methyl-aminolevulinate photodynamic therapy using red light-emitting diode light for treatment of multiple actinic keratoses: a randomized, double-blind placebo-controlled study. J Am Acad Dermatol. 2008;59(4):569–76.
23. Freeman M, Vinciullo C, Francis D, Spelman L, Nguyen R, Fergin P, et al. A comparison of photodynamic therapy using topical methyl aminolevulinate (Metvix) with single cycle cryotherapy in patients with actinic keratosis: a prospective, randomized study. J Dermatol Treat. 2003;14:99–106.
24. Kaufmann R, Spelman L, Weightman W, Reifenberger J, Szeimies RM, Verhaeghe E, et al. Multicentre intraindividual randomized trial of topical methyl aminolaevulinate photodynamic therapy vs. cryotherapy for multiple actinic keratoses on the extremities. Br J Dermatol. 2008;158(5):994–9.
25. Moloney FJ, Collins P. Randomized, double-blind, prospective study to compare topical 5-aminolaevulinic acid methylester with topical 5-aminolaevulinic acid photodynamic therapy for extensive scalp actinic keratosis. Br J Dermatol. 2007;157:87–91.
26. Morton C, Campbell S, Gupta G, Keohane S, Lear J, Zaki I, et al. Intraindividual, right–left comparison of topical methyl aminolaevulinate-photodynamic therapy and cryotherapy in subjects with actinic keratoses: a multicentre, randomized controlled study. Br J Dermatol. 2006;5(155):1029–36.
27. Pariser DM, Lowe NJ, Stewart DM, Jarratt MT, Lucky AW, Pariser RJ, et al. Photodynamic therapy with topical methyl aminolevulinate for actinic keratosis: results of a prospective randomized multicenter trial. J Am Acad Dermatol. 2003;48:227–32.
28. Braathen LR, Paredes BE, Saksela O, Fritsch C, Gardlo K, Morken T, et al. Short incubation with methyl aminolevulinate for photodynamic therapy of actinic keratoses. J Eur Acad Dermatol Venereol. 2008;23:550–5.
29. Kurwa HA, Yong Gee SA, Seed PT. A randomized paired comparison of photodynamic therapy and topical 5 fluorouracil in the treatment of actinic keratosis. J Am Acad Dermatol. 1999;41:414–8.
30. Rud E, Gederaas O, Hogset A. 5-aminolevulinic acid, but not 5-aminolevulinic esters, is transported into adenocarcinoma cells by BETA trabsporter. Photochem Photobiol. 2000;71:640–7.

Methyl Aminolevulinate in Skin Cancers

7

Rolf-Markus Szeimies and Philipp Babilas

Abstract

Methyl aminolevulinate (MAL) is registered in several countries worldwide not only for PDT of actinic keratoses but also for superficial and nodular basal cell carcinoma (sBCC & nBCC) and Bowen's disease. In the following chapter, evidence-based data of MAL-PDT for epithelial skin cancer are reviewed and further use of MAL-PDT is discussed. Cure rates for sBCC and nBCC are comparable to that of other nonsurgical procedures, whereas MAL-PDT for Bowen's disease is as effective as conventional surgery or application of topical 5-FU or cryotherapy, but with much better cosmesis.

Methyl aminolevulinate (MAL) is registered in several countries worldwide not only for PDT of actinic keratoses but also for superficial and nodular basal cell carcinoma (sBCC and nBCC) and Bowen's disease [1–3]. In the following chapter, evidence-based data of MAL-PDT for epithelial skin cancer are reviewed and further use of MAL-PDT is discussed.

Basal Cell Carcinoma

Various studies concerning MAL-PDT for BCC have been performed over the years [4–10]. The weighted average complete clearance rates calculated from 12 studies (follow-up periods: 3–36 months) were 87% for sBCC (n=826) and 53% for nBCC (n=208) [2, 10]. Available compiled data from other trials have shown an average of 87% for sBCC and of 71% for nBCC [11].

Solèr et al. [4] studied the long-term effects of MAL-PDT (59 patients, 350 BCC). Nodular tumors had been curetted before MAL-PDT (160 mg/g) was applied for 24 or 3 h prior to irradiation with a broadband halogen light source (50–200 J/cm^2). The patients were followed for 2–4 years (mean 35 months). Overall cure rate was 79%; cosmetic outcome was excellent or good in 98% of completely responding lesions.

In a recent, open, uncontrolled, prospective, multicenter trial, both patients with superficial and/or nodular BCC who were at risk of complications (poor cosmetic outcome, disfigurement, and/or recurrence) when using conventional therapy were studied. Ninety-four patients were treated with a single cycle of MAL-PDT involving two treatment sessions 1 week apart, and followed up at 3 months, at which time nonresponders were retreated. The clinical lesion remission rate

R.-M. Szeimies (✉)
Department of Dermatology and Allergology, Klinikum Vest Academic Teaching Hospital, 45657, Recklinghausen, Germany
and
Department of Dermatology, Regensburg University Hospital, 93042, Regensburg, Germany
e-mail: Rolf-markus.szeimies@klinikum-vest.de

M.H. Gold (ed.), *Photodynamic Therapy in Dermatology*,
DOI 10.1007/978-1-4419-1298-5_7,

after 3 months was 92% for sBCC and 87% for nBCC. Histological cure rates at this time point were 85% for sBCC and 75% for nBCC. At 2 years after treatment, the overall lesion recurrence rate was 18% [6].

In a comparative trial in Australia, MAL-PDT for nBCC was compared to placebo. Lesions from 66 patients were treated in two sessions of either placebo or MAL-PDT in a randomized, double-blind controlled study. In case there was no complete response 3 months after initial treatment, the lesions were excised. After 6 months, complete remission rate was 73% for MAL-PDT compared to 21% for placebo [12].

In another European multicenter, open, randomized trial, MAL-PDT for nBCC was compared with surgery. A total of 101 patients were included and received either PDT twice 7 days apart (75 J/cm^2 red light) or surgical excision. The primary end point of this trial was the clinically assessed lesion clearance at 3 months after treatment, besides cosmetic outcome. The 3-month cure rate was similar with MAL-PDT or surgery (91 vs. 98%), the 2-year recurrence rate was 10% with MAL and 2% with surgery. The cosmetic result was rated good or excellent in 85% of the patients receiving PDT vs. 33% treated with surgery [7].

In a multicenter, randomized, controlled, open study, Szeimies et al. compared MAL-PDT (two sessions, 1 week apart, repeated 3 months later if there is an incomplete clinical response) to simple excision surgery of sBCC (196 patients, on average 1.4 lesions each). Primary end points were efficacy and cosmetic outcome over a 1-year period. Mean lesion count reduction at 3 months was 92.2% with MAL-PDT vs. 99.2% with surgery, confirming the noninferiority hypothesis (95% confidence interval: −12.1, −1.9). A total of 92.2% lesions showed complete remission at 3 months with MAL-PDT vs. 99.2% with surgery. At 12 months, 9.3% lesions recurred with MAL-PDT and none recurred with surgery. Cosmetic outcome was statistically superior for MAL-PDT at all time points. At 12 months, 94.1% lesions treated with MAL-PDT had an excellent or good cosmetic outcome according to the investigator compared to 59.8% with surgery. This difference was confirmed by self-assessment of the patients. The proportion of excellent cosmetic outcome markedly improved over time with MAL-PDT in contrast to surgery. However, the surgical standard treatment for sBCC is curettage, and this procedure would likely lead to significantly better cosmetic results as compared to simple excision surgery [13].

In a recent study under "real-life" conditions, Caeckelbergh and coworkers treated sBCC with MAL-PDT and checked for clinical response and cosmetic outcome after 6 months [14]. In this prospective, single-arm, open study, a total of 90 patients with sBCC were included. BCCs were mostly located on the face, the back and the chest, and the mean number of lesions per patient was 1.6. The mean number of visits to a dermatologist during a period of 6 months was 4 per patient, including the two treatment sessions. CR rate was 89% after 6 months, and cosmetic outcome was judged as "excellent" or "good" in 96% of patients. The cumulative amount of MAL per treatment was 1.2 g. The total cost of care was $414 per patient ($280 per lesion) (figures based on the specific costs in Belgium) [14].

In a retrospective analysis, Fai and coworkers from Italy treated 228 subjects with 348 BCC, 213 of nodular type and 135 of superficial type [15]. MAL-PDT was performed according to the standard procedures (two treatments 1 week apart, illumination with red light (λ_{em} 630 nm, 37 J/cm^2). Posttreatment assessments were performed over a period of at least 12 months. Independent of the clinical type of BCC, CR was observed in 71% of lesions after 3 months, and recurrence rate after 12 months was 15%. Interestingly, the risks for initial treatment failure and recurrence were both higher for nodular variants of BCC than for superficial types [15].

New treatment modalities try to enhance the efficacy of MAL-PDT. One possible way is to enhance the penetration of MAL into the diseased tissue prior to light activation. In a recent publication, Haedersdahl et al. used ablative fractional resurfacing with a CO_2-laser prior to MAL application in an animal model and studied protoporphyrin IX (PPIX) fluorescence as a parameter of MAL penetration into epidermal tissue [16]. They were able to detect a significantly higher level of PPIX fluorescence within the pretreated tissue vs. the tissue with MAL application alone. So far, this experiment has not been validated in clinical use, as it has been done so far with a microneedling device and ALA [17].

Another option to enhance PDT efficacy is the use of an iron chelator to block the inactivation of PPIX by insertion of ferric ions. Pye and coworkers used the iron chelator CP94 to enhance PPIX accumulation [18]. In an open, dose-escalating study, patients with nBCC were included and treated with conventional MAL-PDT combined with simultaneous CP94 application. Greater reductions in tumor depth were observed in the CP94-coincubated BCC [18].

However, even if all new developments and the so-far published clinical studies qualify PDT as an effective treatment of BCC, Mohs micrographic surgery shows generally higher cure rates as compared to PDT. Besides, the relatively short follow-up of most of the performed studies has to be considered. Mandatory indications for surgical treatment are histological subtypes such as pigmented or morpheic BCC, BCC located in the area of the facial embryonic fusion clefts, and all BCC thicker than 3 mm if no debulking procedure is performed prior to PDT. Clinical examples of BCC are shown in Figs. 7.1 and 7.2.

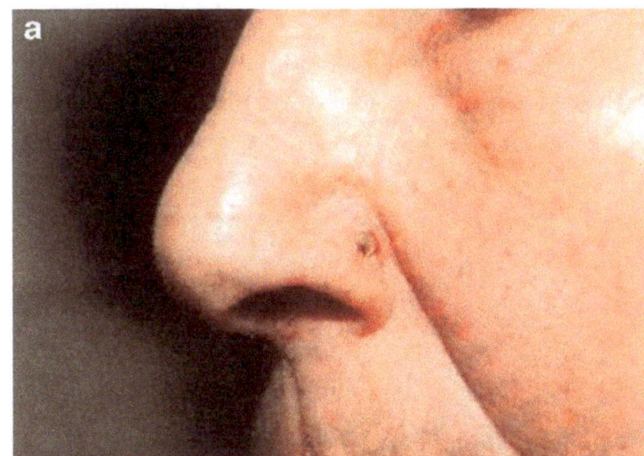

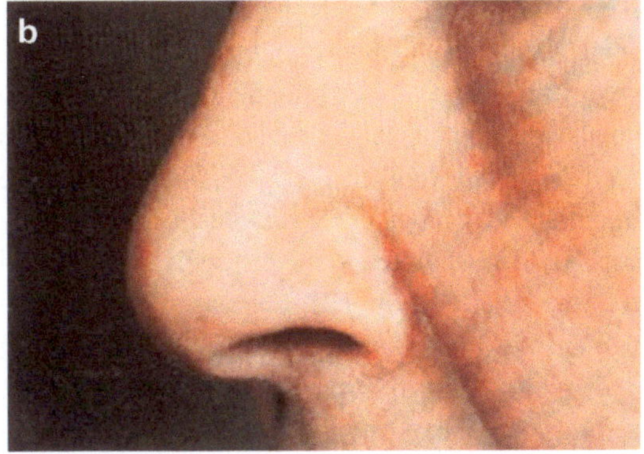

Fig. 7.1 Superficial basal cell carcinoma (BCC) lesion (**a**) before treatment and (**b**) after MAL-PDT treatment (courtesy of Galderma Laboratories, Fort Worth, TX)

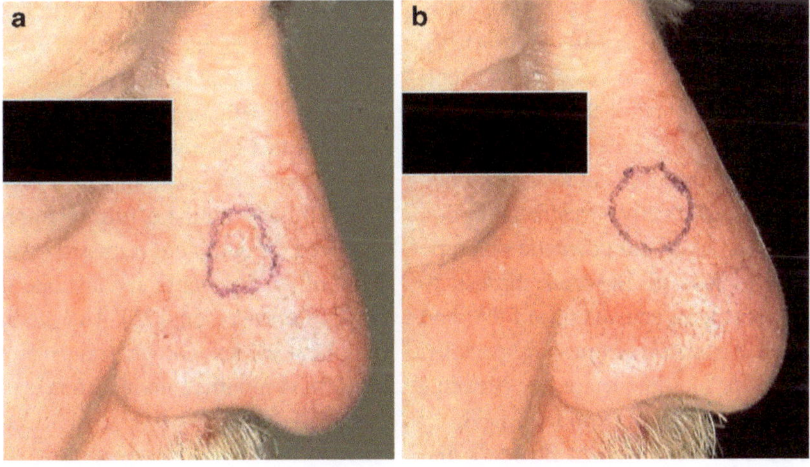

Fig. 7.2 Nodular BCC lesion (**a**) before treatment and (**b**) after MAL-PDT treatment (courtesy of Galderma Laboratories, Fort Worth, TX)

Bowen's Disease and Initial Squamous Cell Carcinoma

Bowen's disease is approved for MAL-PDT since 2006 and is – as a planar epithelial precancerous lesion – highly suitable for PDT and received strong recommendations for use by several guideline publications [19–21]. In a placebo-controlled, randomized multicenter study, Morton et al. [22] compared the effectiveness of MAL-PDT with cryotherapy and 5-FU in the treatment of histologically confirmed in situ squamous cell carcinoma (SCC) (225 patients, 295 lesions, lesion size 6–40 mm) at 3 and 12 months after the last treatment. MAL-PDT or matching placebo cream PDT ($n=17$), cryotherapy ($n=82$), or topical 5-FU (5% cream; $n=30$) was performed. MAL or placebo cream was applied for 3 h before illumination with broadband red light (75 J/cm^2, 570–670 nm). The treatment was repeated 1 week later. Cryotherapy was performed with liquid nitrogen spray. 5-FU was applied for 1 month. Lesions with a partial response at 3 months were re-treated. The primary end point was a clinically verified complete response of lesions and the cosmetic outcome on a 4-point rating scale. The authors reported that at 1 year, the estimated sustained lesion complete response rate with MAL-PDT was superior to that with cryotherapy (80 vs. 67%; odds ratio, 1.77; 95% confidence interval, 1.01–3.12; $p=0.047$) and better than that with 5-FU (80 vs. 69%; odds ratio, 1.64; 95% confidence interval, 0.78–3.45; $p=0.19$). Cosmetic outcome at 3 months was good or excellent in 94% of patients treated with MAL-PDT vs. 66% with cryotherapy and 76% with 5-FU and was maintained for 1 year. The authors concluded that MAL-PDT is an effective treatment option for in situ SCC, with excellent cosmetic outcome [22]. The response rate of Bowen's disease to MAL-PDT is also at least equivalent to 5-FU and cryotherapy, but with superior cosmesis. Especially, patients with large or multiple lesions of Bowen's disease may particularly profit from PDT [23].

Since MAL-PDT works well in Bowen's disease, Calzavara-Pinton and coworkers from Brescia, Italy, studied whether it works also for initial SCC. Patients ($n=55$) with either Bowen's disease or initial invasive SCC (in total 112 biopsy-proven lesions) were included in this trial. After a standard MAL-PDT with red LED light (Aktilite, Galderma, France, 37 J/cm^2), and a repetition after 7 days, the patients were monitored every third month until 2 years of follow-up. The overall complete response rates were 73.2% at 3 months and 53.6% at 2 years. Especially, histological atypia was a statistically robust and significant predictor of response at 3 months. According to their findings, superficial SCC with a microinvasive dermatohistopathological pattern and nodular invasive variants, especially when poorly differentiated keratinocytes are present, are no good indications even for a MAL-PDT [24].

Other Nonmelanoma Skin Cancers

Only a few other indications besides BCC and Bowen's disease have been studied so far with MAL-PDT. One of the interesting indications is cutaneous T-cell lymphoma (CTCL). Especially, unilesional CTCL is characterized by a limited involvement of the skin and a highly chronic course. For solitary lesions, topical corticosteroids help nicely, but in case they are refractory, localized chemotherapy, photochemotherapy either with or without systemic interferons, systemic retinoids, or X-ray therapy are available. MAL-PDT offers an interesting alternative as its level of toxicity is quite low and, in contrast to radiotherapy, repetition is possible [25]. In a pilot study, Zane et al. treated five patients suffering from unilesional CTCL and refractory to the previously mentioned therapeutic modalities with topical MAL-PDT. After a conventional procedure, which was repeated once weekly until total clearance of the lesions appeared, the patients were treated consecutively until no further improvement was achieved. A complete remission was observed in 4 out of the 5 patients, the last one showed only a partial improvement [25]. The median number of treatment cycles was six (range 1–9). At follow-up (12–34 months), no recurrence was seen.

Conclusion

MAL-PDT is effective in treating nonmelanoma skin cancers. This accounts for Bowen's disease and also for superficial and nodular variants

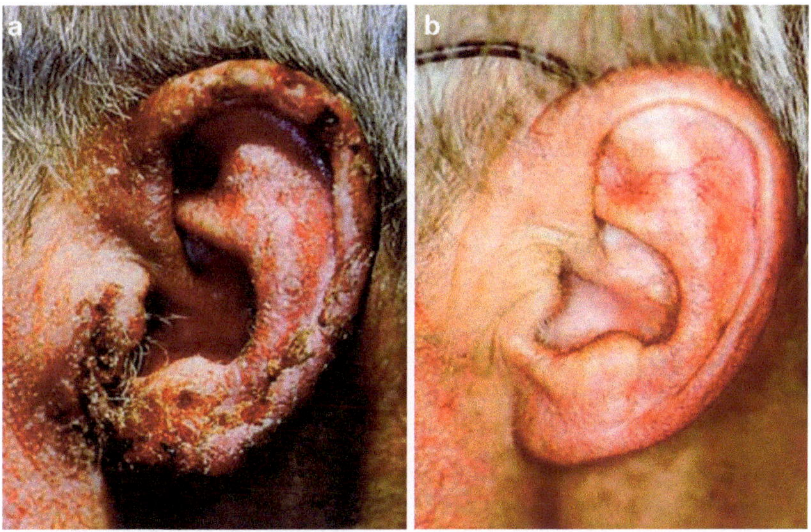

Fig. 7.3 Squamous cell carcinoma of the ear (**a**) before treatment and (**b**) after MAL-PDT treatment (courtesy of Galderma Laboratories, Fort Worth, TX)

of BCC. SCC as well as pigmented or morpheic variants of BCC are no indications for PDT with MAL. Though New technologies such as pretreatments (fractional ablation or microneedling) to improve drug penetration may increase effectivity, so far no studies with a significant study population have been published. A clinical example of SCC is shown in Fig. 7.3.

References

1. Babilas P, Schreml S, Landthaler M, Szeimies RM. Photodynamic therapy in dermatology: state-of-the-art. Photodermatol Photoimmunol Photomed. 2010;26:118–32.
2. Lehmann P. Methyl aminolaevulinate-photodynamic therapy: a review of clinical trials in the treatment of actinic keratoses and nonmelanoma skin cancer. Br J Dermatol. 2007;156:793–801.
3. Christensen E, Warloe T, Kroon S, et al. Guidelines for practical use of MAL-PDT in non-melanoma skin cancer. J Eur Acad Dermatol Venereol. 2010;24:505–12.
4. Soler AM, Warloe T, Berner A, Giercksky KE. A follow-up study of recurrence and cosmesis in completely responding superficial and nodular basal cell carcinomas treated with methyl 5-aminolaevulinate-based photodynamic therapy alone and with prior curettage. Br J Dermatol. 2001;145:467–71.
5. Morton CA, Whitehurst C, McColl JH, et al. Photodynamic therapy for large or multiple patches of Bowen disease and basal cell carcinoma. Arch Dermatol. 2001;137:319–24.
6. Horn M, Wolf P, Wulf HC, et al. Topical methyl aminolaevulinate photodynamic therapy in patients with basal cell carcinoma prone to complications and poor cosmetic outcome with conventional treatment. Br J Dermatol. 2003;149:1242–9.
7. Rhodes LE, de Rie M, Enstrom Y, et al. Photodynamic therapy using topical methyl aminolevulinate vs. surgery for nodular basal cell carcinoma: results of a multicenter randomized prospective trial. Arch Dermatol. 2004;140:17–23.
8. Wang I, Bendsoe N, Klinteberg CA, et al. Photodynamic therapy vs. cryosurgery of basal cell carcinomas: results of a phase III clinical trial. Br J Dermatol. 2001;144:832–40.
9. Basset-Seguin N, Ibbotson SH, Emtestam L, et al. Topical methyl aminolaevulinate photodynamic therapy versus cryotherapy for superficial basal cell carcinoma: a 5 year randomized trial. Eur J Dermatol. 2008;18:547–53.
10. Foley P, Freeman M, Menter A, et al. Photodynamic therapy with methyl aminolevulinate for primary nodular basal cell carcinoma: results of two randomized studies. Int J Dermatol. 2009;48:1236–45.
11. Zeitouni NC, Oseroff AR, Shieh S. Photodynamic therapy for nonmelanoma skin cancers. Current review and update. Mol Immunol. 2003;39:1133–6.
12. Foley P. Clinical efficacy of methyl aminolevulinate (Metvix) photodynamic therapy. J Dermatolog Treat. 2003;14 Suppl 3:15–22.
13. Szeimies RM, Ibbotson S, Murrell DF, et al. A clinical study comparing methyl aminolevulinate photodynamic therapy and surgery in small superficial basal cell carcinoma (8-20 mm), with a 12-month follow-up. J Eur Acad Dermatol Venereol. 2008;22: 1302–11.
14. Caekelbergh K, Nikkels AF, Leroy B, et al. Photodynamic therapy using methyl aminolevulinate in the management of primary superficial basal cell carcinoma: clinical and health economic outcomes. J Drugs Dermatol. 2009;8:992–6.

15. Fai D, Arpaia N, Romano I, et al. Methylaminolevulinate photodynamic therapy for the treatment of actinic keratoses and non-melanoma skin cancers: a retrospective analysis of response in 462 patients. G Ital Dermatol Venereol. 2009;144:281–5.
16. Haedersdal M, Sakamoto FH, Farinelli WA, et al. Fractional CO_2 laser-assisted drug delivery. Lasers Surg Med. 2010;42:113–22.
17. Clementoni MT, Roscher M, Munavalli GS. Photodynamic photorejuvenation of the face with a combination of microneedling, red light, and broadband pulsed light. Lasers Surg Med. 2010;42:150–9.
18. Pye A, Campbell S, Curnow A. Enhancement of methyl-aminolevulinate photodynamic therapy by iron chelation with CP94: an in vitro investigation and clinical dose-escalating safety study for the treatment of nodular basal cell carcinoma. J Cancer Res Clin Oncol. 2008;134:841–9.
19. Cox NH, Eedy DJ, Morton CA. Guidelines for management of Bowen's disease: 2006 update. Therapy Guidelines and Audit Subcommittee, British Association of Dermatologists. Br J Dermatol. 2007;156:11–21.
20. Braathen LR, Szeimies RM, Basset-Seguin N, et al. Guidelines on the use of photodynamic therapy for nonmelanoma skin cancer: an international consensus. International Society for Photodynamic Therapy in Dermatology, 2005. J Am Acad Dermatol. 2007;56:125–43.
21. Morton CA, McKenna KE. British Association of Dermatologists Therapy Guidelines and Audit Subcommittee and the British Photodermatology Group. Guidelines for topical photodynamic therapy: update. Br J Dermatol. 2008;159:1245–66.
22. Morton C, Horn M, Leman J, et al. Comparison of topical methyl aminolevulinate photodynamic therapy with cryotherapy or Fluorouracil for treatment of squamous cell carcinoma in situ: results of a multicenter randomized trial. Arch Dermatol. 2006; 142:729–35.
23. Morton CA. Methyl aminolevulinate: actinic keratoses and Bowen's disease. Dermatol Clin. 2007; 25:81–7.
24. Calzavara-Pinton PG, Venturini M, Sala R, et al. Methylaminolaevulinate-based photodynamic therapy of Bowen's disease and squamous cell carcinoma. Br J Dermatol. 2008;159:137–44.
25. Zane C, Venturini M, Sala R, Calzavara-Pinton P. Photodynamic therapy with methylaminolevulinate as a valuable treatment option for unilesional cutaneous T-cell lymphoma. Photodermatol Photoimmunol Photomed. 2006;22:254–8.

Methyl Aminolevulinate: Photorejuvenation

8

Ricardo Ruiz-Rodriguez and Brian Zelickson

Abstract

There are currently myriad methods that can be used to treat photodamaged skin. For more severe sun damage, chemical peels [Am J Clin Dermatol. 2004;5(3):179–87], dermabrasion, and laser resurfacing [Semin Cutan Med Surg. 1996;15(3):177–88] are found to be very successful.These treatments act by removing or destroying the top layers of skin and allowing new skin to grow and recover the treated areas, but recovery times can be long and scarring can occur. Today, the use of nonablative and fractionated ablative lasers has helped many patients to obtain good cosmetic results with little downtime. Among the novel methods for maximizing the efficacy of nonablative treatment is the concurrent use of a photosensitizing agent. On the other hand, many lasers at different wavelengths and light devices are currently being promoted for photodynamic therapy in rejuvenation.

There are currently myriad methods that can be used to treat photodamaged skin. Topical treatment with tretinoin cream has shown to bemoving the overlying epidermis. The mechanism of action [4] inherent in all such devices is the selective damage to the dermis causing an inflammatory response and resultant collagen repair. The collagen and elastic fiber restoration results in decreased wrinkles. The advantage of nonablative laser resurfacing is that there is no appreciable downtime or recovery period; however, the clinical results are only modest.

R. Ruiz-Rodriguez (✉)
Department of Dermatology, Clínica Ruber of Madrid, Madrid, Spain
and
Clínica Dermatológica Internacional, Madrid, Spain
e-mail: ricardo@ricardoruiz.es

The goal of nonablative rejuvenation is to restore damaged collagen without injuring and/or removing the overlying epidermis. The mechanism of action [4] inherent in all such devices is the selective damage to the dermis causing an inflammatory response and resultant collagen repair. The collagen and elastic fibber restoration results in decreased wrinkles. The advantage of non-ablative laser resurfacing is that there is no appreciable downtime or recovery period, however the clinical results are only modest.

Among the novel methods for maximizing the efficacy of nonablative treatment is the concurrent use of a photosensitizing agent. There are many studies that have showed the superior efficacy of certain lasers and light sources plus a photosensitizer than a laser o light source used alone [5, 6]. On the other hand, many lasers at different wavelengths and light devices are currently being

M.H. Gold (ed.), *Photodynamic Therapy in Dermatology*,
DOI 10.1007/978-1-4419-1298-5_8, © Springer Science+Business Media, LLC 2011

promoted for photodynamic therapy (PDT) in rejuvenation [7].

Nonablative Rejuvenation

Nonablative rejuvenation [8–10] describes technologies that improve aging structural changes in the skin without disruption of cutaneous integrity, minimize downtime, and low risk profile.

The first category is visible light lasers or light sources that have more absorption by hemoglobin and melanin, so they have more influence on the telangiectatic and melanotic components of photoaging. These sources can be subdivided into vascular and pigmented lasers. Intense pulsed light (IPL) is a broadband light source with filters used to limit the emitted spectrum.

Another category is infrared lasers with absorption predominantly by water. Infrared wavelengths are used to create thermal dermal and collagen injury. The most commonly used devices are 1,320 nm Nd:YAG, 1,450 nm diode laser, and 1,540 nm erbium:glass laser.

Fractional resurfacing [11] has revolutionized the approach to nonablative rejuvenation. The concept is, instead of treating the whole surface of the skin, only treat a fraction. This allows for faster healing and significant decrease in side effects. These fractionated devices can be divided into nonablative and ablative. The nonablative devices employ infrared lasers to produce multiple columns of thermal damage, referred to as microthermal treatments zones. The ablative devices use lasers that ablate columns of tissue creating vertical holes into the dermis.

The History of Photodynamic Rejuvenation

The primary goal expected of such nonablative procedures is to accomplish a long-lasting, effective rejuvenation without major side effects or long period of recuperation. Among the novel methods for maximizing, the efficacy of nonablative treatments is the concurrent use of a photosensitizing agent.

In 2002, Ruiz-Rodriguez et al. [12] studied the use of IPL as a light source of PDT in patients with AK, and the technique was called "Photodynamic Photorejuvenation." They treated 17 patients with a combination of AKs and diffuse photodamaged. They applied 20% 5-aminolevulinic acid (5-ALA) mixed in an oil-in-water emulsion and under occlusion for 4 h before treatment (0.2 g/cm^2) with the pulsed-light devise (Lumenis, Inc.), using a 615-nm cutoff filter and a total fluence of 40 J/cm^2 in a double-pulse mode of 4 ms, with a 20 ms interpulse delay.

The results were confirmed by Alexiades-Armenakas and Geronimus [13], who showed that photodynamic treatment of actinic keratosis could be accomplished not only with IPL, but also with a 595-nm pulse-dye-laser (PDL). This device offered the benefits of rapidity of treatment and the comfort and protective epidermal effects associated with cryogen spray cooling. The 5-ALA incubation time was 3 h, and nonpurpuric PDL settings (4.0–7.5 J/cm^2; pulse duration, 10 ms; 10 mm spot size; and 30-ms cryogen spray with a 30-ms delay) were used. In this study, the authors were focused on AK.

In 2005, Dover et al. [5] showed the superior efficacy of IPL-PDT over IPL alone in a prospective, randomized, split-face study. Twenty subjects participated in a series of three split-face treatments 3 weeks apart in which half of the face was pretreated with 5-ALA followed by IPL treatment, while the other half was treated with IPL alone. The incubation time of the 5-ALA was 30–60 min. The adjunctive use of 5-ALA in the treatment of facial photoaging with IPL provided significantly greater improvement in global photodamage, mottled pigmentation, and fine lines than treatment with IPL alone. They showed that this combination treatment enhances the results of photorejuvenation and improves patient satisfaction. Adverse effects and tolerability did not differ significantly between the IPL-only treated areas and the areas treated with 5-ALA plus IPL.

Marmur et al. published in 2005 [14] a small pilot study about the ultrastructural changes seen after ALA-IPL photorejuvenation. They found a greater shift toward type I collagen synthesis in the ALA-IPL treatment group compared to the IPL-only treatment group.

In 2006, Gold et al. [6] performed a split-face comparison study of PDT with 5-ALA and IPL vs. IPL alone for photodamage. He also showed the superior efficacy of IPL-PDT over IPL alone.

Light Sources Used in PDT

Blue light is the most potent wavelength for activation of the PDT effect. The absorption maximum of PpIX around 410 nm makes blue light 40 times more potent that red light and significantly greater than yellow light in term of a photochemical effect. However, for cosmetic skin conditions, blue light ALA-PDT is limited by a lack of cutaneous penetration and superficial melanin absorption. Despite these limitations, nonablative rejuvenation has been reported using blue light.

The two light devices currently most used for photodynamic rejuvenation are IPL and PDL [12, 13]. Deeper penetrating visible wavelengths produced by IPL and PDL not only have enough energy to activate the photochemical process, but also have long enough wavelengths to effectively reach and thermally target multiple chromophores including hemoglobin, melanine, and to a less selective degree, collagen.

We are still far from thorough understanding of the molecular mechanism of rejuvenation with this technique, although the activation of a nonspecific immune response could be involved [15]. It is likely that surface texture and pigmentation improved through mild desquamation. Histological studies have also demonstrated increased fibrosis and new collagen formation in the dermis several months after 5-ALA-PDT for the treatment of basal cell and squamous cell carcinomas [16].

Methyl Aminolevulinate

Methyl aminolevulinate-hydrochloride cream (Metvix® [in Canada] and Metvixia® [in the US], Galderma) in combination with PDT provides an effective treatment option for actinic keratoses (AKs), superficial basal cell carcinoma (sBCC), and Bowen's disease (BD).

Metvix/Metvixia cream contains methyl aminolevulinate (MAL) as the hydrochloride salt in a 20% solution [17]. The optimal regimen for MAL-PDT (as used in all clinical trials) is MAL 160 mg/g applied for 3 h before illumination with red light (570–670 nm) at a total light dose of 75 J/cm^2, as determined in dose-finding trials.

Topically applied MAL penetrates the skin and induces a high production of metabolites in the cells leading to intracellular accumulation of photoactive porphyrins. The underlying mechanism of this induction is not fully understood. However, there is evidence from studies that MAL may enter the heme biosynthetic pathway without hydrolysis to ALA, an endogenous precursor of PpIX. If photoactive porphyrins-loaded cells are exposed to appropriate wavelengths of light, reactive oxygen species are generated which irreversibly oxidize cellular components and cause cell death, tissue injury, and necrosis.

Local phototoxicity reactions were the most common local adverse events in all clinical trials using MAL-PDT, mainly burning sensation, erythema, crusting, and pain. Most of the local events resolve quickly on the same day of treatment and all of them within 2 weeks. There is no increase in the incidence of local adverse events after the second cycle of MAL-PDT.

Higher lipophilicity of the esterified form of ALA permits very effective penetration within the cutaneous tissue. Comparison of ALA and MAL in patients with AK revealed that Metvix cream induced higher accumulation of porphyrins in tumor cells than in normal tissue. Furthermore, ALA induced higher porphyrin level than MAL; however, MAL was more selective for lesional skin than ALA 6 h after application. This might result from different cellular uptake and feedback mechanisms of ALA and MAL. Higher lipophilicity, penetration depth, and selectivity for neoplastic lesions are MAL's desirable characteristics compared with 5-ALA. However, there is no comparison study of these two molecules in rejuvenation.

In a split-faced internal controlled study by Wiegell et al. [18], 20 patients were treated with ALA or MAL on tape-stripped skin of their forearms. ALA generated significantly more pain than MAL during and after illumination. The authors hypothesized that ALA and not MAL may be transported by gamma-aminobutyric acid receptors into peripheral nerve endings, explaining the higher pain scores. There are rare reports of contact eczema induce by MAL confirmed by positive patch test reactions with MAL, but not with ALA [19].

MAL-Red Light Rejuvenation

In Europe, the most widely used PDT protocol is Metvix and red light. Ruiz-Rodriguez et al. recently published a prospective, randomized split-face study [20] of Metvix-PDT rejuvenation using red light comparing 1–3 h exposure time. In this comparison study, ten patients with moderate photodamage and no AK had two tubes of Metvix applied to the whole face. One hour later, red light was administered using the Aktilite lamp (630 nm) in a dose of 37 J/cm^2 to one side of the face; the other side received the same treatment, but 3 h after the Metvix application.

The study resulted in moderate improvement in skin quality, fine wrinkling, and skin tightness which was statistically significant. The authors observed no improvement in mottled pigmentation or telangiectasias. The improvement was superior on the 3-h-incubation-time side in most of the patients compared to the 1-h-incubation-time side.

The authors observed more erythema, edema and scaling on the 3-h side compared to the 1-h side (Figs. 8.1 and 8.2). They also performed UV-B photos and greater fluorescence of the 3-h-incubation-time side compared to the 1-h-incubation-time side was observed.

In conclusion, Metvix-PDT using red light is effective for skin rejuvenation (fine lines and skin tightness), and 3 h of exposure to Metvix produces better results than 1 h of exposure, but with a significant increase in adverse effects (erythema and edema) (Figs. 8.3 and 8.4).

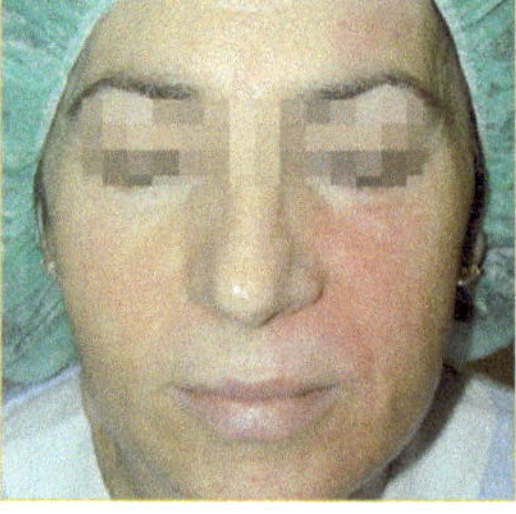

Fig. 8.1 Difference of erythema between 3-h (*left side*) and 1-h (*right side*) incubation time

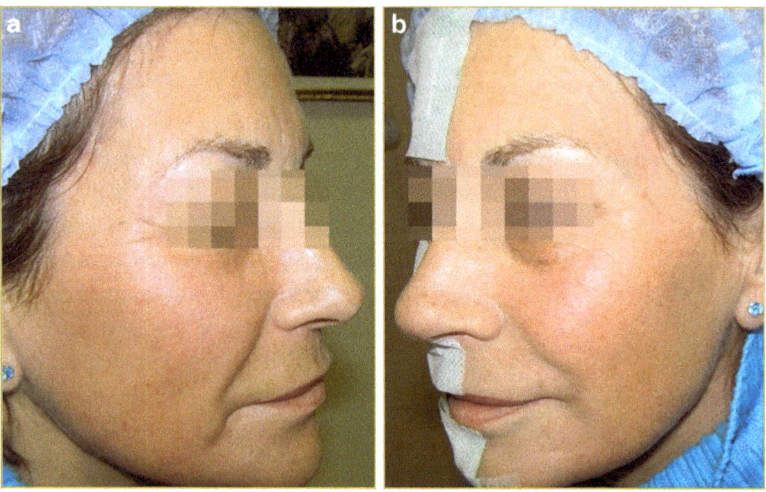

Fig. 8.2 (**a**) No edema in the 1-h incubation side and (**b**) edema in the 3-h incubation side

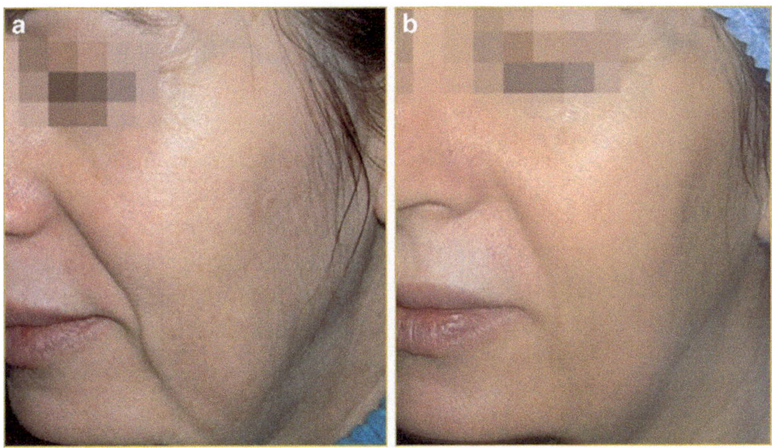

Fig. 8.3 (**a**) Before and (**b**) after 2 months after three treatments in the 3-h incubation side

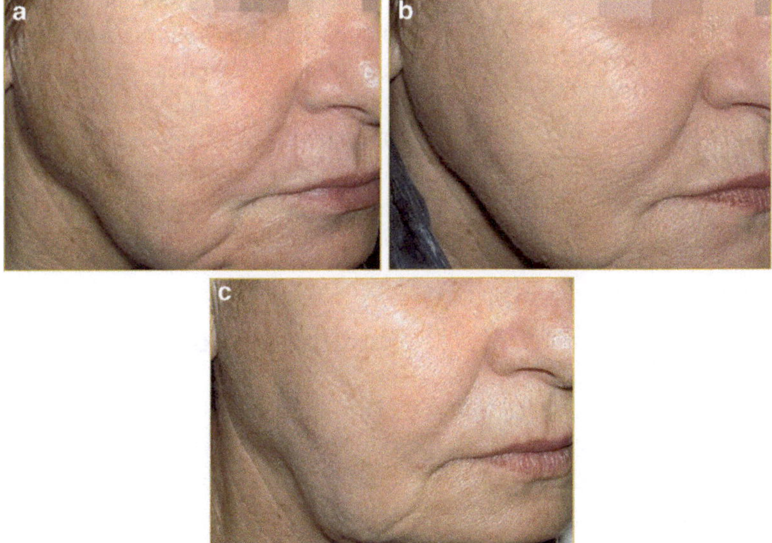

Fig. 8.4 (**a**) Before treatment, (**b**) 2 months after three treatments, and (**c**) 1 year after three treatments

How to Improve Penetration

One of the limitations of PDT is its capacity to penetrate deep into the skin. One possibility is to facilitate the penetration of the photosensitizer through fractional resurfacing or microneedling.

Fractional resurfacing has greatly enhanced the ability to improve sun-induced skin texture with minimal downtime and risks of side effects. Fractional resurfacing prior to the application of methyl 5-aminolevulinate (MAL) has been shown to give a synergistic response [21].

These results might support the use of fractional resurfacing or any physical microneedling [22] prior to PDT in skin rejuvenation. Perhaps, the prior use of fractional technology or microneedling might enhance the absorption of the photosensitizer in the PDT treatment. This combination technique might also be used in noncosmetic conditions that can be treated with PDT as nonmelanoma skin cancer, refractory warts, or acne. Further studies are needed to verify this hypothesis.

Molecular Changes

There are few studies that have showed the histological and molecular changes in PDT rejuvenation [14]. Recently, a study has been published [23] to quantitatively examine the epidermal and dermal cellular and molecular changes that occur after PDT of photodamaged human. The authors performed serial in vivo biochemical and immunohistochemical analyses after PDT using topical 5-ALA and pulsed-dye laser treatment. They used a volunteer sample of 25 adults with clinically apparent photodamage of the forearm skin.

Three-hour application of 5-ALA followed by pulsed-dye laser therapy using nonpurpura-inducing settings to focal areas of photodamaged forearms and serial biopsy specimens taken at baseline and various times after treatment was performed.

They showed that epidermal proliferation was stimulated as demonstrated by increases in Ki67 and epidermal thickness. Up-regulation of collagen production was demonstrated with increases in procollagen I messenger RNA, procollagen III messenger RNA, and procollagen I protein levels detected. In comparison with historical data, using pulsed-dye laser therapy alone suggests that use of the photosensitizer may enhance dermal remodeling.

Overview of Treatment Strategy

Before Treatment

Some authors recommend microdermabrasion immediately before treatment to remove stratum corneum and allow more uniform and rapid penetration of the photosensitizer. Other techniques that improve absorption of the photosensitizer are vibradermabrasion, urea 40% cream, or just cleaning the skin with either alcohol or acetone. Fractional resurfacing and microneedling could be used before the procedure to favor penetration.

During Treatment

A forced cool-air device (Cryo 5 Zimmer; SmartCool, Cynosure) can be very helpful in alleviating pain during light exposure especially on the scalp with multiple AKs. Application of topical analgesics prior to irradiation is not recommended as their high Ph might chemically inactivate the photosensitizer. When treating the full face, sometimes it is necessary to divide the face in two or more areas for illumination (with the Aktilite lamp we divide the face in two areas). It is very important to cover the side that is not being treated during the illumination to avoid activation of the photosensitizer prior to treatment.

After Treatment

Strict avoidance of sun and bright lights is essential to limit the redness, swelling, and crusting associated with phototoxicity. Invariably, a certain amount of PpIX remains in situ following treatment. Careful patient selection, patient education, and careful sun avoidance for up to 2 days after treatment are essential for successful photodynamic rejuvenation [24].

Indications for PDT Rejuvenation

The initial approach to the patient requesting nonablative rejuvenation should be of a conservative realistic motive. One must set patient expectations as to the expected results and side effects. Also, the patient should understand that maintenance treatments may be necessary.

Understanding the laser–tissue interactions associated with PDT is crucial in selecting patients which will most likely benefit. Shorter wavelengths are more valuable in the management of pigmented dyschromia, vascular ectasias, and pilosebaceous irregularities, while longer, more deeply penetrating wavelengths are more effective in wrinkle reduction and prophylaxis. Depending on the type of photodamage of the patient, we should use different procedures:

1. Photodamage type I: Lentigines, telangiectasias, increased coarseness, symptoms of rosacea. In these cases, we can use IPL and/or a combination of q-switch and vascular lasers.

2. Photodamage type II: Wrinkles, laxity, dermatochalasis. We have been using midinfrared lasers for these patients, although now our treatments of choice are nonablative and ablative fractional resurfacing. Radiofrequency and focused ultrasound technology can produce tightening of dermal collagen and can be combined with other procedures that improve the more superficial changes associated with photoaging.
3. Photodamage type III: Actinic keratosis, nonmelanoma skin cancers. Photodynamic rejuvenation is the treatment of choice, sometimes in combination with other nonablative treatments. The risk of temporarily masking nonmelanoma skin cancer makes it prudent to maintain a low threshold to biopsy any suspicious lesions. The approach of this type III group of patients can be divided in:
   - Patients with multiple actinic keratosis and diffuse facial redness: PDT rejuvenation using PDL as the preferred light device, using purpura free fluences of 5–7.5 J/cm^2, 10 ms pulse width and a 10 mm spot. The ideal immediate treatment endpoint is visible spasm of vessels without purpura, sometimes using 2 or 3 passes.
   - Patients with multiple actinic keratosis and multiple lentigines and telangiectasias: IPL is the light of choice for PDT in these patients. When using the Quantum IPL, 560-nm cutoff filter and parameters between 24 and 32 J/cm^2 with pulse duration setting of 2.4 and 4.0 ms for the first and second pulses in the pulse sequence, respectively, should be applied.
   - According to the aforementioned study (in press), Metvix-PDT using red light is effective for skin rejuvenation (mottled pigmentation, fine lines, and skin tightness). Patients with AK can benefit cosmetically from this technique. If telangiectasias or lentigines are present, we might treat these lesions additionally with PDL or Q-switch laser, respectively, as red light-PDT has no effect on these conditions. We have found that the results on AK are much better using red light than using IPL or PDL as a light source of PDT.

Future of Photodynamic Rejuvenation

As public demand grows for less invasive, highly effective cosmetic procedures, dermatologists must continue to explore and develop new treatments options and combinations. Further studies with multiples patients and conditions, different time exposures, different light source, and in vivo fluorescence microscopy analysis are warranted.

It is our opinion that we are facing the beginning of a promising technology for treating cutaneous aging that results from UV exposure. This future might go forward with fractionated PDT rejuvenation alone or most likely in combination with other minimally invasive procedures. This should be done judiciously to avoid unnecessary risk for the patient. Conservative parameters should be used when more than one treatment is provided at the same time.

Photodynamic rejuvenation could theoretically prevent skin cancer appearance by inducing a phototoxic reaction in nonvisible lesions [25, 26]. Weekly large surface ALA-PDT performed on hairless mice has been shown to delay the appearance of UV-induced actinic keratosis. Therefore, photodynamic rejuvenation can be the bridge between cosmetic and medical dermatology. With the use of this procedure, our skin becomes more beautiful and healthier.

References

1. Phillips TJ, Gottlieb AB, Leyden JJ, Lowe NJ, Lew-Kaya DA, Sefton J, Walker PS, Gibson JR. Efficacy of 0.1% tazarotene cream for the treatment of photodamage: a 12-month multicenter, randomized trial. Arch Dermatol. 2002;138(11):1486.
2. Fulton JE, Porumb S. Chemical peels: their place within the range of resurfacing techniques. Am J Clin Dermatol. 2004;5(3):179–87.
3. Dover JS, Hruza GJ. Laser skin resurfacing. Semin Cutan Med Surg. 1996;15(3):177–88.
4. Grema H, Raulin C, Greve B. "Skin rejuvenation" by non-ablative laser and light systems. Literature research and overview. Hautarzt. 2002;53(6):385–92.
5. Dover JS, Bhatia AC, Stewart B, Arndt KA. Topical 5-aminolevulinic acid combined with intense pulsed

light in the treatment of photoaging. Arch Dermatol. 2005;141(10):1247–52.

6. Gold MH, Bradshaw VL, Boring MM, Bridges TM, Biron JA. Split-face comparison of photodynamic therapy with 5-aminolevulinic acid and intense pulsed light versus intense pulsed light alone for photodamage. Dermatol Surg. 2006;32(6):795–801. discussion 801–3.
7. Gold MH. Photodynamic therapy update 2007. J Drugs Dermatol. 2007;6(11):1131–7.
8. Ruiz-Rodriguez R, López-Rodriguez L. Nonablative skin resurfacing: the role of PDT. J Drugs Dermatol. 2006;5(8):756–62.
9. Zelickson BD, Kilmer SL, Bernstein E, Chotzen VA, Dock J, Mehregan D, Coles C. Pulsed dye laser therapy for sun damaged skin. Lasers Surg Med. 1999;25:229–36.
10. Sadick NS. Update on nonablative light therapy for rejuvenation: a review. Lasers Surg Med. 2003;32: 120–8.
11. Manstein D, Herron GS, Sink RK, Tanner H, Anderson RR. Fractional photothermolysis: a new concept for cutaneous remodeling using microscopic patterns of thermal injury. Lasers Surg Med. 2004;34(5):426–38.
12. Ruiz-Rodriguez R, Sanz-Sanchez T, Córdoba S. Photodynamic photorejuvenation. Dermatol Surg. 2002;28:742–4.
13. Alexiades-Armenakas MR, Geronimus RG. Laser-mediated photodynamic therapy of actinic keratosis. Arch Dermatol. 2003;139:1313–20.
14. Marmur ES, Phelps R, Goldberg DJ. Ultrastructural changes seen after ALA-IPL photorejuvenation: a pilot study. J Cosmet Laser Ther. 2005;7:21–4.
15. Nowis D, Makowski M, Stoklosa T, Legat M, Issat T, Golab J. Direct tumor damage mechanisms of photodynamic therapy. Acta Biochim Pol. 2005;52:339–52.
16. Van den Akker JTHM, de Bruijn HS, Beijersbergen van Henegouwen GMJ, Star WM, Sterenborg HJCM. Protoporphyrin IX fluorescence kinetics and localization after topical application of ALA pentyl ester and ALA on hairless mouse skin with UVB-induced early skin cancer. Photochem Photobiol. 2000;72:399–406.
17. Siddiqui MA, Perry CM, Scott LJ. Topical methyl aminolevulinate. Am J Clin Dermatol. 2004;5(2): 127–37.
18. Wiegell SR, Stender IM, Na R, Wulf HC. Pain associated with photodynamic therapy using 5-aminolevulinic acid or 5-aminolevulinic acid methylester on tape-stripped normal skin. Arch Dermatol. 2003;139: 1173–7.
19. Wulf HC, Philipsen P. Allergic contact dermatitis to 5-aminolevulinic acid methylester but not to 5-aminolevulinic acid after photodynamic therapy. Br J Dermatol. 2004;150:143–5.
20. Ruiz-Rodríguez R, López L, Candelas D, Pedraz J. Photorejuvenation using topical 5-methyl aminolevulinate and red light. J Drugs Dermatol. 2008;7(7): 633–7.
21. Ruiz-Rodriguez R, López L, Candelas D, Zelickson B. Enhanced efficacy of photodynamic therapy after fractional resurfacing: fractional photodynamic rejuvenation. J Drugs Dermatol. 2007;6(8):818–20.
22. Badran MM, Kuntsche J, Fahr A. Skin penetration enhancement by a microneedle device (Dermaroller) in vitro: dependency on needle size and applied formulation. Eur J Pharm Sci. 2009;36(4–5):511–23.
23. Orringer JS, Hammerberg C, Hamilton T, Johnson TM, Kang S, Sachs DL, Fisher G, Voorhees JJ. Molecular effects of photodynamic therapy for photoaging. Arch Dermatol. 2008;144(10):1296–302.
24. Gilaberte Y, Serra-Guillén C, de las Heras ME, Ruiz-Rodríguez R, Fernández-Lorente M, Benvenuto-Andrade C, González-Rodríguez S, Guillén-Barona C. Photodynamic therapy in dermatology. Actas Dermosifiliogr. 2006;97(2): 83–102.
25. Stender IM, Bech-Thomsen N, Poulsen T, Wulf HC. Photodynamic therapy with topical ALA delays UV photocarcinogenesis in hairless mice. Photochem Photobiol. 1997;66:493–6.
26. Bissonette R, Bergeron A, Liu Y. Large surface photodynamic therapy with ALA: treatment of actinic keratosis and beyond. J Drugs Dermatol. 2004;3: S26–31.

Photodynamic Therapy of Acne

9

Carin Sandberg, Ann-Marie Wennberg, and Olle Larkö

Abstract

Topical therapies may be used for treating mild to moderate acne. In the recent years, antibiotics, especially tetracyclines, have been used for the treatment of acne. For very severe cases, isotretinoin is still probably the therapy of choice. Photodynamic therapy (PDT) may be an alternative to antibiotic treatment in selected cases. However, the exact treatment scheme is not established yet. We know neither the relevant concentration of the prodrug nor the proper intensity of the light or the total light dose. PDT may be used in selected cases, but much more research has to be done before PDT of acne can be used in routine clinical practice.

Acne is a common disease involving the pilosebaceous duct. It affects majority of young people and may be very troublesome for the individual patient. The therapy is usually efficient ranging from topical preparations such as benzoyl peroxide, topical antibiotics, retinoic acid to more advanced treatments [1–3].

For more severe cases, oral antibiotics are usually used, especially tetracyclines. The effect of antibiotics is good on moderate acne, but there is an increasing problem with bacterial resistance [4–6], and the environmental problems are cumbersome as the half-life in the environment is rather long, and tetracyclines can affect other organisms in nature. Only recently, this pollutant effect has been discussed [7, 8].

Acne can be graded in various ways such as by Pilbury et al. [9] and O'Brien et al. [10]. The etiology of acne is not entirely known, but overproduction of sebum is essential. Follicular hyperkeratosis occurs, which makes it hard for sebum to be evacuated. The anaerobic bacterium *Propionibacterium acnes* degrades triglycerides into fatty acids, which causes inflammation [11–13]. The therapy against acne is usually directed against follicular hyperkeratosis, sebum production, and *P. acnes*. *P. acnes* excretes porphyrins. The treatment steps for acne usually involves self-treatment, topical treatment with monotherapy or combination therapy, tetracyclines, and isotretinoin for the most severe cases [12].

C. Sandberg (✉)
Department of Dermatology, Sahlgrenska University Hospital, Gothenburg, Sweden
e-mail: Carin.sandberg@vgregion.se

M.H. Gold (ed.), *Photodynamic Therapy in Dermatology*,
DOI 10.1007/978-1-4419-1298-5_9, © Springer Science+Business Media, LLC 2011

Photodynamic Therapy

PDT has been used for many years and was first described by von Tappeiner and Jesionek [14]. PDT typically involves the application of a precursor to a photosensitizer, i.e., ALA, which is converted into protoporphyrin IX (Pp IX) inside and outside mitochondria (Fig. 9.1). Pp IX is usually accumulated in rapidly proliferating tissues, such as tumors or sebocytes [15].

Recently, the methyl ester of ALA, MAL has been introduced. It has been shown to penetrate more easily into target lesions and be more selective in the accumulation [16]. However, Sandberg et al. [17] showed that there is no significant difference in the penetration of ALA and MAL in tumor tissue. Microdialysis has been used to study the penetration.

Absorption Spectrum of Pp IX

Porphyrins typically absorb light at the Soret band around 400 mm, but also at longer wavelengths such as yellow and red. The net effect is highest when red light used as the absorption of Hb is not disturbing the result. Also, red light penetrates deep into the skin. When Pp IX is irradiated, photobleaching occurs. It has recently been showed by Ericson et al. [18] that at least for tumor treatment, doses above 40 J/cm^2 are not necessary.

Fluorescence

When irradiated with UVA or blue light, porphyrins fluoresce. This can also be seen in acne treatment [19], but its major use is for delineating tumors [20].

Light Sources for PDT

Different light sources may be used. Originally, halogen lamps were used with broad band emission. Lasers have also been used and have the advantage of emitting monochromatic light. They may also be used together with fiber optics. The specific effects of laser light are not necessary

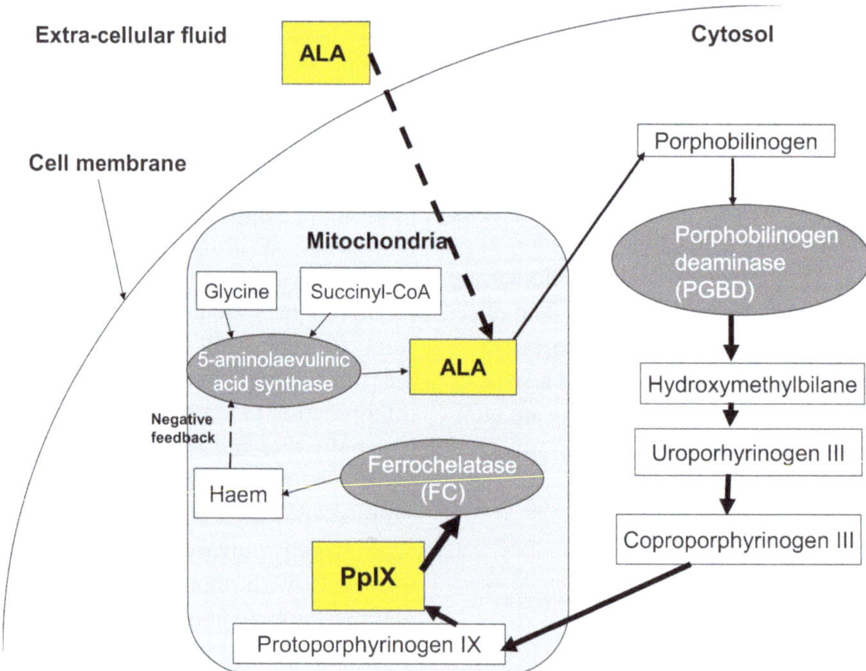

Fig. 9.1 Heme biosynthesis. PDT typically involves the application of a precursor to a photosensitizer, i.e., ALA, which is converted to protoporphyrin IX inside and outside mitochondria

for acne treatment. The most common light sources today are light emitting diodes (LEDs). Compared to filtered lamps, the wavelength band is narrower. They are also reliable and relatively cheap.

Acne Vulgaris and Sun Exposure

Cunliffe has reported that solar radiation may be beneficial for acne. Sunlight may exert an anti-inflammatory effect on the Langerhans cells [21]. UVB kills bacteria, and UVA may be absorbed by *P. acnes* as *P. acnes* excretes porphyrins. Visible light may also have an effect on acne through the same mechanism [1].

Earlier Studies of PDT and Acne

Hongcharu et al. [22] used ALA for the treatment of acne. They reported significant effect on acne 10 weeks after a single treatment and 20 weeks after four treatments. The use of PDT for acne was further studied by Pollock et al. [23]. Red laser light was used, and the clinical effect was good, but they could not demonstrate any reduction in *P. acnes* number or sebum excretion.

Wiegell and Wulf [24] have introduced the treatment of acne with MAL-PDT. They could not demonstrate any difference between ALA and MAL. However, ALA-PDT resulted in more severe adverse effects. Blue light would theoretically be the light of choice for PDT of acne, but as red light penetrates deeper the net effect is probably greater using red light for PDT.

Hörfelt et al. used MAL for treatment of facial acne vulgaris in a randomized controlled study. They demonstrated a statistically significant reduction in acne with MAL-PDT compared to placebo PDT. MAL-PDT was associated with relatively severe pain [25].

In another study, Hörfelt et al. studied dose response and the mechanism of action. Fifteen patients were studied using ALA-PDT. The light source was an incoherent Waldmann PDT 1200. 30 J/cm^2 was compared to 50 J/cm^2 on the face, and on the back 50 J/cm^2 was compared to 70 J/cm^2. No difference could be seen between the light doses. Interestingly, no reduction in sebum excretion or *P. acnes* number was noted [26]. Maybe, there is an alternative mechanism for PDT on acne. Cunliffe et al. [21] discuss whether UV-radiation has an anti-inflammatory effect on follicular Langerhans cells. Sigurdsson et al. [1] describes that UV-radiation except its anti-inflammatory effect might have an effect on the comedonal cytokines. There are also reports that the UV radiation can induce changes to surface lipids and subsequently enhance comedogenesis [27].

Besides these, there is the effect of ALA-PDT itself on the cells. All cells that have accumulated Pp IX and become photosensitized will, after radiation, produce ROS (reactive oxygen species), and therefore, the sebaceous gland cells will be damaged and killed [15, 22].

When performing ALA-PDT on acne, the standard procedure has been taken from the treatment schedule of nonpigmented skin cancer. The ALA/MAL cream has been topically applied for 3 h under occlusion, and thereafter, either blue or red light has been used to illuminate the treated area.

Blue light might be a more effective wavelength to activate both the *P. acnes* porphyrin and PpIX. The disadvantage of poor penetration (<2 mm) in the skin will make red light more attractive. The red light has also a wavelength that can activate the porphyrins, but its ability to penetrate deeper into the skin is advantageous. There has also been reports that a combination of both blue and red light can be used [28, 29]. Though it has not yet been investigated whether or not this is more effective, theoretically, by combining anti-inflammatory actions with antibacterial actions, it could be more effective.

Using the standard procedure of treating acne, the adverse events with pain and inflammation of the skin are quite severe. Both Hörfelt et al. [25] and Wiegell et al. [25] report on very severe pain after treatment for inflammation and also pustule formation. Though MAL seems to give somewhat lesser adverse events than ALA, there have also been investigations made to change the treatment schedule both by reducing the intensity used and by modifying the pretreatment of the topical MAL/ALA [26, 30].

Though many attempts to control the pain has been done, no topical anesthesia has shown to be effective [31–34]. Grapengiesser et al. [35] and Sandberg et al. [32] performed studies to find the risk factors for pain. They found that the larger the area treated the more pain inflicted. Also, the redness (inflammation) was a risk factor. Wiegell et al. [36] showed that the pain was dependent on how much fluorescence was built up (i.e., porphyrin accumulation). Subcutaneous infiltration anesthesia could be effective but with the disadvantage of very large edema [37]. Nerve block is very effective but with the disadvantage that not all areas can be blocked; for instance, the lateral part of the cheeks and the back are today some areas that will be difficult to block [38, 39]. In these areas, nothing but the standard procedures such as pauses, cold water spraying, and fans are used as pain-relieving strategies.

Practical Aspects of PDT Treatment

Often, percutaneous penetration of MAL or ALA is a problem. Generally, the documentation of MAL is better than that of ALA. A very obvious way of increasing percutaneous penetration is by curettage. This is often performed before treating nonmelanoma skin cancer. However, with acne this is not necessary. Before treatment, an opaque dressing should be used to avoid a phototoxic reaction. Also, an opaque dressing should be utilized for at least 24 h after treatment. The amount of topical compound applied is usually to cover the whole treatment area to a 1-mm thick layer. The proper application time has yet to be established, but currently it is 3 h, although this is probably too long a time.

Also, there has been one study reporting that only a single low dose of red light is efficient without any pretreatment of MAL or ALA [30]; the reason for this is supposed to be that the red light is activating the porphyrins excreted by the bacterium *P. acnes* itself.

When using the pretreatment with MAL and ALA, after the 3-h application time, the cream is gently removed, and the treatment area is irradiated with red light at an intensity varying in different studies between 30 and 63 mW/cm^2, and a light dose between 15 and 37 J/cm^2 [25, 26, 30]. The extent of area that is possible to treat is dependent on pain as the limiting factor. After the treatment, the treated area should be protected from sun exposure for 24 h. Sunscreens are usually of very little help as the action spectrum extends into the visible range (Fig. 9.2).

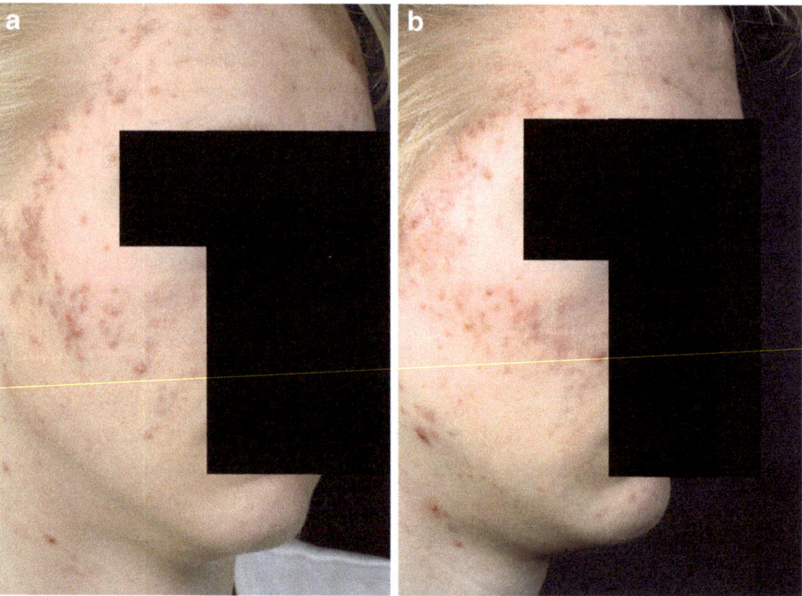

Fig. 9.2 (**a**) Before and (**b**) after acne treatment with PDT

Pain Management

As shown by our group previously, the pain is normally distributed. EMLA as well as local anesthetics has been used, but the only effective treatment against the pain is nerve blocks [32, 39]. The experience from treatment of actinic keratosis reveals that the pain is more intense when lesions are located in the face than when located on the trunk. Also, treatment of large skin areas results in more pain than treatment on small areas [35].

Where Does PDT Stand in the Armamentarium of Acne Treatment?

Topical therapies may be used for treating mild to moderate acne. In the recent years, antibiotics, especially tetracyclines, have been used for the treatment of acne. However, increasing concern regarding antimicrobial resistance has been discussed. Few new antibiotics have been on the market in recent years.

For very severe cases, isotretinoin is still probably the therapy of choice. PDT may be an alternative to antibiotic treatment in selected cases. However, the exact treatment scheme is not established yet. We know neither the relevant concentration of the prodrug nor the proper intensity of the light or the total light dose. This has to be elaborated further. PDT may be used in selected cases, but much more research concerning the parameters described above has to be done before PDT of acne can be used in routine clinical practice.

References

1. Sigurdsson V, Knulst AC, van Weelden H. Phototherapy of acne vulgaris with visible light. Dermatology. 1997;194:256–60.
2. Leyden JJ, McGinley K, Mills OH, et al. Topical antibiotics and topical antimicrobial agents in acne therapy. Acta Derm Venereol Suppl (Stockh). 1980;Suppl 89:75–82.
3. Leyden JJ, Shalita AR. Rational therapy for acne vulgaris: an update on topical treatment. J Am Acad Dermatol. 1986;15:907–15.
4. Leyden JJ, McGinley KJ, Cavalieri S, et al. *Propionibacterium acnes* resistance to antibiotics in acne patients. J Am Acad Dermatol. 1983;8:41–5.
5. Oprica C, Emtestam L, Lapins J, et al. Antibiotic-resistant *Propionibacterium acnes* on the skin of patients with moderate to severe acne in Stockholm. Anaerobe. 2004;10:155–64.
6. Eady EA, Gloor M, Leyden JJ. *Propionibacterium acnes* resistance: a worldwide problem. Dermatology. 2003;206:54–6.
7. Batt AL, Bruce IB, Aga DS. Evaluating the vulnerability of surface waters to antibiotic contamination from varying wastewater treatment plant discharges. Environ Pollut. 2006;142:295–302.
8. Kong WD, Zhu YG, Fu BJ, et al. The veterinary antibiotic oxytetracycline and Cu influence functional diversity of the soil microbial community. Environ Pollut. 2006;143:129–37.
9. Pillsbury DM, Shelly WB, Kligman A. A manual of cutaneous medicine, vol. 1. Philadelphia: WB Saunders; 1961.
10. O'Brien SC, Lewis JB, Cunliffe WJ. The Leeds revised acne grading system. J Dermatol Treat. 1998;9:215–20.
11. Eady EA, Cove JH. Is acne an infection of blocked pilosebaceous follicles? Implications for antimicrobial treatment. Am J Clin Dermatol. 2000;1:201–9.
12. Cunliffe WJ, Holland DB, Jeremy A. Comedone formation: etiology, clinical presentation, and treatment. Clin Dermatol. 2004;22:367–74.
13. Tan HH. Topical antibacterial treatments for acne vulgaris: comparative review and guide to selection. Am J Clin Dermatol. 2004;5:79–84.
14. Tappeiner H, Jesionek A. Therapeutische versuche mit fluoreszierenden stoffen. Münch Med Wochenschr. 1903;47:2042–4.
15. Divaris DX, Kennedy JC, Pottier RH. Phototoxic damage to sebaceous glands and hair follicles of mice after systemic administration of 5-aminolevulinic acid correlates with localized protoporphyrin IX fluorescence. Am J Pathol. 1990;136:891–7.
16. Peng Q, Soler AM, Warloe T, et al. Selective distribution of porphyrins in skin thick basal cell carcinoma after topical application of methyl 5-aminolevulinate. J Photochem Photobiol B. 2001;62:140–5.
17. Sandberg C, Halldin CB, Ericson MB, et al. Bioavailability of aminolaevulinic acid and methylaminolaevulinate in basal cell carcinomas: a perfusion study using microdialysis in vivo. Br J Dermatol. 2008;159:1170–6.
18. Ericson MB, Sandberg C, Stenquist B, et al. Photodynamic therapy of actinic keratosis at varying fluence rates: assessment of photobleaching, pain and primary clinical outcome. Br J Dermatol. 2004;151: 1204–12.
19. Ashkenazi H, Malik Z, Harth Y, et al. Eradication of *Propionibacterium acnes* by its endogenic porphyrins after illumination with high intensity blue light. FEMS Immunol Med Microbiol. 2003;35:17–24.

20. Redondo P, Marquina M, Pretel M, et al. Methyl-ALA-induced fluorescence in photodynamic diagnosis of basal cell carcinoma prior to Mohs micrographic surgery. Arch Dermatol. 2008;144:115–7.
21. Cunliffe WJ, Goulden V. Phototherapy and acne vulgaris. Br J Dermatol. 2000;142:855–6.
22. Hongcharu W, Taylor CR, Chang Y, et al. Topical ALA-photodynamic therapy for the treatment of acne vulgaris. J Invest Dermatol. 2000;115:183–92.
23. Pollock B, Turner D, Stringer MR, et al. Topical aminolaevulinic acid-photodynamic therapy for the treatment of acne vulgaris: a study of clinical efficacy and mechanism of action. Br J Dermatol. 2004;151:616–22.
24. Wiegell SR, Wulf HC. Photodynamic therapy of acne vulgaris using 5-aminolevulinic acid versus methyl aminolevulinate. J Am Acad Dermatol. 2006;54:647–51.
25. Horfelt C, Funk J, Frohm-Nilsson M, et al. Topical methyl aminolaevulinate photodynamic therapy for treatment of facial acne vulgaris: results of a randomized, controlled study. Br J Dermatol. 2006;155: 608–13.
26. Horfelt C, Stenquist B, Larko O, et al. Photodynamic therapy for acne vulgaris: a pilot study of the dose-response and mechanism of action. Acta Derm Venereol. 2007;87:325–9.
27. Mills OH, Porte M, Kligman AM. Enhancement of comedogenic substances by ultraviolet radiation. Br J Dermatol. 1978;98:145–50.
28. Papageorgiou P, Katsambas A, Chu A. Phototherapy with blue (415 nm) and red (660 nm) light in the treatment of acne vulgaris. Br J Dermatol. 2000;142:973–8.
29. Sadick NS. Handheld LED array device in the treatment of acne vulgaris. J Drugs Dermatol. 2008;7:347–50.
30. Horfelt C, Stenquist B, Halldin CB, et al. Single low-dose red light is as efficacious as methyl-aminolevulinate–photodynamic therapy for treatment of acne: clinical assessment and fluorescence monitoring. Acta Derm Venereol. 2009;89:372–8.
31. Skiveren J, Haedersdal M, Philipsen PA, et al. Morphine gel 0.3% does not relieve pain during topical photodynamic therapy: a randomized, double-blind, placebo-controlled study. Acta Derm Venereol. 2006;86:409–11.
32. Sandberg C, Stenquist B, Rosdahl I, et al. Important factors for pain during photodynamic therapy for actinic keratosis. Acta Derm Venereol. 2006;86: 404–8.
33. Holmes MV, Dawe RS, Ferguson J, et al. A randomized, double-blind, placebo-controlled study of the efficacy of tetracaine gel (Ametop) for pain relief during topical photodynamic therapy. Br J Dermatol. 2004;150:337–40.
34. Langan SM, Collins P. double-blind, placebo-controlled prospective study of the efficacy of topical anaesthesia with a eutetic mixture of lignocaine 2.5% and prilocaine 2.5% for topical 5-aminolaevulinic acid-photodynamic therapy for extensive scalp actinic keratoses. Br J Dermatol. 2006;154:146–9.
35. Grapengiesser S, Ericson M, Gudmundsson F, et al. Pain caused by photodynamic therapy of skin cancer. Clin Exp Dermatol. 2002;27:493–7.
36. Wiegell SR, Skiveren J, Philipsen PA, et al. Pain during photodynamic therapy is associated with protoporphyrin IX fluorescence and fluence rate. Br J Dermatol. 2008;158:727–33.
37. Borelli C, Herzinger T, Merk K, et al. Effect of subcutaneous infiltration anesthesia on pain in photodynamic therapy: a controlled open pilot trial. Dermatol Surg. 2007;33:314–8.
38. Paoli J, Halldin C, Ericson MB, et al. Nerve blocks provide effective pain relief during topical photodynamic therapy for extensive facial actinic keratoses. Clin Exp Dermatol. 2008;33:559–64.
39. Halldin CB, Paoli J, Sandberg C, et al. Nerve blocks enable adequate pain relief during topical photodynamic therapy of field cancerization on the forehead and scalp. Br J Dermatol. 2009;160:795–800.

10 Photodynamic Therapy for the Treatment of Verrucae, Condylomata Acuminata, and Molluscum Contagiosum Lesions

Michael H. Gold

Abstract

The use of ALA-PDT has been shown to be successful for the treatment of recalcitrant verrucae, condylomata acuminata, and molluscum contagiosum lesions. Studies have shown that ALA-PDT is a useful modality for these lesions and that it should be considered when confronted with a patient with any of these viral conditions. Additional studies are warranted to further evaluate protocols used, light sources, and incubation times, to determine how to make the therapy even more appealing to clinicians and patients alike.

Photodynamic therapy (PDT) has been used for a variety of dermatologic skin concerns, which have been demonstrated throughout this textbook. The use of PDT for some of the more intriguing dermatologic disorders that have been described in the medical literature involves its role in the treatment of recalcitrant verrucae, condylomata acuminata, and molluscum contagiosum lesions. Various case reports and series have been published with regard to the use of PDT for these conditions, and this chapter reviews these reports and shows how PDT can be used for these conditions.

As is the case with many of the entities PDT is commonly used for, this remains an off-label use with commonly used photosensitizers, both ALA and methyl ALA (MAL). The Food and Drug Administration's (FDA) approval for 20% 5-ALA in USA is for the treatment of nonhyperkeratotic AKs of the face and scalp, utilizing a blue light source and a drug incubation time of 14–18 h [1]. And the FDA approval for MAL is for the nonhyperkeratotic AKs of the face and scalp after a 3-h under-occlusion-drug incubation period and treatment with red light [1].

M.H. Gold (✉)
Gold Skin Care Center, Tennessee Clinical Research Center, 2000 Richard Jones Road, Suite 220, Nashville, TN, USA
and
Department of Dermatology, Vanderbilt University School of Medicine and Nursing, Nashville, TN, USA
e-mail: goldskin@goldskincare.com

Verrucae, Condylomata, and Molluscum Lesions

Verrucae are double-stranded DNA viral entities that are caused by the human papilloma virus, commonly known as HPV. HPV is a member of the papova viral family. HPV infections, or verrucae, are seen almost every day in dermatology offices and have been identified to occur in virtually all parts of the body. Over 70 genotypes of verrucae have been identified; however, it is beyond the scope of this chapter to cover all of them, but many references exist that describe the genotypes in great detail. Both skin and mucosal surfaces can be affected by these lesions.

M.H. Gold (ed.), *Photodynamic Therapy in Dermatology*,
DOI 10.1007/978-1-4419-1298-5_10,

Verrucae, commonly referred to as warts, are clinically identified as being either papular or nodular structures that have a horny layer on their surface; they can range in size from 1 to 2 mm to several centimeters and may even become confluent forming even larger lesions. These lesions may be asymptomatic, but pain and functional abnormalities have been reported especially with those verrucous lesions that occur on the hands and feet. Epidemiologic studies have shown that up to 22% of school age children may develop verrucous lesions and that upward of 50–95% of renal transplant patients may develop verrucous lesions, some of which may progress toward squamous cell carcinomas, and therefore, require aggressive treatment strategies, of which PDT may play an important role [2].

The histology of verrucous lesions shows epidermal hyperplasia with acanthosis and papillomatosis, hyperkeratosis with parakeratosis, as well as thrombosed capillaries within the dermal papillae. Elongated rete ridges curve, in most incidences, to the center of the lesion. Viral replication takes place in differentiated keratinocytes in or above the stratum granulosum. Vacuolated cells, known as koilocytotic cells, are found in the mid upper dermis [2].

Treatments for verrucae are numerous and varied, and oftentimes discouraging to both the patient receiving them and to the clinician performing them. Numerous manuscripts have summarized treatment options for verrucae and are not reviewed here. Treatment modalities usually focus on the physical destruction of the individual lesion, i.e., the viral cell, and include cryotherapy [3], curettage, excision, carbon dioxide laser ablation [4], pulsed dye laser (PDL) therapy [5], liquid nitrogen, electrosurgery, and the application of a variety of topical acid preparations [6, 7]. Other modalities reported in the dermatologic literature include the use of infrared coagulation [8], alpha-interferon, topically applied 5-fluorouracil [9], intralesional bleomycin [10], and the use of topically applied DNCB [11]. Despite these treatment modalities, some lesions remain recalcitrant to the therapies, and some of these therapies are so painful that they are not practical in everyday clinical practice.

Condylomata acuminata are anogenital verrucous lesions caused by the HPV virus as described above. It has been related to genital carcinomas, and so treatment is essential to prevent the conversion into carcinoma. Treatment options are similar to what has been described for recalcitrant verrucae [12].

Molluscum contagiosum lesions are also caused by viruses, and many clinicians consider these lesions to be "cousins" of verrucae, although we know that they are caused by a different family of viruses. They are large DNA pox viruses. Molluscum lesions are commonly seen in children and have shown resurgence in those afflicted with HIV disease, especially when the viral load in these individuals is low [13–18]. They are clinically described as being discrete skin-colored smooth papules with an umbilicated center. These lesions occur on both the skin and mucous membranes. In children, the lesions are reported to occur on all body surfaces; those in HIV-positive individuals are more commonly described on the skin surfaces of the head and neck area. They are also reported to be larger than the typical small papular lesions seen in children and are, in general, more recalcitrant to therapeutic options [19].

The incidence of molluscum lesions is reported to be as high as 5% in children and up to 5–18% in the HIV and immunocompromised population. Histologic examination shows a hypertrophied and hyperplastic epidermis. Above the basal layer, there are lobules of enlarged epidermal cells with inclusion bodies, commonly known as molluscum bodies. The inclusion bodies contain the viral particles [17, 20–25].

Treatment options for molluscum are numerous and are similar to those described for verrucous lesions. Typical treatment modalities include liquid nitrogen, cantharidin, tretinoin cream, podophyllin 20–25%, salicylic acid, tincture of iodine, silver nitrate, trichloroacetic acid, and surgery with curettage with or without electrical desiccation. In HIV-positive individuals, antiretroviral therapy, intralesional alpha interferon, and injection of streptococcal antigen OK-432 have been reported to be useful in treating molluscum lesions. Despite these modalities, recalcitrant lesions are also often reported [16].

PDT and its Use in Verrucae, Condylomata, and Molluscum Lesions

Verrucae

PDT has been used in the treatment of recalcitrant verrucous lesions and molluscum lesions over the past 10 years. The remainder of this chapter reviews the various published case reports and series using ALA and MAL for treating verrucae and molluscum lesions, showing their value in treating recalcitrant disease.

In the first pilot series published in 1995, Ammann et al. [26] reported findings utilizing PDT in a total of six patients with refractory verrucae vulgaris lesions of the hands. All the patients reported failure with conventional modalities. The duration of their recalcitrant verrucous lesions varied from 2 to 10 years. They utilized a 20% ALA oil-in-water emulsion, which was applied under occlusion for 5–6 h before being illuminated utilizing a slide projector light source for 30 min. The patients were followed for up to 2 months following their therapy. The treated areas in all the patients studied showed an acute inflammatory skin reaction following the treatment. In five of the individuals, there was no change in the verrucae; however, in one patient, complete resolution was achieved. The authors noted that PDT was not a success in the treatment of verrucae, but they were encouraged by the one case of treatment success and encouraged further research into the field of study.

Several years later, in 1997, Smetana et al. [27] reported on their experiences with both an in vivo and an in vitro analyses utilizing PDT for both verrucae and molluscum lesion patients. In their verrucae case report, a 15-year kidney transplant patient presented with recalcitrant verrucae on the hands. A 20% ALA cream containing 2% EDTA and 2% DMSO was applied to the affected areas and incubated for a period of 4 h. Red light was used to activate the photosensitizer, at 120 J/cm^2. They noted dramatic improvement at the 1-month follow-up period. No recurrence was noted 2 years later. Their second patient, an HIV-positive individual, presented with numerous molluscum lesions on the face. Utilizing a similar protocol, the authors achieved similar clearance at the 1-month follow-up period. The authors concluded that ALA-PDT may be a useful modality for recalcitrant verrucae and molluscum lesions, especially with the unique ingredients that were added to the ALA preparation.

Stender et al. [28], in 2000, published findings in 232 hand and foot verrucous lesions found in 45 individuals in what is the first placebo-controlled clinical trial for ALA-PDT in the treatment of verrucous lesions. They randomized 117 verrucous lesions to receive ALA-PDT and 115 to receive placebo-PDT. Each lesion was treated with occlusion of the affected area for 4 h, and the lesions were irradiated with a red light source (Waldman PDT 1200, Waldmann-Medizin-Technik, Villingen-Schwenningen, Germany) with a wavelength range of 590–700 nm. The lesions were exposed to 50 J/cm^2 for 23 min and 20 s, yielding a total dose of 70 J/cm^2. All of the verrucae were treated at baseline, at 1 and 2 weeks, with another treatment regimen of three treatments given 1 month later if clearance was not achieved. Follow-up was at 1 and 2 months following the last treatment. Their results were as follows: at week 14, there was a relative reduction in wart area of 98% in the ALA group vs. 52% in the placebo group. At week 18, the relative reduction in the ALA group was 100 vs. 71% in the placebo group. Pain was more evident in the ALA-treated group compared to the placebo group. The authors concluded their study supported the use of ALA-PDT in the treatment of recalcitrant verrucae.

In 2001, Fabbrocini et al. [29] reported their experience with recalcitrant plantar warts in a controlled placebo clinical trial. They evaluated 67 patients utilizing PDT for these recalcitrant lesions. Each lesion was pretreated for 7 days with a topical ointment containing 10% urea and 10% salicylic acid to remove the superficial hyperkeratotic layers commonly seen in these lesions. A gentle curettage was also used prior to the application of the ALA; the ALA was a 20% cream preparation utilizing Eucerin® cream as its base. The ALA preparation was occluded for 5 h prior to light therapy. Sixty-four lesions received the ALA cream, while 57 verrucae received only the Eucerin® cream base. The photoactivator utilized was a tungsten lamp that emitted a spectrum of light from 400 to 700 nm, with a peak at 630 nm. The power incidence was 50 mW/cm^2, at a distance of 10 cm. The patients received one treatment, and if not clear, received up to two more therapies at 1 week intervals. The patients were then followed for 22 months following their last therapy. The results showed that 48 of the 64 warts (75%) completely healed in the ALA group compared to 13 out of the 57 lesions in the placebo group (22.8%). Of interest, 47.9% of the ALA lesions cleared following one treatment, 31.3% required two treatments, and only 20.8% needed three treatments for clearance to occur. The authors concluded that ALA was successful in the treatment of recalcitrant verrucae.

Stender et al. [30], in 1999, reported further work on the use of ALA-PDT in the treatment of recalcitrant verrucae of the hands and feet. They evaluated 30 individuals with a total of 250 verrucous lesions and randomized patients to receive one of the five following treatment protocols: ALA-PDT with white light 3 times in 10 days, ALA-PDT with white light for one treatment, ALA-PDT with red light for three treatments in 10 days, ALA-PDT with blue light for three treatments in 10 days, and cryotherapy up to four treatments within a 2-month period. The ALA utilized was a 20% ALA preparation; each lesion was incubated for 5 h under occlusion. The areas treated were illuminated with light from slide projectors (halogen lamp) at a distance of 15 cm, with a given total dose of 40 J/cm^2. The treatments were repeated if the lesions were not completely cleared after the first course. The results from the study showed complete clearance of 73% with white light with three treatments, 71% after one white light treatment, 42% after red light therapy, 23% after blue light therapy, and 20% after cryotherapy. Of the areas that cleared, no recurrences were noted after a 12-month follow-up period. The authors concluded that ALA-PDT is a useful modality for the treatment of recalcitrant verrucae of the hands and feet.

Mizuki et al. [31], in 2003, reported on the use of ALA-PDT in a 13-year-old Japanese boy who had a 2-year history of multiple "plane" warts of the face, unresponsive to previous therapies. They used a 20% ALA oil-in-water emulsion and a single 500-W metal halide lamp with peaks of 630 and 700 nm. The ALA was incubated for 6 h under occlusion; illumination was for 20 min for an energy of 120 J/cm^2. The patient underwent two ALA-PDT sessions. Five months after the final treatment, the areas remained disease free. This suggested that ALA-PDT is useful for the treatment of recalcitrant plane warts.

In 2005, Smucler and Jatsova [32], reported on the use of a PDL with ALA in the treatment of verrucous lesions. They compared PDL alone vs. PDL plus PDT as well as PDT and an LED light source. They found that all three of their protocols were effective in treating these recalcitrant lesions, but the combination of PDL plus PDT resulted in the highest cure rate with the shortest number of treatments. PDL cured 81% of the lesions treated ($n=112$), with a mean number of sessions being 3.34. PDL plus PDT cured 100% ($n=86$), with a mean number of sessions being 1.95. PDT plus LED cured 96% of the lesions ($n=76$), with a mean number of sessions being 2.53. The authors strongly suggested this combined modality to become a treatment of choice for viral warts.

Gold and Pope [33] reported a case of fractional laser resurfacing and the use of ALA-PDT in treating a recalcitrant verrucous lesion of the foot in 2008. The patient had presented with a verrucous lesion on the heel of the foot that did not respond to conventional therapy, including the use of topical medications, liquid nitrogen, PDL treatments, and even conventional PDT using both short- and long-contact ALA and treatment with the PDL. The patient was successfully treated with an erbium:YAG fractional laser, which served as an enhancement mechanism for delivery of ALA into the skin. 20% 5-ALA solution was then applied and occluded for 24 h. After two PDL treatments, the verrucous lesion had resolved. The use of the erbium:YAG fractional laser delivered microscopic holes to the skin, which, as noted, enhanced the delivery of ALA into the thick skin of the foot, making the ALA efficacious with the PDL. This is shown in Fig. 10.1.

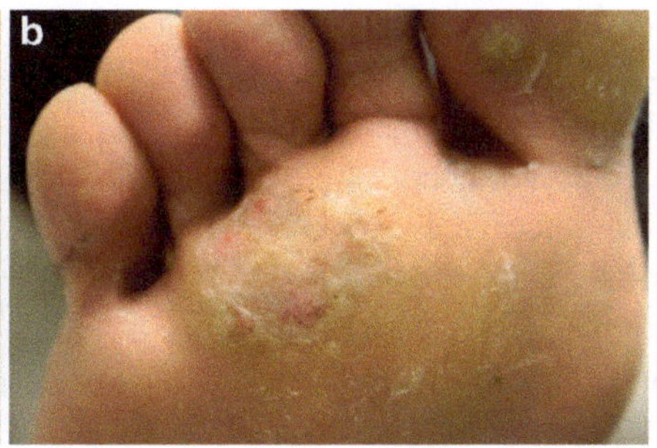

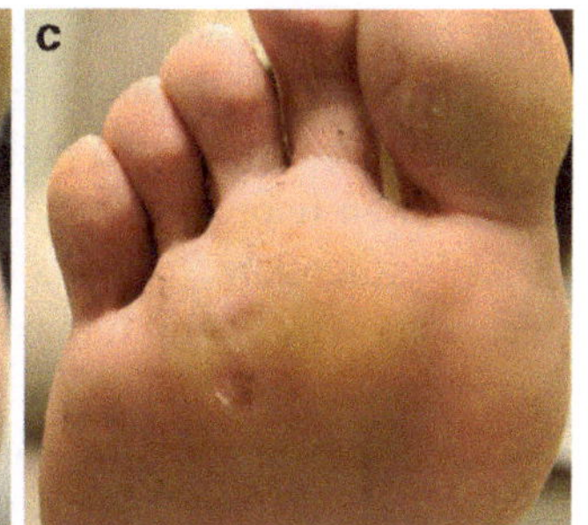

Fig. 10.1 Clinical example of fractional laser resurfacing and the use of ALA-PDT in treating a recalcitrant verrucous lesion of the foot; before treatment (**a**) and 1 month following the first treatment with marked reduction in size (**b**); 1 month after second treatment with complete resolution of lesion (**c**)

Condylomata

Several reports have shown the successes of PDT in the treatment of condylomata acuminata. In 2002, Stefanaki et al. [34] reported on the use of ALA-PDT in the treatment of 12 male patients with condylomata acuminata. The lesions were treated with 20% ALA and irradiated with optimal doses of red light at 70 and 100 J/cm^2. The overall cure rate reported was 72.9% at the 12-month follow-up period. Wang et al. [35], in 2004, reported on 164 patients with urethral condylomata acuminata treated with 10% ALA. Complete response rates at 6–24 months were 95.12% with recurrence rates of 5.13%. Chen et al. [36], in 2007, reported their experiences with ALA-PDT vs. conventional CO_2 laser therapy in patients with condylomata acuminata. Sixty-five patients received ALA-PDT, and 21 patients received CO_2 laser therapy. The complete response was 95% after one treatment, with a recurrence rate noted to be 6.3% at 12 weeks. This was better than conventional CO_2 laser therapy, and adverse events were also noted to be lower in the PDT group. Liang et al. [37], in 2009, reported on 90 patients treated with ALA-PDT ($n=67$) or conventional CO_2 laser therapy ($n=23$). In this study, 20% ALA was used with a 3-h drug incubation. Light irradiation with red light of 100 J/cm^2 at 100 mW was applied to the lesions, and up to 3 weekly treatments were given. Complete clearance was noted in 95.93% of the ALA group and 100% in the CO_2 laser group 1 week after the last treatment, but recurrence rates and adverse events were much less in the ALA treated group.

Molluscum Lesions

Gold [38], reported on the successful use of ALA-PDT in the treatment of recalcitrant molluscum contagiosum lesions in an HIV patient in 2004. They treated an HIV-positive individual who had numerous large face and neck molluscum lesions with four sessions of ALA-PDT utilizing the original FDA treatment protocol, which is covered elsewhere in this textbook. The ALA was applied to individual lesions and allowed to incubate for 16 h before exposure to a blue light source (ClearLight, CureLight, Yokneam, Israel) for 16 min and 40 s. The therapy was reported painful during the illumination, so cool water and a fan was utilized to ease this discomfort. There was a significant inflammatory response following each treatment, which required systemic and topical corticosteroids for relief. The treatments were performed at 2 week intervals, and a dramatic response was seen after the fourth treatment. The patient was then able to take a long trip, which he had planned, to visit lands that he had always dreamed of visiting. Unfortunately, he succumbed to his HIV disease during the travels, but his friends credited this therapy for allowing him to leave home and go on the journey.

Moiin and Gold [39] reviewed charts from a total of 40 patients with molluscum lesions treated with ALA-PDT and a blue light source, the BluU® (Dusa Pharmaceuticals, Wilmington, MA). Six of the individuals had a history of HIV infection and were the basis of this report. The ALA was applied broadly to the affected areas, incubated from 14 to

24 h, and treated with the blue light for 16 min and 40 s. All of the patients studied improved in their lesion count. In two patients, one treatment produced an improvement in the lesion count of 60%. Furthermore, patients who received 3–5 treatments were found to have a 75–80% reduction in the number of lesions counted. The therapy did have adverse events, including erythema, edema, vesiculation, hyperpigmentation, hypopigmentation, pain, stinging/burning, and itching. The only deliberately intense side effect was a burning sensation described by one patient when placed under the blue light source. Only one child did not tolerate the procedure fully due to erythema formation. The conclusion is that PDT is a viable option for treating molluscum contagiosum in HIV-positive patients and immunocompromised children. All of the patients expressed preference of ALA-PDT over previous therapies for their molluscum lesions.

Conclusion

In conclusion, the use of ALA-PDT has been shown to be successful for the treatment of recalcitrant verrucae, condylomata acuminata, and molluscum contagiosum lesions. Studies have shown that ALA-PDT is a useful modality for these lesions and that it should be considered when confronted with a patient with any of these viral conditions. Additional studies are warranted to further evaluate protocols used, light sources, and incubation times, to determine how to make the therapy even more appealing to clinicians and patients alike.

References

1. Jeffes EW, McCullough JL, Weinstein GD, Kaplan R, Glazer SD, Taylor JR. Photodynamic therapy of actinic keratoses with topical aminolevulinic acid hydrochloride and fluorescent blue light. J Am Acad Dermatol. 2001;45:96–104.
2. Stender IM. Treatment of human papilloma virus. In: Goldman MP, editor. Photodynamic therapy. Munich: Elsevier; 2005. p. 77–88.
3. Bourke JF, Berth-Jones J, Hutchinson PE. Cryotherapy of common viral warts at intervals of 1, 2, and 3 weeks. Br J Dermatol. 1995;132:433–6.
4. Logan RA, Zachary CB. Outcome of carbondioxide laser therapy for persistent cutaneous viral warts. Br J Dermatol. 1989;121:99.
5. Tan OT, Hurwitz TM, Stafford TJ. Pulsed dye laser treatment of recalcitrant verrucae, a premliminary report. Lasers Surg Med. 1993;13:127–37.
6. Hirose R, Hori M, Shukuwa R, Udono M, Yamada M, Koide T, et al. Topical treatment of resistant warts with glutaraldehyde. J Dermatol. 1994;21:248–53.
7. Bunney MH, Nolan MW, Williams DA. An assessment of methods of treating viral warts by comparative treatment trials based on standard design. Br J Dermatol. 1976;94:667–80.
8. Halasz CL. Treatment of common warts using the infrared conagulator. J Dermatol Surg Oncol. 1994;20: 252–6.
9. Brodell RT, Breadle DL. The treatment of palmar and plantar warts using natural alpha interferon and a needleless injector. Dermatol Surg. 1995;21:213–8.
10. James MP, Collier PM, Aherne W, Hardcastle A, Lovegrove S. Histologic, pharmacologic and immunocytochemical effects of injection of bleomycin. J Am Acad Dermatol. 1993;28:933–7.
11. Shah KC, Patel RM, Umrigar DP. Dinitroclorobenzene treatment of verrucae plana. J Dermatol. 199118(11): 639–42.
12. Schneede P. Genital human papillomarvirus infections. Curr Opin Urol. 2002;12:57–61.
13. Siegfried EC. Warts and molluscum contagiosum on children: an approach to therapy. Dermatol Ther. 1997;2:51–67.
14. Verbov J. How to manage warts. Arch Der Child. 1999;80:97–9.
15. Lewis EJ, Lam M, Crutchfield CE. An update on molluscum contagiosum. Cutis. 1997;60:29–34.
16. Husar K, Skerlev M. Molluscum contagiosum from infancy to maturity. Clin Dermatol. 2002;20:170–2.
17. Coldiron BM, Bergstresser PR. Prevalence and clinical spectrum of skin disease in patients infected with human immunodeficiency virus. Arch Dermatol. 1989;125:357–61.
18. Czelasta A, Yen-Moore A, Vander Straten M, Carrasco D, Tyring SK. An overview of sexually transmitted diseases. Part III. Sexually transmitted diseases in HIV-infected patients. J Am Acad Dermatol. 2000;43:409–32.
19. Schwartz JJ, Myskowsk PL. Molluscum contagiosum in patients with humanimmunodeficiency virus infection: a review of twenty-seven patients. J Am Acad Dermatol. 1992;27:583–8.
20. Lowy DR. Molluscum contagiosum. In: Freedberg IM, Eisen AZ, Wolff K, et al., editors. Dermatology in general medicine. New York: McGraw-Hill; 1999. p. 2478–81.
21. Matis WL, Triana A, Shapiro R, Eldred L, Polk BF, Hood AF. Dermatologic findings associated with human immunodeficiency virus infection. J Am Acad Dermatol. 1987;17(5 Pt 1):746–51.
22. Goodman DS, Teplitz ED, Wishner A, Klein RS, Burk PG, Hershenbaum E. Prevalence of cutaneous disease in patients with acquired immunodeficiency syndrome

(AIDS) or AIDS-related complex. J Am Acad Dermatol. 1987;17(2 Pt 1):210–20.

23. Schwartz JJ, Myskowski PL. Molluscum contagiosum in patients with human immunodeficiency virus infection. A review of twenty-seven patients. J Am Acad Dermatol. 1992;27(4):583–8.
24. Epstein WL, Senecal I, Krasnobrod H. Viral antigens in human epidermal tumors: localization of an antigen to molluscum contagiosum. J Invest Dermatol. 1963;40:51.
25. Kwittken J. Molluscum contagiosum: some new histologic observations. Mt Sina J Med. 1980;47:583.
26. Ammann R, Hunziker T, Braathen LR. Topical photodynamic therapy in verrucae. Dermatology. 1995;191: 346–7.
27. Smetana Z, Malik Z, Orenstein A, et al. Treatment of viral infections with 5-aminolevulinic acid and light. Lasers Surg Med. 1997;21:351–8.
28. Stender IM, Na R, Fogh H, et al. Photodynamic therapy with 5-aminolevulinic acid or placebo for recalcitrant foot and hand warts: randomized double-blind trial. Lancet. 2000;355:963–6.
29. Fabbrocini G, Costanzo M, Riccardo A, et al. Photodynamic therapy with topical 5-aminolevulinic acid for the treatment of plantar warts. J Photochem Photobiol B. 2001;61(1–2):30–4.
30. Stender IM, Lock-Andersen J, Wulf HC. Recalcitrant hand and foot warts successfully treated with photodynamic therapy with topical 5-aminolaevulinic acid: a pilot study. Clin Exp Dermatol. 1999;24(3): 154–9.
31. Mizuki D, Kaneko T, Hanada K. Successful treatment of topical photodynamic therapy using 5-aminolevulinic acid for plane warts. Br J Dermatol. 2003;149(5): 1087–8.
32. Smucler R, Jatsova E. Comparative study of aminolevulic acid photodynamic therapy plus pulsed dye laser versus pulsed dye laser alone in treatment of viral warts. Photomed Laser Surg. 2005;23(2):202–5.
33. Gold MH, Pope A. Fractional resurfacing aiding photodynamic therapy of a recalcitrant plantar verruca – a case report & review of the literature. J Clin Aesthet Dermatol. 2008;1(1):30–3.
34. Stefanaki IM, Georgiou S, Themelis GC, et al. In vivo fluorescence kinetics and photodynamic therapy in condylomata acuminate. Br J Dermatol. 2003;149:972–6.
35. Wang XL, Wang HW, Wang HS, et al. Topical 5-aminovaevulinic clylomata acuminate. Br J Dermatol. 2004;151:880–5.
36. Chen K, Chang BZ, Ju M, et al. Comparative study of photodynamic therapy vs CO2 laser vaporization in treatment of condylomata acuminate, a randomized clinical trial. Br J Dermatol. 2007;156:516–20.
37. Liang J, Lu XN, Tang H, et al. Evaluation of photodynamic therapy using topical aminolevulinic acid hydrochloride in the treatment of condylomata acuminata: a comparative, randomized clinical trial. Photodermatol Photoimmunol Photomed. 2009;25(6): 293–7.
38. Gold MH. The Use of ALA-PDT in the treatment of recalcitrant molluscum contagiosum in HIV/AIDS affected individuals. J Laser Surg Med. 2003;15 (Suppl):40.
39. Moiin A, Gold MH. Treatment of verrucae vulgaris and molluscum contagiosum with photodynamic therapy. Dermatol Clin. 2007;25:75–80.

Photodynamic Therapy and Inflammatory Disorders

11

Cara Garretson and Amy Forman Taub

Abstract

While still in its infancy, photodynamic therapy is becoming a prominent treatment option in a number of dermatological diseases, such as psoriasis, lichen planus, lichen sclerosis, morphea/scleroderma, vitiligo, necrobiosis, lipoidica diabeticorum, sarcoidosis, granuloma annulare, alopecia areata, and Darier's disease. Given the breadth of clinical implications, it is clear that both basic science and clinical studies are still needed to learn more about the mechanism of action, efficacy, and optimal treatment regimens in many of these inflammatory disorders.

As photodynamic therapy (PDT) has been found to be an excellent tool to treat nonmelanoma skin cancer, actinic keratoses, and acne, it has been continually evaluated to determine its effectiveness in the treatment of a number of other skin conditions. Given the success of PDT in the treatment of acne vulgaris [1–4], it has been increasingly utilized in the treatment of many other inflammatory disorders of the skin in the hopes of recreating this success in these often difficult-to-treat disease states. Variable photosensitizers and light sources were examined and it should be noted that none of these forms of PDT are currently FDA-approved at this time for these disorders. However, these studies provide great insight not only into many of these inflammatory conditions, but also into PDT itself.

A.F. Taub (✉)
Advanced Dermatology, 275 Parkway Drive, Suite 521, Lincolnshire, IL 60069, USA
and
Department of Dermatology, Northwestern University Medical School, Chicago, IL, USA
e-mail: drtaub@skinfo.com

Psoriasis

There is a substantial amount of literature devoted to the treatment of psoriasis with PDT. Attempting to establish mechanism of action, specificity of uptake of photosensitizer, and clinical efficacy has been the main focus of these studies.

Mechanism of Action

Psoriasis in now known to be an inflammatory disorder with altered immune system function. Particularly, psoriasis involves an infiltrate of T lymphocytes and excessive T-cell helper activation, with a predominance of Th1 pattern of cytokines [5]. Boehncke et al. [6] established that PDT with red light (630 nm) caused a decrease in inflammatory cytokines (Interleukin(IL)-6, tumor necrosis factor (TNF)-α, and IL-1β) associated with psoriasis, although to a lesser extent than that caused by PUVA (oral psoralen plus UVA light).

M.H. Gold (ed.), *Photodynamic Therapy in Dermatology*,
DOI 10.1007/978-1-4419-1298-5_11, © Springer Science+Business Media, LLC 2011

These cytokines are secreted by mononuclear cells that were isolated after irradiation. They also demonstrated that progressive photobleaching correlated with higher energy irradiations, thus establishing that there was a dose dependency of PDT for skin affected with psoriasis vulgaris. Another study [7] showed that systemic PDT (oral aminolevulinic acid [ALA]-blue light at 417 nm) induces apoptosis in lesional T lymphocytes in psoriatic plaques, which is a feature that may predict a longer-lasting therapeutic effect [8]. A study evaluating topical ALA-PDT found that histological specimens of the PDT-treated side showed a decrease in CD8+ and CD45RO cells and Ki67+ nuclei as well as an increase in epidermal K10 expression and CD4+ cells. This indicates that PDT works via normalization of epidermal proliferation, keratinization, and differentiation, as well as by changing the T-cell population of the treated skin [9]. In the above-mentioned study, Boehncke et al. [6] also noted there was preferential accumulation of PpIX in psoriatic plaques, greater improvement with higher doses, and minimal pain with administration of oral ALA leading them to conclude that this modality warranted further study (Table 11.1).

Specificity of Uptake

Many studies focused on evaluating if there was preferential photosensitizer uptake in psoriatic plaques, and if so, how to increase it and make it more uniform. Stringer et al. [10] first addressed this by showing an increase of protoporphyrin IX (PpIX) accumulation in psoriatic plaques after application of 5-ALA and exposure to a 488-nm laser [10]. However, he also noted significant variability of fluorescence between plaques, as well as accumulation of photosensitizer in distant sites that did not receive application of ALA. Bissonnette et al. [11] studied the fluorescence of oral ALA at doses of 10, 20, and 30 mg/kg in psoriatic plaques, normal skin, and inflammatory skin cells in 12 patients. They found a tenfold increase in fluorescence of lesional psoriatic skin 3–5 h after a single 30 mg/kg dose of ALA, though also noted some fluorescence of noninvolved facial skin. The Bisonette study mentioned previously [7] also supports that there was preferential accumulation of PpIX in psoriatic plaques after administration of oral ALA, pointing to some specificity of the photosensitizer to the psoriatic plaques.

Kleinpenning et al. [12] sought to further evaluate the heterogeneity of fluorescence in psoriasis after ALA application. After a week of pretreatment with 10% salicylic acid in petrolatum, fourteen patients with plaque psoriasis were treated with 20% 5-ALA under occlusion of 3 h and were then biopsied for further evaluation. Twelve of fourteen lesions showed nonhomogenous fluorescence, despite equal metabolic activity across psoriatic plaques and no significant difference in epidermal thickness between the plaques. However, the low fluorescent plaques had significantly thicker stratum corneum compared to the high fluorescent plaques (Fig. 11.1). Thus, the authors concluded that keratolytic pretreatment was essential to obtain the most efficacious results with PDT. Kleinpenning et al. [13] took this one step further in another attempt to elucidate the best pretreatment for PDT of psoriasis lesions. His group evaluated two psoriatic plaques in ten patients. One side was treated with either retinoic acid or a hydrocolloid dressing, with the latter providing the best results while the former was associated with irritation and point bleeding. In a second arm, eight patients were pretreated with a hydrocolloid dressing or salicylic acid in petrolatum during the 6 weeks the patients received PDT, followed by histological evaluation. Both the salicylic acid and the hydrocolloid dressing were found to decrease hyperkeratosis with the authors concluding both regimens could be used in the keratolytic pretreatment algorithm of PDT treatment for psoriasis.

Smits et al., having previously found more fluorescence of PpIX in psoriasis vs. actinic keratosis [14], evaluated the intrinsic protoporphyrin IX accumulating capabilities of lesional and nonlesional skin in psoriasis and actinic keratoses in comparison to normal skin ex vivo. Overall, they found no significant differences in PpIX synthesis in the various skin types. The authors attributed this to the fact that in explants of skin tissue, the

Table 11.1 Study results of PDT for psoriasis mechanism of action and specificity

References	Study objective/summary	Results
Boehncke et al. [6]	Analysis of effects of PDT on cytokine secretion in plaque psoriasis patients compared to PUVA	The combination of PDT and 630 nm light decreased TNF-α, IL-1β, and IL-6 in dose-dependent manner. This was less than PUVA for IL-1β and IL-6 on peripheral mononuclear cells. There was a preferential increase in fluorescence/PpiX in psoriatic plaques
Bissonnette et al. [7]	Evaluate the effects of PDT with blue light after oral ALA administration on psoriatic plaques and determine if systemic ALA-PDT induces apoptosis on lesional T lymphocytes	Oral ALA induces preferential accumulation of PpIX in psoriatic plaques and oral ALA-PDT does induce apoptosis in lesional CD3+ T lymphocytes
Stringer et al. [10]	Evaluate accumulation of protoporphyrin IX in 42 psoriatic plaques of 15 patients after application of 5-ALA and exposure to 488 nm light source	Psoriatic plaques showed preferential uptake of PpIX with increasing intensity up to 6 h after application. There was great variability of fluorescence between plaques; occlusion did not appear to make a significant difference. Days after the procedure, photosensitization was noted in some untreated areas of psoriasis
Smits et al. [9]	Determine the PpIX accumulating capabilities of skin explants in patients with psoriasis, actinic keratosis, and normal skin	No significant differences in PpIX accumulation were found in the different cell types. There was increased PpIX in B-1 integrin negative (suprabasal) cells. Authors conclude in vivo importance of stratum corneum in affecting accumulation capabilities of the different lesions
Kleinpenning et al. [12]	Evaluate the heterogeneity in fluorescence of PpIX in plaque psoriasis. One plaque in 14 patients treated with 20% 5-ALA for 3 h after 1 week of salicylic acid pretreatment, then evaluated for fluorescence and biopsied for comparative differences	12 of 14 plaques showed inhomogenous fluorescence despite no differences in epidermal proliferation, keratinization, and inflammation. However, the lesions with a thicker stratum corneum exhibited lower fluorescence as compared to those with less hyperkeratosis
Kleinpenning et al. [13]	Determine the ideal keratolytic pretreatment of psoriatic plaques to obtain the best results with PDT. In one arm, two plaques in ten patients were treated with a retinoid or a hydrocolloid dressing; in another arm, salicylic acid or a hydrocolloid dressing were used, all followed by histological analysis	Both the salicylic acid and hydrocolloid dressings provided decreases in hyperkeratosis with less irritation as compared to retinoids
Bissonnette et al. [11]	Determine if oral ALA could be a viable option in treatment of plaque psoriasis. Fluorescence was evaluated in psoriatic plaques, normal skin, and peripheral blood cells in 12 patients after treatment with 10, 20, or 30 mg/kg of oral ALA	The 20 and 30 mg/kg doses induced preferential accumulation of PpIX in psoriatic plaques as compared to surrounding normal skin, with ratios up to 10 with the 30 mg/kg dose of oral ALA. Visible PpIX fluorescence was noted on normal facial skin and nonspecific photosensitivity occurred in patients who received the 20 or 30 mg/kg doses
Smits et al. [9]	Evaluate clinical effectiveness, immunohistochemical changes, and accumulation of PpIX in psoriatic lesions after treatment with topical 5-ALA and photodynamic therapy (PDT) 600–750 nm light exposure	The histological specimens of the PDT-treated side showed a decrease in CD8+ and CD45RO lymphocytes and Ki67+ nuclei as well as an increase in epidermal K10 expression and CD4+ lymphocytes. This indicates that PDT works via normalization of epidermal proliferation, keratinization, and differentiation, as well as by changing the T-cell population to that typical of normal skin

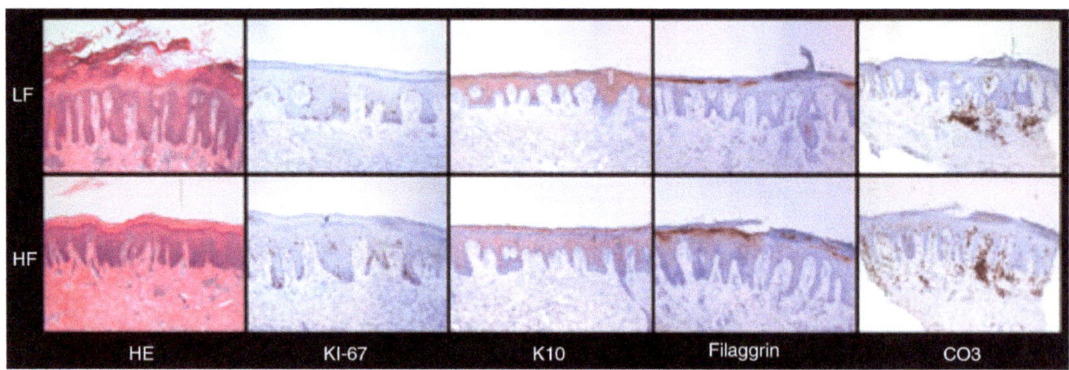

Fig. 11.1 Morphological and immunohistochemical images of both low- and high-fluorescent psoriatic skin. Hematoxylin and eosin, Ki-67, keratin 10 (K10), and filaggrin stainings of heterogeneous fluorescent lesional skin are displayed at 100× magnification. CD3 is displayed at 50× magnification. Hematoxylin and eosin sections showed a significantly thicker stratum corneum in low-fluorescent psoriatic skin. Immunohistochemically, no differences in epidermal proliferation, differentiation, and inflammation were found between high- and low-fluorescent skin (from Kleinpenning et al. [12], with permission)

penetration of ALA through the stratum corneum is bypassed, thus suggesting that the stratum corneum is an important route of – and possible barrier to – penetration of ALA into psoriatic plaques. This finding is a bit at odds with previous literature showing that there is preferential uptake of both actinic keratosis tissue and psoriasis lesions even with oral ALA absorption [7].

Clinical Studies

Given some evidence of mechanism of action and specificity of uptake for PDT's effect on psoriasis, studies were initiated to determine the efficacy of PDT in a clinical setting. An initial study by Collins et al. [15] investigated the response of psoriasis to PDT as well as protoporphyrin fluorescence before, during, and after treatment. Twenty-two patients were divided into two equal groups with one group receiving 2, 4, 8, and 16 J/cm^2 at 25 mW/cm^2, while the other group receiving 8 and 16 J/cm^2 at 10 and 40 J/cm^2 on four focal areas of psoriasis, with one square on each patient receiving ALA but no illumination. Using the scale, erythema and index (SEI) score, 35% showed clearance of some plaques. By measuring the protoporphyrin levels before, during, and after treatment, they were able to determine rate and degree of photo-oxidation at the light doses given. There was considerable variability in pre-illumination fluorescence between patients and between sites on the same patients. Based on the results, it appeared that it is the intensity of preillumination PpIX fluorescence rather than light dose that determines the rate and degree of photo-oxidation and thus the photodynamic dose. While rate of the light dose, i.e., 10, 25, or 40 mW/cm^2, seemed to affect photo-oxidation, it was not to a statistically significant degree. Also, they found that the majority of oxidation was complete at 16 J/cm^2 concluding that higher light doses would not confer any further benefit. Overall, this study suggested that the photosensitizers' ability to engender fluorescence in plaques, i.e., specificity of uptake, is the key feature to achieving efficacious results with PDT for psoriasis. Multiple treatments could also be expected to increase efficacy, which is what a subsequent study explored. Robinson et al. [16] evaluated ten patients with plaque psoriasis, each treated 3 times weekly with topical 5-ALA (4 h incubation) and broadband visible radiation at dosage of 8 J/cm^2. Eight out of ten patients showed clinical response, but only 1 of 19 sites cleared completely and 5 sites showed no improvement. More concerning was that, upon histological evaluation, fluorescence showed little consistency of uptake, even within the same plaque. Finally, there was so much discomfort with the treatments that the investigators concluded PDT was not a practical therapy for psoriasis. In Germany, a prospective randomized intrapatient comparison study was completed by Schleyer et al. [17] who evaluated 12 patients with psoriasis, exposing three plaques each to 0.1, 1, and 5% 5-ALA, respectively (occlusion time of 4–6 h), to 20 J/cm^2 of a filtered metal halide light (600–740 nm) twice weekly for up to 12 irradiations. There was dose-dependent improvement, but there was no complete clearance. Unfortunately, pain was also dose-dependent. One patient showed flare of a healing plaque after a very painful treatment. Another larger study [18] evaluated 29 patients with plaque psoriasis treated twice weekly for 6 weeks. Three plaques in each patient were pretreated with 10% salicylic acid in petrolatum for 2 weeks followed by 1% ALA under occlusion for 4–6 h. Treatments with a filtered metal halide using light dosimetries of 5, 10, or 20 J/cm^2 were assessed for their efficacy in clearing psoriatic lesions. Complete clearance was noted in 8 of 63 treated lesions, with best results seen at 20 J/cm^2. Although they demonstrated a clear decrease in PASI (46–49%) in more than 95% of plaques, the slow pace, pain during therapy, and only partial results led the investigators to deem this form of PDT a less than optimal treatment option for psoriasis. They concluded that oral ALA and blue light or verteporfin and red light may be a more practical and efficacious method of treatment. The significance of keratolytic pretreatment was again highlighted, as the pretreatment alone decreased the PASI by 25%. Another study of 12 patients was completed using topical 5-ALA 20% solution with red light at 10–30 J/cm^2 to psoriatic plaques once weekly for 2–5 treatments [19]. Four patients dropped out of the study due to pain during treatments. Of the eight remaining patients, statistically significant improvement in the clinical appearance of the lesions was noted. Immunohistochemical evaluation correlated with this clinical improvement, showing a decreased inflammatory infiltrate and near disappearance of Keratin 16 staining, which is normally found in significantly elevated levels in psoriatic plaques [20].

In a placebo-controlled randomized study [9], eight patients with symmetric plaque psoriasis were studied for clinical response and evaluation of immunohistochemical markers. Ten percent ALA ointment under occlusion was used on one plaque, whereas the vehicle alone was used on the contralateral plaque; both were occluded for 4 h then exposed to fractionated light (Waldman PDT 1200L, 650–700 nm) at 2 J/cm^2 then 2 dark hours, followed by 8 J/cm^2, as there is some evidence in the literature that fractionated PDT can be more effective than single-exposure PDT [21, 22].The PDT-treated side exhibited clinical improvement as well as histological improvement with a decrease in CD4+, CD8+, and CD45RO cells and Ki67+ nuclei as well as an increase in epidermal K10 expression. This correlated with normalization of epidermal proliferation and differentiation, and as stated above, change in the T-cell population of the treated skin. These biological changes were absent in the placebo-treated sides. Of importance, two patients developed new psoriatic lesions in a treated area implying that a Koebner phenomenon could occur. The risk of a Koebner phenomenon occurring may be dependent on the dose and photosensitizer used. Also, heterogeneity of plaques in fluorescent staining was still seen as an obstacle to practical therapy, despite pretreatment with salicylic acid cream. Even with this modest clinical result, the investigators remained hopeful that protocols could be optimized for psoriatic therapy, since desired molecular changes were clearly documented on the treated side. The findings in this study highlight the potential immune-related mechanism of action in photodynamic treatment of psoriasis.

As noted above in the specificity of uptake section, Kleinpenning's group worked on two different studies to determine if salicylic acid or hydrocolloid dressings were optimal and if they were necessary to decrease heterogeneity of uptake and improve clinical outcome [13]. These studies clearly document that these pretreatments may not be enough to provide homogenous uptake and may provide a barrier to consistently effective treatment. However, potential improvements could be made by addressing other variables.

Salah et al. [23] sought to investigate the use of a different photosensitizer, methylene blue, in PDT treatments for psoriasis. This study evaluated topical methylene blue with a 565 mW light-emitting diode (LED, 670 nm) to treat resistant plaque psoriasis. The rationale was that methylene blue has better absorption at longer wavelengths, which are known to penetrate more deeply into tissue. The increased absorption of long wavelengths may be necessary for optimal penetration of thick plaques of psoriasis. Of 23 patients enrolled, 18 completed this intrapatient placebo-controlled study. Each lesion received topical application of either methylene blue 0.1% gel or placebo vehicle occluded for 30 min followed by twice weekly irradiation for 8 min (5 J/cm^2) for up to 12 sessions. The methylene blue-treated lesions resulted in a nearly 84% decrease in PASI score, while the placebo group showed no improvement. Histological examination exhibited normalization of the epidermis after treatment. Also of great importance, there was no associated pain with this treatment. The authors propose that the improved efficacy of methylene blue is due in part to its higher accumulation in mitochondria, which is an important target in PDT to induce apoptosis [24]. They also note the low tissue toxicity and strong absorption of methylene blue at more optimal wavelengths for tissue penetration as reasons to further investigate this photosensitizing method in PDT for psoriasis. This different methodology may open a new door for PDT treatment of psoriasis.

Several recent studies sought to evaluate PDT for palmoplantar and nail psoriasis. In one case report [25], a patient with recalcitrant palmoplantar pustular psoriasis was treated with topical 20% ALA (5 h occlusion) followed by illumination with 632 nm diode laser (15 J/cm^2). After 11 weekly treatments, the patient was found to be nearly clear. The patient subsequently received maintenance therapy every other week for three treatments, then every third week for two treatments. Three months after the final treatment, the patient remained clear. In a second case report [26], three intractable cases of palmoplantar pustular psoriasis were treated with PDT using 20% 5-ALA (4 h occlusion) and 630±50 nm LED device (fluence 15 J/cm^2 and power density 30 mW/cm^2) with variable results from mild to marked improvement. One patient showed marked improvement on palms and soles, one showed mild improvement on palms and soles, and one patient had mild improvement on soles and marked improvement on palms, all after different number of treatment sessions. The authors speculated the results were less favorable due to the difference in light source from the first to the second case report, suggesting the 632 nm light may provide better results. This could also potentially be due to the nature of pulsed light vs. continuous wave light also. Finally, a recent study [27] evaluated Methylaminolevulinic acid (MAL)-PDT with pulsed dye laser (PDL, 595 nm) vs. PDL in the treatment of refractory nail psoriasis in 14 patients. Specifically, 61 nails were treated with PDL and 60 nails were treated with MAL (occlusion for 3 h) followed by PDL monthly for 3 months. There was statistical significance in the Nail Psoriasis Severity Index (NAPSI) at months 3 and 6 in both nail bed and nail matrix with no statistical significance between groups. The authors concluded that PDL is an effective treatment for nail psoriasis and that the photosensitizer MAL doesn't appear to improve the clinical response.

Overall, there is still much to be determined before a definitive statement can be made about the efficacy of PDT for psoriasis. There is clear evidence that PDT can alter biochemical markers of psoriatic plaques to be more consistent with normal skin. Clinical studies have demonstrated success, albeit not consistently or without pain or inconvenience. Strategies have been mapped out to reduce heterogenous uptake and yield a more consistent response (Table 11.2). Perhaps further studies can get us closer to making PDT a practical and widely utilized treatment for psoriasis.

Lichen Planus

Oral lichen planus (OLP) is a difficult disease to treat; currently, topical steroids remain the mainstay of treatment with many recent studies also focusing on calcinuerin immunomodulators [28].

Table 11.2 Clinical studies of PDT for psoriasis

References	Study/objective	Photosensitizer and occlusion time	Light source and duration of exposure	Frequency of treatment	Results
Collins et al. [15]	5 squares in psoriatic plaques of 22 patients received varying doses of broadband visible light delivered at variable rates and evaluated via the scale, erythema and induration (SEI) index. Fluorescence of protoporphyrin was evaluated	Topical 5% ALA × 4 h under occlusion	Broadband light: 2, 4, 8, 16 J/cm^2 at 25 mW/cm^2 or 8 and 8 J/cm^2 at 10 and 40 mW/cm^2	1 treatment	+ Variability of fluorescence/protoporphyrin IX between plaques and between patients. Unpredictable efficacy: 35% of patients showed clearing of psoriasis of some sites. Of 36 sites, 10 cleared, 4 showed 30–50% improvement, and 22 had minimal or no improvement as measured by SEI. Only in patients whose psoriasis improved was there a relationship between photodynamic dose and clinical response + variability in discomfort levels
Robinson et al. [16]	19 plaques of psoriasis treated in ten patients treated with multiple applications of 5-ALA and broadband light. Also evaluated protoporphyrin fluorescence	5% ALA × 4 h under occlusion	Broadband light: 2 and 4 J/cm^2 (first 3 patients), 8 J/cm^2 (remaining patients) at rate of 15 mW/cm^2	3× weekly up to 12 treatments	Of 19 sites, 4 cleared completely, 10 responded without complete clearance, 5 did not respond + variability in PpIX fluorescence within and between patients + fluorescence at distant sites that did not receive 5-ALA. Increased discomfort with increased photodynamic dose
Radakovic-Fijan et al. [18]	29 patients are randomized within patient comparison topical ALA-PDT at various doses + keratolytic pretreatment with 10% salicylic acid 2 weeks prior to start of treatment	1% topical ALA × 4–6 h under occlusion	Filtered metal halide lamp 600–740 nm, at 5, 10, and 20 J/cm^2	2× weekly for up to 12 treatments	Keratolytic pretreatment decreased PASI by 25% alone. 20 J/cm^2 more efficacious than 10 and 5, with PASI decreased by 59% + pain during treatment
Franson and Ros [19]	1 psoriatic plaque treated in 12 patients at various energy doses	20% topical ALA × 4–5 h under occlusion	Red light (630 nm) at 10–30 J/cm^2	Once weekly for 2–5 weeks	Four patients dropped out due to pain during treatment; scale, erythema, and induration index (SEI) decreased for 7–1.5 in remaining patients. Average pain score 7/10 on Visual Analog Scale
Schleyer et al. [17]	Randomized double blind w/in patient study of 12 patients with topical ALA	0.1, 1, 5% topical ALA × 4–6 h under occlusion	Filtered metal halide lamp 600–740 nm at 20 J/cm^2	2× weekly for up to 12 treatments	Greatest improvement with 5% ALA at 51.2%; therapy interrupted frequently due to severe burning and pain. Authors conclude disappointing and time-consuming

(continued)

Table 11.2 (continued)

References	Study/objective	Photosensitizer and occlusion time	Light source and duration of exposure	Frequency of treatment	Results
Smits et al. [9]	8 patients in randomized placebo-controlled intrapatient study. Pretreated for 1 week with 10% salicylic acid	10% topical ALA or placebo	600–750 nm light at 2 J/cm^2 then occluded for 2 more hours then exposed to 8 J/cm^2	Once weekly for up to 4 weeks	Authors noted clinical and histological improvement in psoriatic plaques, two patients developed koebnerization
Salah et al. [23]	Single blinded placebo-controlled randomized intrapatient comparison of methylene blue vs. placebo in 16 patients with treatment-resistant plaque psoriasis	0.1% methylene blue or placebo for 30 min under occlusion	LED 670 nm at 5 J/cm^2 for 8 min	2× weekly for upto 12 treatments	89% reduction in PASI in methylene blue-treated lesions vs. no statistically significant improvement in placebo lesions. Treatment was considered painless
Kim et al. [26]	Case report of 1 patient with palmoplantar pustular psoriasis	20% ALA for 5 h	632 nm diode laser	Once weekly for 11 weeks then maintenance	Cleared after 11 weeks then received less frequent maintenance treatments for ~12 weeks, remained clear for 3 months; only minor burning sensation reported
Kim et al. [25]	Three cases of intractable palmoplantar pustular psoriasis with PDT	20% ALA for 4 h under occlusion	LED at 15 J/cm^2	Once weekly for 7–23 treatments	Patient 1 had good response at 10 treatments (palms > soles), patient 2 had mild improvement at 7 sessions, but stopped due to time commitment. Patient 3 had marked improvement after 10 treatments
Fernández-Guarino et al. [27, 46, 56]	Comparison of PDT vs. PDL for nail psoriasis in 121 nails; one nail treated with photosensitizer only and the other treated with photosensitizer followed by PDL	MAL for 3 h with bioadhesive patch	Pulsed dye laser 595 nm (9 J/cm^2, 7 mm, 6 ms)	Monthly for 6 months	Improvement in NAPSI score in both nail bed and nail matrix. No statistical significance between PDL vs. MAL. No adverse events, slight pain during treatments, but none significant enough to interrupt light sessions

However, these treatments are not always efficacious and can result in intolerable side effects like chronic thrush and immunosuppression. Two publications for the treatment of OLP with PDT were noted. The first is a case report of two patients with five lesions of OLP who were treated by gargling methylene blue for 5 min, then receiving irradiation to each area with 632 nm diode laser at 100 J/cm^2 [29]. One patient had complete resolution after one treatment and remained in remission for at least 9 months. The second patient had reduction in the size of buccal cheek lesions which was stable for 2 months, while the tongue lesions did not respond at all. The same author also conducted a similar study in which 26 lesions of OLP were treated with gargling 5% methylene blue followed by irradiation with 632-nm laser at 120 J/cm^2. Signs and symptoms were decreased significantly at weeks 1 and 12 in 16 of the 26 lesions. There were no adverse events and subjects tolerated the procedure well, with only a "few" patients experiencing a mild burning sensation. These findings led the investigators to conclude that this was a promising treatment for OLP [30].

Lichen Sclerosis

There has been interest in the use of PDT for lichen sclerosis, another difficult-to-treat entity. An early study by Hillemanns et al. [31] sought to determine if PDT could be a treatment option for vulvar lichen sclerosis. Twelve women underwent 1–3 cycles of PDT with an argon ion-pumped dye laser (630 nm) at 80 J/cm^2, irradiance of 40–70 mW/cm^2 for up to 40 min. Prior to irradiation, the area was occluded with 20% 5-ALA for 4–5 h. Ten of the 12 women had significant improvement in symptoms of pruritus that lasted from 3 to 9 months. The procedure was tolerated well overall, though 25% of patients did require opioid analgesia. The authors did not see significant changes in the clinical appearance of the skin; histological examination was not completed. However, they did use a xenon lamp with a yellow filter to evaluate the specificity of uptake and found PpIX fluorescence diffused throughout vulvar skin, not just affected areas. The authors concluded PDT could be a promising steroid-sparing treatment option for vulvar lichen sclerosis, although not altogether specific for lesional skin. In a more recent case using MAL, fluorescence was increased in the erosive areas of one patient's vulvar lichen sclerosis [32], signifying potential for some specificity or increased uptake in affected areas that are ulcerated. It is also possible that this might have a destructive effect on preclinical lesions of squamous cell carcinoma in situ, which might reduce the risk for development of this potential sequelae of LSA.

Subsequent case reports and small case series since Hillemans' initial study [31] have followed, evaluating PDT for recalcitrant vulvar lichen sclerosis. Romero et al. [33] reported improvement in a single patient with severe recalcitrant LS after 2 monthly treatments of 20% ALA-PDT 2 h occlusion followed by red light (633 nm) at 30 J/cm^2 and 80 mW/cm^2. Vulvar lesions healed well with a decrease in symptoms, though vaginal lesions were less responsive, which is unsurprising given no exposure to the light. Sotiriou et al. [34] reported symptomatic improvement in five patients treated once with 20% 5-ALA × 3 h followed by red light (570–670 nm, 40 J/cm^2, 80 mW/cm^2). In all cases in this series, there was minimal change in clinical appearance and no resolution on histological evaluation. In both reports, however, patients tolerated the procedure well and had a sustained response of 3–6 months, with minimal symptoms that were now able to be controlled with (and previously had been refractory to) topical steroids. In another series, ten patients [35] were treated with 20% ALA and PDT at 2-week intervals with significant improvement in symptoms, but again minimal change in the clinical appearance of the affected areas. Another study evaluated the use of a bioadhesive patch impregnated with ALA followed by red light for the use in LS and Squamous hyperplasia of the vulva [36]. Ten patients received 4–6-h application of the ALA patch and were then treated with red light for 1–2 treatments at varying intervals. In this case, topical anesthesia was used during the treatment due to the intense burning sensation several patients experienced.

Nine out of ten patients had symptomatic relief, but no changes in the histological features of LS, corroborating previous research. However, it was noted that the apoptotic index was increased and that low levels of bcl-2, an antiapoptotic protein, was detected in the "majority" of the posttreatment biopsies, though they were absent in pretreatment biopsies. These findings suggest that perhaps PDT in lichen sclerosis works at least in part via an apoptotic pathway.

Successful treatment of PDT for extragenital lichen sclerosis (shoulders, axillae, and abdomen) has also been reported [37]. In an initial case report, a patient served as an internal control with half of her lesions treated with 20% 5-ALA (occlusion time of 1 h) followed by two passes of PDL (fluence of 7/5 J/cm^2, 10 ms pulse duration and 10 mm spot size) vs. just PDL alone. After 3 monthly treatments, the patient had resolution of pruritus as well as clinical improvement in measurements of erythema, scaling, and atrophy on the ALA-PDL-treated sides, but not on the areas treated with PDL alone. The patient tolerated the procedure well with minimal discomfort. The authors hypothesized the mechanism of action could involve up-regulation of collagen formation and targeting the dilated vessels that allow passage of the lymphocytes that contribute to the underlying disorder. In a second case report of a patient with two plaques of extragenital LS, one lesion on the abdomen was treated with 595 nm PDL, while the breast lesion was treated with MAL-PDL for 2 monthly sessions [38]. The authors noted marked improvement in the MAL-PDL-treated side, and unlike the previous case, there was some moderate improvement in the PDL-only-treated lesion. Overall, though, this again suggests the need for a photosensitizer to ensure better efficacy.

As in the case with psoriasis, further studies are needed to learn more about the mechanism and determine the ideal regimen of PDT for lichen sclerosis, but the results of the studies thus far are promising (Table 11.3). Not only would this be an alternative treatment for both extragenital as well as genital LS where there are few alternatives, but it may even reduce the potential for transformation of LS into squamous cell carcinoma, a relatively common and potentially lethal complication.

Morphea/Scleroderma

Given the many often unsuccessful treatments of scleroderma, a trial study was completed on five patients to determine if PDT would provide a more satisfactory option [39]. One plaque in each of five patients with localized scleroderma was treated with 3% ALA for 6 h, then exposed to incoherent light (580–740 nm, 40 mW/cm^2, 10 J/cm^2) once or twice weekly for 3–6 months. All patients tolerated the procedure well and treated lesions showed significant improvements both clinically and with objective durometer scores. Two patients also showed increased joint mobility at the corresponding treated sites following the procedure. The untreated lesions did not show any improvement. In the 2-year follow-up, there was no recurrence or flare of the disease.

Having achieved successful results, Karrer sought to determine the mechanism of action of PDT for scleroderma. Given that scleroderma is a disease process with increased collagen production and decreased collagen breakdown, Karrer began her studies using an initial observation by Herrmann et al. [40] which showed an increase in matrix metalloproteinases (MMPs) after photosensitization of fibroblasts. Given that MMPs break down collagen, Karrer sought to evaluate the effects of photosensitization on scleroderma fibroblasts in vitro [41]. After culturing fibroblasts from both normal and sclerodermatous skin, the cells were treated with ALA and then irradiated with red light (580–740 nm). There was a time-dependent increase (maximum at 12 h) in MMP-1 and MMP-3 in the cells from both the normal and the scleroderma-affected skin, as well as a decrease in type I collagen mRNA, signifying decreased collagen production. These findings did appear to be transient, which could be correlated clinically with the need for multiple treatments prior to resolution. Tissue inhibitors of metaloproteinases (IMPs), which normally inhibit MMPs and therefore decrease collagen breakdown, did not seem to be affected.

Table 11.3 Clinical studies of PDT for lichen sclerosus

References	Study/objective	Photosensitizer and occlusion time	Light source	Frequency of treatment	Results
Hillemans et al. [31]	Prospective pilot study to evaluate the effect of PDT on 12 women with vulvar lichen sclerosis	20% solution of 5-ALA	635 nm argon ion-pumped dye laser at 80 J/cm^2 and 40–70 mW/cm^2	1–3 treatments 1–3 weeks apart	Significant improvement in pruritus in 10/12 women with results lasting mean of 6.1 months + burning sensation to treatment with three patients given IV opioids. No necrosis or scarring from PDT
Alexiades-Armenakas [37]	Case report of 1 patient with extragenital lichen sclerosus with some lesions treated with ALA-pulsed dye laser (PDL) and other lesions treated with PDL only	20% 5-ALA × 1 h	Long-pulsed PDL 595 nm, 10 mm spot size, 10 ms pulse duration, 7.5 J/cm^2, + dynamic cooling	3 monthly treatments	Resolution of pruritus plus significant improvement in erythema, scaling, and atrophy in the ALA-PDL-treated lesions, but not in the PDL-only control lesions. Absent to slight pain reported during and immediately after treatment
Romero et al. [33]	Case report of recalcitrant erosive vulvar lichen sclerosis with PDT	20% 5-ALA × 2 h	633 nm red light at 30 J/cm^2 and 80 mW/cm^2	2 monthly treatments	Reepithelialization of vulvar erosions and near resolution of burning, pruritus, and pain after two treatments. At 3- and 6-month follow-ups patient had mild symptoms controlled with topical clobetasol ointment. Moderate pain during and up to 4 days after each treatment
Vano-Galvan et al. [32]	Case report of one patient with recalcitrant erosive vulvar lichen sclerosis	Topical methyl-aminolaevulinic acid (MAL) under occlusion × 2 h	595 nm PDL at mm, 6 ms, and 9 J/cm^2	3 monthly treatments	Marked improvement of genital lesions and almost complete disappearance of pruritus. Relapse at 4 months + pain during procedure requiring intralesional mepivacaine. Fluorescence was noted to concentrate in affected areas, particularly erosions and decreased as affected areas improved
Sotiriou et al. [34]	Evaluation of therapeutic effect of PDT for 5 patients with biopsy-proven vulvar lichen sclerosus	20% 5-ALA under occlusion for 3 h	Noncoherent red light (570–670 nm) at 40 J/cm^2 and 80 mW/cm^2	One treatment	Histological examination of two patients showed no resolution of LS features, but all patients had significant reduction in pruritus and burning pain lasting 3–6 months with moderate topical steroids able to control residual symptoms. No patients interrupted procedure due to pain

(continued)

Table 11.3 (continued)

References	Study/objective	Photosensitizer and occlusion time	Light source	Frequency of treatment	Results
Sotiriou et al. [35]	Evaluation of therapeutic effect of PDT for 10 patients with biopsy-proven vulvar lichen sclerosus	20% 5-ALA under occlusion for 4 h	Noncoherent red light (570–670 nm) at 40 J/cm^2 and 80 mW/cm^2	Two treatments 2 weeks apart	Remission or reduction in subjective symptoms of pruritus burning and pain, but only minor improvement in clinical scores of atrophy, depigmentation, sclerosis, and hyperkeratosis. No patients interrupted procedure due to pain
Zawislak et al. [36]	Evaluation of vulval lichen sclerosus and squamous hyperplasia to PDT with administration of ALA via a bioadhesive patch in ten patients with total of 17 treatment sessions	ALA dissolved into a poly (methylvinylether/maleic anhydride) copolymer (PMVE/MA) bioadhesive patch × 4–6 h	630 nm red light 100 J/cm^2	Two treatments 2–15 weeks apart depending on initial response to therapy	6/9 patients returned to a 6-week follow-up had significant relief in pruritus. There was no statistical difference in atrophy between pre- and posttreatment histological specimens. Significant increase in the apoptotic index in post-PDT-treated lesional biopsies. Patients reported intense burning pain with treatment with local analgesia administered during 8/17 treatment sessions
Passeron et al. [38]	Case report comparison of MAL-PDL vs. PDL alone to treat extragenital lichen sclerosus in one patient	MAL for 3 h	595 nm PDL (10 mm spot) size, 40 ms duration, 10 J/cm^2 fluence	2 monthly treatments	Marked improvement in the PDT-PDL-treated lesion and moderate improvement in the PDL-only-treated lesion per patient assessment. Significantly better improvement with PDT-PDL on objective assessment via photographs. Decrease in ivory color of lesions

When a singlet-oxygen quencher was used on some of these cells, the MMP levels did not increase significantly, suggesting that ALA-PDT produces its effects on MMP-1 via (at least in part) singlet oxygen. The positive control group of fibroblasts exposed to UVA light showed similar increases in MMP-1. The authors ponder the potentially negative implications of this finding on photoaging and carcinogenesis, particularly that ALA-PDT might enhance photoaging. However, PDT light has not been found to have the carcinogenic potential that UVA light is known to have and might in fact have anticarcinogenic capability [42, 43]. There has been little to no data on negative effects of ALA-PDT on photoaging thus far. In a follow-up study, Karrer et al. [44] sought to evaluate the effects of ALA-PDT on keratinocytes and their subsequent effects on dermal fibroblasts via the cytokine milieu. The ALA-PDT (red light, 580–740 nm)-treated keratinocytes produced significantly increased amounts of IL-1α and TNF-α, but not increases in IL-6, MMP-1, or MMP-3. When fibroblasts were exposed to these keratinocytes, as in the previous study, there was an increase in MMP-1 and MMP-3. If an IL-1 receptor antagonist is added to the keratinocyte-conditioned media prior to fibroblast stimulation, the increase in MMPs was not seen. This implies that the effects of ALA-PDT act in a paracrine manner from keratinocytes to fibroblasts and that IL-1α is the main mediator of this reaction. Another photosensitizer, ATX-S10(Na)-PDT utilizing a diode laser (LD670-05) as the light source, had an even more potent decrease in type I collagen and increase in MMP-1 and MMP-3 as compared to ALA-PDT (with pulsed excimer-dye laser as light source) with similar time to maximum effect on both fibroblasts and mouse skin. Further clinical studies are warranted to evaluate in vivo effects.

Another study [45] sought to replicate the clinical results in seven patients with scleroderma. One plaque in each of these patients was treated weekly with 20% 5-ALA cream for 5 h and then exposed to a noncoherent broadband halogen light source filtered to 570–670 nm (25 J/cm^2, 90 mW/cm^2) for 6 weeks. The six patients who completed the study had variable responses: four patients had improvement in treated lesions, and two remained the same; however, four of these patients had improvement in untreated areas as well. The durometer readings were not consistent, showing both increases and decreases in sclerosis in treated lesions. Histological examination of the treated lesions did not show significant changes in the collagen bundles of the sclerotic skin. The authors cited the short duration, small numbers, and possibly limited reliability of measuring devices as possible limitations of the study, concluding further studies are needed.

Overall, the studies show promise for improvement of scleroderma with PDT. It is difficult to assemble a large group of patients with this disease, but hopefully future investigations will point the way to consistent protocols for these patients.

Vitiligo

An initial report of three cases of facial vitiligo [46] who received 6–8 monthly sessions of MAL occluded for 1.5 h followed by irradiation with 630 nm red light (at 37.5 J/cm^2) for 7.5 min. Each patient served as an internal control. No patients experienced pain, burning, or erythema. There was no evidence of repigmentation after the series of treatments. The authors encouraged further studies given the unpredictable response to treatment of vitiligo. In a recent study, Serrano et al. [47] sought to evaluate PDT with repeated application of low strength ALA in acne, photoaging, and vitiligo. Six patients with vitiligo of face, hands, and trunk received four treatments 3–4 weeks apart with follow-up evaluation 16 weeks after treatment cessation. Patients were first treated with a salicylic acid peel followed by 2% ALA applied every 10 min 4–6 times followed by "several light sources" in the yellow-red spectrum of 550–630 nm for 4–14 min at 100 mW/cm^2. Four of six patients experienced partial repigmentation (noted to be 25–40% total area), two patients had >55% repigmentation. As might be expected, best responses were on chest, neck, and face. Again, further studies are needed to determine the value of PDT for vitiligo.

Necrobiosis Lipoidica Diabeticorum

In more recent literature, references to PDT for necrobiosis lipoidica diabeticorum (NLD), another difficult-to-treat disease, have surfaced. An initial case report [48] evaluated PDT for biopsy-proven recalcitrant NLD. A single patient received 6 weekly treatments of MAL under occlusion for 3 h followed by red light for 8 min. Halfway through the treatment, this patient had significant improvement in lesions; after six treatments, the lesions appeared resolved both clinically and histologically with remission lasting at least 2 years. The authors speculated the mechanism of action may be due to cytokine alteration and their role in the inflammatory changes of NLD. In another case of recalcitrant necrobiosis lipoidica, a patient was treated with 10% ALA occluded for 3 h, then underwent an 8-min exposure to red light 632 nm (37 J/cm^2) every 4 weeks for four sessions at which time "total healing" was noted. As a follow-up to the above cases [49], Berking et al. completed a study on 18 patients with NLD. These patients underwent 9 cycles of PDT with MAL-red LED. A complete response was seen in only patient, while one third of patients had a partial response, with the remaining patients not responding. It remains unclear what subpopulation of NLD may respond to PDT, but it warrants further study in yet another often recalcitrant progressive disease state.

Sarcoidosis

There were two reports of treatment for cutaneous sarcoidosis with PDT. An initial case report of recalcitrant cutaneous sarcoidosis noted complete resolution of the granulomatous lesions after 22 treatments. The patient was treated with 3% ALA in 40% dimethyl sulfoxide under occlusion for 6 h followed by incoherent metal halogen lamp (PDT 1200, 580–740 nm at 20 J/cm^2 or 40 mW/cm^2) twice weekly for 8 weeks, then once weekly. The patient did experience transient burning, erythema, and edema, and later hyperpigmentation that resolved. Upon biopsy, there was no histological evidence of sarcoidosis remaining and the patient stayed in remission 18 months after her last treatment [50] (Fig. 11.2).

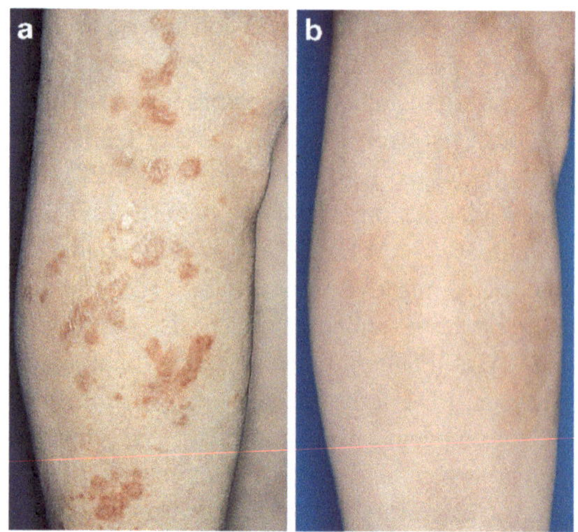

Fig. 11.2 (**a**) Two days after the first photodynamic therapy (PDT) session, inflammatory reaction is sharply restricted to the affected areas. (**b**) Two months after a 3-month course of PDT using 5-aminolevulinic acid, complete remission of the skin lesions is seen, with only a slight hyperpigmentation in the former lesional area, which resolved within another 4 weeks (from Karrer et al. [50]. Copyright 2002 American Medical Association. All rights reserved)

In a more recent case report, two patients with single sarcoid lesions were treated with MAL followed by red light and broadband light, respectively, both with complete resolution by 8 weeks and no recurrence at 4–6 months after last treatment [51]. A unique case of sarcoid tenosynovitis successfully treated with ALA-PDT has also been reported. In this case, 10% ALA solution was injected into the affected area and then treated with an excimer-dye laser (pulsed light at 630 nm, 100 J/cm^2) for six treatments. MRI confirmed the clinically noted decrease in swelling; the patient remained clear at 2-year follow-up.

Granuloma Annulare

Positive results were seen in a case report of a patient with granuloma annulare (GA) of the fingers treated with PDT. This patient was treated with

4 weekly treatments of 20% ALA (5 h occlusion) followed by 630 nm LED at 120 J/cm^2. The lesions were "almost completely clear" after the fourth treatment and the patient did not have recurrence at 7 months of follow-up [52]. In a case series, seven patients with GA of the extremities were treated with a red-light PDT source at 100 J/cm^2 after a 5 h occlusion with 20% ALA every 2–4 weeks for 2–3 sessions. Two of the seven patients had lesions on both hands and thus served as an internal control with one hand treated with ALA-red light and the other receiving just the red light. The red light-only lesions did not respond. Of the treated areas in all seven patients, two patients had resolution of lesions with remission during the 6-month follow-up, 2 patients markedly improved, and 3 patients did not respond. The authors noted that patients who responded reported more pain than the nonresponders. Many of these patients received either oral or subcutaneous anesthesia. Though the mechanism of action is yet to be elucidated, the authors speculated that for PDT in GA, it may again involve the apoptotic pathway [53].

Alopecia Areata

In a small pilot study, six patients with alopecia areata (AA) were treated with 5–20% ALA lotion and vehicle to separate areas of the scalp and were then exposed to red light [54]. The treated areas of the scalp (excluding vehicle) developed erythema, indicating clinical response. However, after the 3-h occlusion, fluorescent microscopy showed diffuse uptake of PpIX in the epidermis and sebaceous glands, but not in the hair follicles or in areas of the inflammatory infiltrate. After twice-weekly treatments for 10 weeks, no patients had significant hair regrowth, leading the authors to conclude that PDT is not a successful therapy for AA.

While the initial authors suggested that the absence of PpIX fluorescence in the inflammatory infiltrate around hair follicles explains the failed results [55], Lee et al. hypothesized that it was a failure of the photosensitizer to get to the affected area. Therefore, another series of six patients with stable AA was treated with MAL-red light PDT once monthly for 3 months. In this study, a microneedle roller was placed on part of area to be treated in order to allow product to better enter the affected area by creating small channels. Despite the use of the microneedle technique, no patients experienced regrowth – either in treated or untreated areas. The authors noted that bleeding caused by the needles may hinder absorption of the photosensitizer.

Another study of six patients with recalcitrant AA confirmed the initial study's conclusion with one exception [56]. Each patient, serving as own control, was treated with MAL-red light once monthly for an average of 8 months. Five patients with scalp AA had no to sparse regrowth over less than 10% of affected area. However, one patient with beard AA had complete regrowth after only four sessions, suggesting that the beard area may respond better to PDT and could possibly be considered a treatment modality, although AA does have a tendency to spontaneously remit. PDT does not appear to be especially effective for AA with the parameters chosen by these researchers.

Darier's Disease

In a series, six patients with this acantholytic dyskeratotic disease were treated with PDT [57]. They served as internal controls with half of their lesions treated with 20% 5-ALA occluded for 4 h, then exposed to an incoherent light source at 580–740 nm (150 J/cm^2, 110–150 mW/cm^2) for 16 min 40 s to 22 min 44 s. Patients received treatments every 4–12 weeks and were followed 6 months to 3 years after treatment. Of the six patients, one could not tolerate the procedure and the remaining patients all experienced an inflammatory reaction for several weeks after PDT. The authors did not consider this reaction to be a flare of the light-sensitive Darier's disease, as biopsies revealed an increased neutrophilic infiltrate. All of the remaining patients showed both clinical and histological improvement after the initial inflammatory reaction with 4 of 5 having a sustained response; however, these four also remained on oral retinoids. This suggests that PDT may have some benefit as an adjunctive treatment, but should not be considered monotherapy. In a case report of recalcitrant Darier's disease [58], a patient was treated with one dose of ALA-PDT (6 h occlusion) with continuous light at 420 nm (5.4 J/cm^2, 6 mW/cm^2). This patient experienced initial improvement, but then flared both in involved and previously uninvolved treated skin. This patient was then phototested and found to develop new lesions with continued photoprovocation to UVB, but no flares with UVA, PUVA, or normal light. Also, MEDs to all types of light were normal. This finding suggests that caution should be used with any form of light-based treatment for Darier's disease.

Conclusion

While still in its infancy, PDT is becoming a prominent treatment option in a number of dermatological diseases. Given the breadth of clinical implications, it is clear that both basic science and clinical studies are still needed to learn more about the mechanism of action, efficacy, and optimal treatment regimens in many of these inflammatory disorders.

References

1. Hongcharu W, Taylor C, Chang Y, et al. Topical ALA-photodynamic therapy for the treatment of acne vulgaris. J Invest Dermatol. 2000;115:183–92.
2. Pollock B, Turner D, Stringer M, et al. Topical aminolaevulinic acid-photodynamic therapy for the treatment of acne vulgaris: a study of clinical efficacy and mechanism of action. Br J Dermatol. 2004;151:616–22.
3. Goldman M, Boyce S. A single-center study of aminolevulinic acid and 417 NM photodynamic therapy in the treatment of moderate to severe acne vulgaris. J Drugs Dermatol. 2003;2:393–6.
4. Taub AF. Photodynamic therapy for the treatment of acne: a pilot study. J Drugs Dermatol. 2004;3(6 Suppl):S10–4.
5. Bos JD. The pathomechanisms of psoriasis; the skin immune system and cyclosporin. Br J Dermatol. 1988;118(2):141–55.
6. Boehncke WH, Konig K, Kaufmann R, et al. Photodynamic therapy in psoriasis: suppression of cytokine production in vitro and recording of fluorescence modification during treatment in vivo. Arch Dermatol Res. 1994;286(6):300–3.
7. Bissonnette R, Tremblay JF, Juzenas P, et al. Systemic photodynamic therapy with aminolevulinic acid induces apoptosis in lesional T lymphocytes of psoriatic plaques. J Invest Dermatol. 2002;119(1): 77–83.
8. Wrone-Smith T, Mitra RS, Thompson CB, et al. Keratinocytes derived from psoriatic plaques are resistant to apoptosis compared with normal skin. Am J Pathol. 1997;151:1321–9.
9. Smits T, Kleinpenning MM, van Erp PE, van de Kerkhof PC, Gerritsen MJ. A placebo-controlled randomized study on the clinical effectiveness, immunohistochemical changes and protoporphyrin IX accumulation in fractionated 5-aminolaevulinic acid-photodynamic therapy in patients with psoriasis. Br J Dermatol. 2006;155(2):429–36.
10. Stringer MR, Collins P, Robinson DJ, Stables GI, Sheehan-Dare RA. The accumulation of protoporphyrin IX in plaque psoriasis after topical application of 5-aminolevulinic acid indicates a potential for superficial photodynamic therapy. J Invest Dermatol. 1996;107(1):76–81.
11. Bissonnette R, Zeng H, McLean DI, et al. Oral aminolevulinic acid induces protoporphyrin IX fluorescence in psoriatic plaques and peripheral blood cells. Photochem Photobiol. 2001;74(2):339–45.
12. Kleinpenning MM, Smits T, Ewalds E, van Erp PE, van de Kerkhof PC, Gerritsen MJ. Heterogeneity of fluorescence in psoriasis after application of 5-aminolaevulinic acid: an immunohistochemical study. Br J Dermatol. 2006;155(3):539–45.
13. Kleinpenning MM, Kanis JH, Smits T, Van Erp PE, Van de Kerkhof P, Gerritsen RM. The effects of keratolytic pretreatment prior to fluorescence diagnosis and photodynamic therapy with aminolevulinic acid-induced porphyrins in psoriasis. J Dermatolog Treat. 2010;21:245–51.
14. Smits T, Robles CA, van Erp PE, et al. Correlation between macroscopic fluorescence and protoporphyrin IX content in psoriasis and actinic keratosis following application of aminolevulinic acid. J Invest Dermatol. 2005;125:833–9.
15. Collins P, Robinson DJ, Stringer MR, Stables GI, Sheehan-Dare RA. The variable response of plaque psoriasis after a single treatment with topical 5-aminolavelulinic acid photodynamic therapy. Br J Dermatol. 1997;137:743–9.
16. Robinson DJ, Collins P, Stringer MR, et al. Improved response of plaque psoriasis after multiple treatments with topical 5-aminolaevulinic acid photodynamic therapy. Acta Derm Venereol. 1999;79(6):451–5.
17. Schleyer V, Radakovic-Fijan S, Karrer S, Zwingers T, Tanew A, Landthaler M, et al. Disappointing results and low tolerability of photodynamic therapy with topical 5-aminolaevulinic acid in psoriasis. A randomized, double-blind phase I/II study. J Eur Acad Dermatol Venereol. 2006;20(7):823–8.
18. Radakovic-Fijan S, Blecha-Thalhammer U, Schleyer V, et al. Topical aminolaevulinic acid-based photodynamic therapy as a treatment option for psoriasis?

Results of a randomized, observer blinded study. Br J Dermatol. 2005;152(2):279–83.
19. Fransson J, Ros AM. Clinical and immunohistochemical evaluation of psoriatic plaques treated with topical 5-aminolaevulinic acid photodynamic therapy. Photodermatol Photoimmunol Photomed. 2005;21(6): 326–32.
20. Leigh IM, Navsaria H, Purkis PE, McKay IA, Bowden PE, Riddle PN. Keratins (K16 and K17) as markers of keratinocyte hyperproliferation in psoriasis in vivo and in vitro. Br J Dermatol. 1995;133:501–11.
21. Robinson DJ, de Bruijn HS, de Wolf WF, et al. Topical 5-aminolevulenic acid-photodynamic therapy of hairless mouse skin using two-fold illumination schemes: PpIX fluorescence kinetics, photobleaching and biological effect. Photochem Photobiol. 2000;72:794–802.
22. de Bruijn HS, van der Veen N, Robinson DJ, Star WM. Improvement of systemic 5-minolevulinic acid photodynamic therapy in-vivo using light fractionation with a 75-minute interval. Cancer Res. 1999;59:901–4.
23. Salah M, Samy N, Fadel M. Methylene blue mediated photodynamic therapy for resistant plaque psoriasis. J Drugs Dermatol. 2009;8(1):42–9.
24. Kessel D, Luo Y. Mitochondrial photodamage and PDT-induced apoptosis. J Photochem Photobiol B. 1998;42(2):89–95.
25. Kim JY, Kang HY, Lee ES, Kim YC. Topical 5-aminolaevulinic acid photodynamic therapy for intractable palmoplantar psoriasis. J Dermatol. 2007;34(1): 37–40.
26. Kim YC, Lee ES, Chung PS, Rhee CK. Recalcitrant palmoplantar pustular psoriasis successfully treated with topical 5-aminolaevulinic acid photodynamic therapy. Clin Exp Dermatol. 2005;30(6):723–4.
27. Fernández-Guarino M, Harto A, Sánchez-Ronco M, García-Morales I, Jaén P. Pulsed dye laser vs. photodynamic therapy in the treatment of refractory nail psoriasis: a comparative pilot study. J Eur Acad Dermatol Venereol. 2009;23(8):891–5.
28. Thongprasom K, Dhanuthai K. Steroids in the treatment of lichen planus: a review. J Oral Sci. 2008;50(4):377–85.
29. Aghahosseini F, Arbabi-Kalati F, Fashtami LA, Fateh M, Djavid GE. Treatment of oral lichen planus with photodynamic therapy mediated methylene blue: a case report. Med Oral Patol Oral Cir Bucal. 2006;11(2):E126–9.
30. Aghahosseini F, Arbabi-Kalati F, Fashtami LA, Djavid GE, Fateh M, Beitollahi JM. Methylene blue-mediated photodynamic therapy: a possible alternative treatment for oral lichen planus. Lasers Surg Med. 2006;38(1):33–8.
31. Hillemanns P, Untch M, Pröve F, Baumgartner R, Hillemanns M, Korell M. Photodynamic therapy of vulvar lichen sclerosus with 5-aminolevulinic acid. Obstet Gynecol. 1999;93(1):71–4.
32. Vano-Galvan S, Fernandez-Guarino M, Beà-Ardebol S, Perez B, Harto A, Jaen P. Successful treatment of erosive vulvar lichen sclerosus with methylaminolaevulinic acid and laser-mediated photodynamic therapy. J Eur Acad Dermatol Venereol. 2009;23(1):71–2.
33. Romero A, Hernández-Núñez A, Córdoba-Guijarro S, Arias-Palomo D, Borbujo-Martínez J. Treatment of recalcitrant erosive vulvar lichen sclerosus with photodynamic therapy. J Am Acad Dermatol. 2007; 57(2 Suppl):S46–7.
34. Sotiriou E, Apalla Z, Patsatsi A, Panagiotidou D. Recalcitrant vulvar lichen sclerosis treated with aminolevulinic acid-photodynamic therapy: a report of five cases. J Eur Acad Dermatol Venereol. 2008;22(11): 1398–9.
35. Sotiriou E, Panagiotidou D, Ioannidis D. An open trial of 5-aminolevulinic acid photodynamic therapy for vulvar lichen sclerosus. Eur J Obstet Gynecol Reprod Biol. 2008;141(2):187–8.
36. Zawislak AA, McCluggage WG, Donnelly RF, Maxwell P, Price JH, Dobbs SP, et al. Response of vulval lichen sclerosus and squamous hyperplasia to photodynamic treatment using sustained topical delivery of aminolevulinic acid from a novel bioadhesive patch system. Photodermatol Photoimmunol Photomed. 2009;25(2):111–3.
37. Alexiades-Armenakas M. Laser-mediated photodynamic therapy of lichen sclerosus. J Drugs Dermatol. 2004;3(6 Suppl):S25–7.
38. Passeron T, Lacour JP, Ortonne JP. Comparative treatment of extragenital lichen sclerosus with methylaminolevulinic acid pulsed dye laser-mediated photodynamic therapy or pulsed dye laser alone. Dermatol Surg. 2009;35(5):878–80.
39. Karrer S, Abels C, Landthaler M, Szeimies RM. Topical photodynamic therapy for localized scleroderma. Acta Derm Venereol. 2000;80(1):26–7.
40. Herrmann G, Wlaschek M, Lange TS, Prenzel K, Goerz G, Scharffetter-Kochanek K. UVA irradiation stimulates the synthesis of various matrix metalloproteinases (MMP) in cultured human dermal fibroblasts. Exp Dermatol. 1993;2:92–7.
41. Karrer S, Bosserhoff AK, Weiderer P, Landthaler M, Szeimies RM. Influence of 5-aminolevulinic acid and red light on collagen metabolism of human dermal fibroblasts. J Invest Dermatol. 2003;120(2):325–31.
42. Berg K. Mechanism of cell damage in photodynamic therapy. In: Honigsmann H, Jori G, Young AR, editors. The fundamental bases of phototherapy. Milano: OEMF; 1996. p. 181–207.
43. Stender IM, Bech-Thomsen N, Poulsen T, Wulf HC. Photodynamic therapy with topical d-aminolevulinic acid delays UV photocarcinogenesis in hairless mice. Photochem Photobiol. 1997;66:493–6.
44. Karrer S, Bosserhoff AK, Weiderer P, Landthaler M, Szeimies RM. Keratinocyte-derived cytokines after photodynamic therapy and their paracrine induction of matrix metalloproteinases in fibroblasts. Br J Dermatol. 2004;151(4):776–83.
45. Batchelor R, Lamb S, Goulden V, Stables G, Goodfield M, Merchant W. Photodynamic therapy for the treatment of morphoea. Clin Exp Dermatol. 2008;33(5): 661–3.

46. Fernández-Guarino M, Harto A, Jaén P. Photodynamic therapy does not induce repigmentation in three cases of facial vitiligo. J Eur Acad Dermatol Venereol. 2008;22(12):1498–500.
47. Serrano G, Lorente M, Reyes M, Millán F, Lloret A, Melendez J, et al. Photodynamic therapy with low-strength ALA, repeated applications and short contact periods (40–60 minutes) in acne, photoaging and vitiligo. J Drugs Dermatol. 2009;8(6):562–8.
48. Heidenheim M, Jemec GB. Successful treatment of necrobiosis lipoidica diabeticorum with photodynamic therapy. Arch Dermatol. 2006;142(12):1548–50.
49. Berking C, Hegyi J, Arenberger P, Ruzicka T, Jemec GB. Photodynamic therapy of necrobiosis lipoidica – a multicenter study of 18 patients. Dermatology. 2009;218(2):136–9.
50. Karrer S, Abels C, Wimmershoff MB, Landthaler M, Szeimies RM. Successful treatment of cutaneous sarcoidosis using topical photodynamic therapy. Arch Dermatol. 2002;138(5):581–4.
51. Wilsmann-Theis D, Bieber T, Novak N. Photodynamic therapy as an alternative treatment for cutaneous sarcoidosis. Dermatology. 2008;217(4):343–6.
52. Kim YJ, Kang HY, Lee ES, Kim YC. Successful treatment of granuloma annulare with topical 5-aminolaevulinic acid photodynamic therapy. J Dermatol. 2006;33(9):642–3.
53. Weisenseel P, Kuznetsov AV, Molin S, Ruzicka T, Berking C, Prinz JC. Photodynamic therapy for granuloma annulare: more than a shot in the dark. Dermatology. 2008;217(4):329–32.
54. Bissonnette R, Shapiro J, Zeng H, McLean DI, Lui H. Topical photodynamic therapy with 5-aminolaevulinic acid does not induce hair regrowth in patients with extensive alopecia areata. Br J Dermatol. 2000;143(5):1032–5.
55. Lee JW, Yoo KH, Kim BJ, Kim MN. Photodynamic therapy with methyl 5-aminolevulinate acid combined with microneedle treatment in patients with extensive alopecia areata. Clin Exp Dermatol. 2010;35:548–9.
56. Fernández-Guarino M, Harto A, García-Morales I, Pérez-García B, Arrazola JM, Jaén P. Failure to treat alopecia areata with photodynamic therapy. Clin Exp Dermatol. 2008;33(5):585–7.
57. Exadaktylou D, Kurwa HA, Calonje E, Barlow RJ. Treatment of Darier's disease with photodynamic therapy. Br J Dermatol. 2003;149(3):606–10.
58. van't Westeinde SC, Sanders CJ, van Weelden H. Photodynamic therapy in a patient with Darier's disease. J Eur Acad Dermatol Venereol. 2006;20(7):870–2.

Photodynamic Therapy for Other Uses

12

George Martin

Abstract

Over the course of the last two decades, the scope of PDT has expanded to include a broad spectrum of neoplastic, inflammatory, and infectious cutaneous and noncutaneous diseases. Four drugs have been approved for these other uses: porfimer sodium, verteporfin, aminolevulinic acid, and methyl aminolevulinic acid.

This chapter discusses the cutaneous and extracutaneous applications for photodynamic therapy (PDT) not covered in other chapters. Over the course of the last two decades, the scope of PDT has expanded to include a broad spectrum of neoplastic, inflammatory, and infectious cutaneous and noncutaneous diseases [1–4].

A variety of photosensitizing agents [2] and light sources [5] have been studied in efforts to enhance target selectivity, optimize treatment efficacy, and maintain therapeutic safety. This research has led to the commercial development of four approved drugs: porfimer sodium (Photofrin®, 1995. Axcan Pharma, Inc.), verteporfin (Visudyne®, 2000. Novartis/QLT Phototherapeutics, Inc.), aminolevulinic acid (ALA) (20% ALA solution; Levulan Kerastick®; 1999; DUSA Pharmaceuticals, Wilmington, Massachusetts), and methyl aminolevulinic acid (MAL) (16.8% methyl aminolevulinate cream; Metvixia Cream®; 2004 PhotoCure ASA, Oslo, Norway; Galderma, Fort Worth, Texas).

G. Martin (✉)
Dermatology and Laser Center of Maui, 41 East Lipoa Street, Suite 21, Kihei, HI 96753, USA
e-mail: drgeorgemartin@aol.com

Most of the research for "other uses" has been limited to early investigational in vitro and ex vivo/in vivo animal model studies. This investigational work has in some instances led to a limited number of "off label" individual or small group case studies presented herein. In the cases of certain extracutaneous diseases such as age-related macular degeneration (ARMD) and Barrett's esophagus (BE), the culmination of these early studies resulted in FDA approval of PDT for both disorders.

Approved Drugs and Light Sources

PDT is a two-step process requiring the presence of a photosensitizing agent followed by its photoactivation. The photosensitizer can be either endogenously present, delivered exogenously, or created by delivery of a prodrug which uses the metabolic pathways of the target tissue to produce the photosensitizer. Photosensitizers can be delivered either topically or systemically. Photosensitizers that absorb visible or near infrared light tend to have large conjugated structures, and because of this, they do not easily penetrate the skin barriers. Because of this physical property,

M.H. Gold (ed.), *Photodynamic Therapy in Dermatology*,
DOI 10.1007/978-1-4419-1298-5_12, © Springer Science+Business Media, LLC 2011

large molecules such as porphyrins are introduced via the blood stream. Systemic drug selectivity for the target tissue depends on many variables, the most important of which is how the drug is partitioned between the target tissues vs. surrounding tissue. A negative aspect systemic administration is the resulting prolonged phototoxicity, which in the case of certain porphyrins can last 3–4 weeks.

The most commonly used class of photosensitizers, the porphyrins, are present in many tissues and organisms endogenously, can be delivered exogenously, or created by the delivery of a prodrug such as ALA or MAL. Both ALA and MAL bypass the rate-limiting enzyme ALA-synthase in the heme synthesis pathway resulting in porphyrins, particularly protoporphyrin IX (PpIX), accumulating in certain tissues. Oxygen is required to produce reactive oxygen species (ROS; singlet oxygen) responsible for the cellular damage caused by PDT. The rate at which light is delivered directly affects the amount of ROS produced [6]. Lower rates of light delivery produce higher levels of tissue ROS during in vivo mouse animal model studies.

There are two topical preparations approved by the US FDA for PDT: 20% ALA solution (Levulan Kerastick®; DUSA Pharmaceuticals, Wilmington, Massachusetts), approved in 1999, and 16.8% methyl aminolevulinate cream (Metvixia Cream®; PhotoCure ASA, Oslo, Norway; Galderma, Fort Worth, Texas), approved in 2004. Levulan ALA has an FDA approval for the treatment of actinic keratoses (AKs). Metvixia has been FDA-approved for the treatment of AKs in the US and for AKs and basal cell carcinoma in the EU [6]. The approved activating light source for the Levulan Kerastick® is the BluU® blue light (417–432 nm) (DUSA Pharmaceuticals, Wilmington, Massachusetts) and for Metvixia Cream® it is the Aktilite® red light (610–650 nm; peak 630 nm) (PhotoCure ASA, Norway; Galderma, Fort Worth, Texas).

Topical application of either ALA or MAL bypasses the rate-limiting enzyme in the heme synthesis pathway, ALA-synthase, resulting in the intracellular accumulation of PpIX and other porphyrins (Fig. 12.1). The relative selectivity of both drugs for producing photosensitizing porphyrins in diseased compared to normal tissues has been attributed to enhanced penetration through the stratum corneum and altered porphyrin metabolism in diseased tissue [7]. PpIX has several absorption peaks with the major one in the Soret band (blue light).

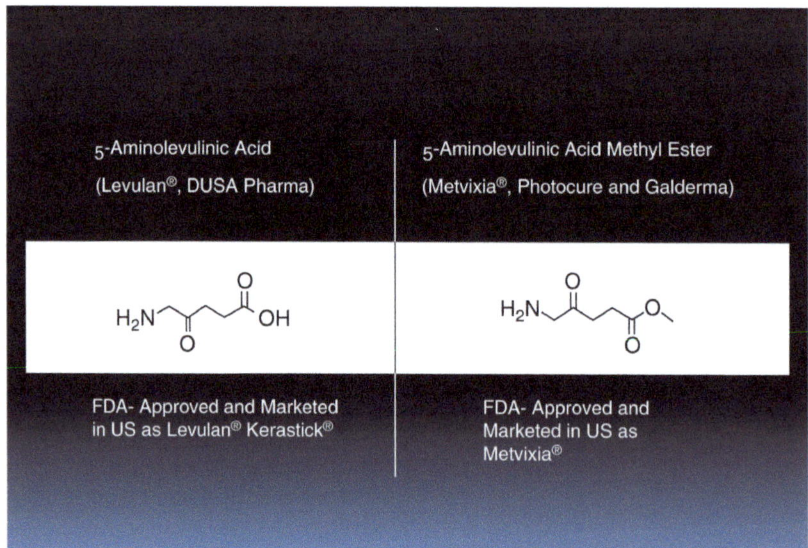

Fig. 12.1 Topical application of either aminolevulinic acid (ALA) or methyl aminolevulinic acid (MAL) bypasses the rate-limiting enzyme in the heme synthesis pathway, ALA-synthase, resulting in the intracellular accumulation of PpIX and other porphyrins

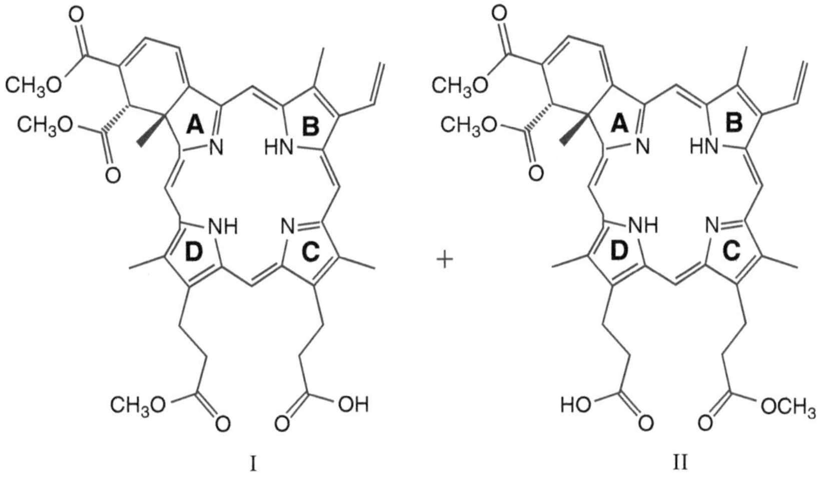

Fig. 12.2 Photofrin is not a single chemical entity, but rather a mixture of oligomers formed by ether and ester linkages of up to eight porphyrin units

Systemic Photosensitizers

There are two approved systemic photosensitizers: Photofrin and Vetoporfin. Photofrin is not a single chemical entity, but rather a mixture of oligomers formed by ether and ester linkages of up to eight porphyrin units (Fig. 12.2). Verteporfin is a 1:1 mixture of two regioisomers (I and II), represented in Fig. 12.3a, b. The chemical names for the verteporfin regioisomers are: 9-methyl (I) and 13-methyl (II) trans-(±)-18-ethenyl-4,4a-dihydro-3,4-bis(methoxycarbonyl)-4a,8,14,19-tetramethyl-23H, 25H-benzo[*b*]porphine-9,13-dipropanoate.

Photofrin is indicated for the palliation of patients with partial or completely obstructing esophageal cancer who are not candidates for Nd:YAG laser therapy. It has also been approved for the treatment of BE which will be covered later in this chapter [8].

It is also indicated for the treatment of obstructing endobronchial lesions of nonsmall-cell lung cancer (NSCLC) and palliation of associated symptoms in patients who are not candidates for surgery or radiotherapy [9].

PDT with Photofrin is a two-stage process requiring drug delivery and activation by light. It is administered as a single intravenous injection over 3–5 min at 2 mg/kg. This is followed by illumination of the target tissue 40–50 h later with laser light (630 nm). A second illumination may be given 96–120 h after injection. Lesions are often debrided between treatment sessions. In cases of esophageal cancer, the light dose of 300 J/cm^2 is recommended [10].

Verteporfin is indicated for the treatment of patients with predominantly classic subfoveal choroidal neovascularization due to ARMD, pathologic myopia, or presumed ocular histoplasmosis. PDT with Verteporfin, like Photofrin, is a two-stage process involving drug delivery and activating light. The drug is dosed at 6 mg/m^2 infused over 10 min. Photoactivation is initiated by a 689-nm wavelength laser light delivered 15 min after the start of the 10 min infusion. In the treatment of choroidal neovascularization, the recommended light dose is 50 J/cm^2 of neovascular lesion administered at an intensity of 600 mW/cm^2 over 83 s.

The role of the light sources in PDT is critical. An extensive review of light sources used in PDT is present in a previous chapter. As a general principle [5], wavelengths in the near and far infrared region have tissue penetration in mammalian skin in the range of 5 mm. Photosensitizers with absorption in this range are capable of targeting deeper tissue elements. Blue light has a more superficial depth of penetration (approximately 0.5 mm) in mammalian skin and is more suited to treating diseases limited to the stratum corneum and superficial epidermis. In addition to the FDA-approved red and blue light sources, the long-pulsed dye laser (LP PDL; 595 nm) and intense pulsed light sources (IPL; 500–1,200 nm) are commonly used to activate PpIX.

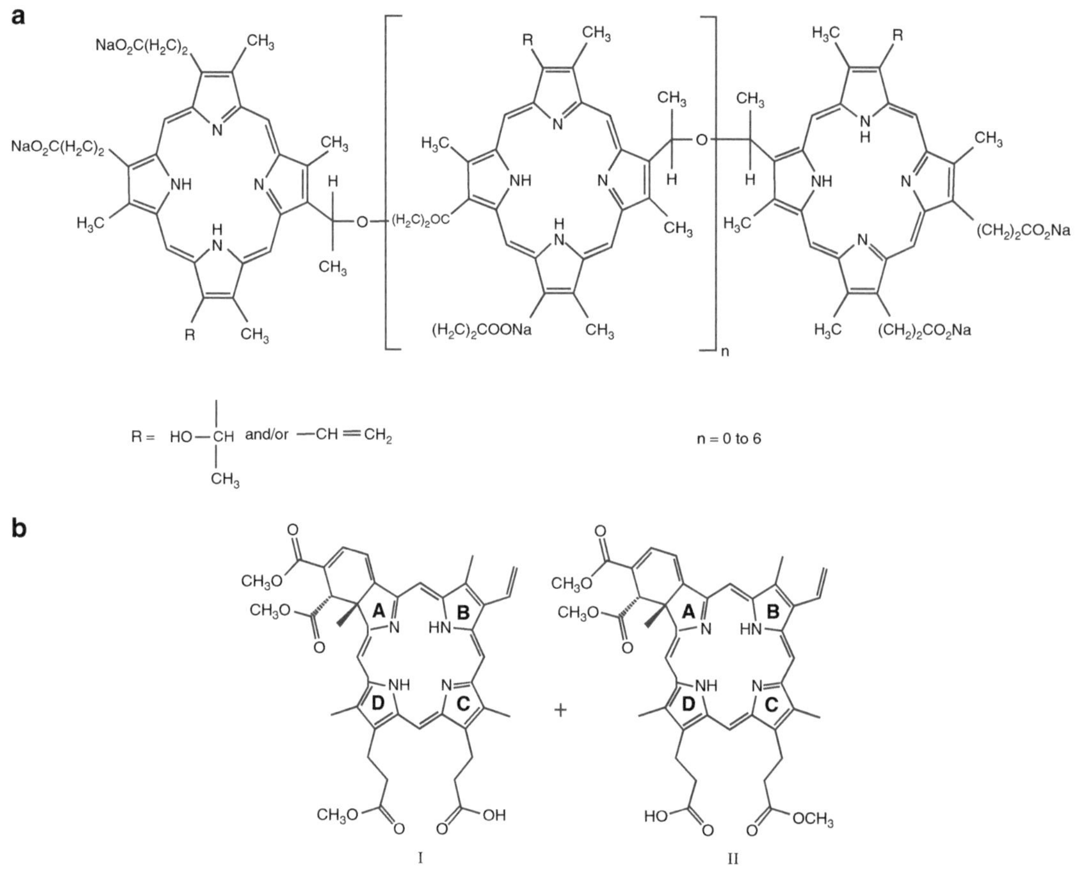

Fig. 12.3 Verteporfin is a 1:1 mixture of two regioisomers (I and II). The chemical names for the verteporfin regioisomers are (**a**) 9-methyl (I) and (**b**) 13-methyl (II) trans-(±)-18-ethenyl-4,4a-dihydro-3,4-bis(methoxycarbonyl)-4a,8,14,19-tetramethyl-23H, 25H-benzo[*b*]porphine-9, 13-dipropanoate

LP PDL and IPL have been demonstrated in clinical studies to be less efficient light sources in performing PDT compared to blue light [11].

Ambient lights including fluorescent light as well as sunlight are also capable of activating porphyrins. Although blue light is most efficient, longer wavelengths penetrate more deeply into skin and thus offer a potential advantage for treating dermal lesions.

PDT in Cutaneous Infections

Bacterial Infections

Worldwide, multidrug-resistant microbial infections have led to the search for new antimicrobial therapies. The observation that an organism can accumulate photosensitizing compounds which when exposed to low levels of visible light result in its destruction has been known since the early 1900s [12]. Oscar Raab discovered the photosensitizing properties of acridine orange while studying the effects of this dye on paramecia. Subsequently, Von Tappeimer and Jesionek used topical eosin (5%) as a photosensitizer. Von Tappeiner and Jodlbauer later determined that oxygen must be present for the photosensitizing reactions to occur.

The advent of antibiotics and their widespread usage overshadowed the development of PDT as a viable antimicrobial therapy. However, the emergence of multidrug microbial resistance has brought about a resurgence of interest in PDT as an antimicrobial therapy. PDT has several features that make it a practical and effective modality to treat microbial pathogens which include [13]: broad spectrum of antimicrobial activity including equal activity against multiple drug-resistant microbes compared to naïve bacteria; bactericidal activity due to its mechanism of action; low mutagenic potential thereby minimizing selection for photo-resistant strains of microbes; and the treatment field within the target tissue can be localized and isolated.

Over the last two decades, there have been a number of published reports which have investigated the bactericidal effects of PDT using various photosensitizers and light sources. To date, this work has been mostly limited to in vitro and in vivo or ex vivo animal models. The development of genetically modified bioluminescent bacteria to follow the effect of PDT in infected wounds, burns, and soft tissue infections in mice has aided research in this area [14].

Research on the antimicrobial effects of PDT has yielded several observations [15]. Gram (+) bacteria are more sensitive to PDT when compared to Gram (−) bacteria. To achieve optimal cytocidal activity against not only bacteria but also fungi and protozoa, the photosensitizer has to maintain a positive charge at physiological pH which is accomplished by the presence of quaternized amino or polylysine groups. Positively charged photosensitizers have increased permeability through the outer membrane of the negatively charged Gram (−) bacteria resulting in increased cellular concentration of the photosensitizer. This allows for greater selectivity compared to the host tissue. Additionally, the molecule has to be moderately hydrophobic (n-octanol/water partition coefficient around 10). When used in micromolar concentrations, these types of photosensitizers resulted in a >4–5 log decrease in the microbial population following short incubation (5–10 min) and irradiation with fluences of 50 mW/cm^2 irradiated for less than 15 min. This has led to the investigation of different classes of molecules that fit this profile and they include: porphyrins, phthalocyanines, phenothiazines, and fullerenes.

The Role of Biofilm in Bacterial Resistance to Therapy

Bacterial virulence is in large part attributable to the formation of a biofilm which provides a microenvironment capable of protecting the microbe from antibiotics, clearance by the immune system, and phagocytosis. In order to kill bacterial pathogens, a strategy had to be developed to specifically target and clear the biofilm. In the case of *Staphylococcus epidermidis*, a commensal bacteria responsible for a significant number of nosocomial infections, a strategy was developed specifically aimed at clearing the biofilm [16].

A marked reduction in the population of *S. epidermidis* was achieved when the biofilm was targeted with the cationic porphyrin, tetra-substituted N-methyl-pyridyl-porphine (TMP) followed by visible light. When the PDT-treated biofilms were then exposed to either vancomycin or the phagocytic action of whole blood, they were nearly completely eradicated. Immature biofilms were more susceptible to PDT destruction than established biofilms.

Investigational Studies in Bacteria

A number of in vitro and animal model in vivo studies over the last 20 years have laid the foundation for future clinical studies in humans involving the use of PDT in antimicrobial therapy. These key studies are briefly summarized.

Escherichia coli when photosensitized with methylene blue (MB) in vitro was killed by white light [17].

Heliobacter could be eradicated in an ex vivo ferret gastric mucosa model without damaging the mucosal tissue when treated with toludine and MB and exposed to a copper vapor-pumped dye laser [18].

Methicillin-resistant *Staphylococcus aureus* (MRSA) in an ex vivo porcine animal model was killed by a porphyrin-based photosensitizer (XF73) without damage to keratinocytes or eukaryotic cells [19].

Vibrio vulnificus is a Gram (−) highly invasive bacteria responsible for opportunistic infections. When inoculated into a mouse model at 100× LD-50 levels, PDT using toluidine blue O followed by broad spectrum red light (150 J/cm^2 at 80 mW/cm^2) resulted in a 50% reduction in mortality despite the presence of septicemia [20].

S. aureus-colonized third-degree burn wounds in a mouse model were treated with meso-mono-phenyl-tri(N-methyl-4-pyridyl)-porphyrin (PTMPP) followed by red light. More than 98% of the bacteria were eradicated; however, bacterial regrowth was observed. Both light alone and PDT delayed wound healing. Treatment optimization by preventing recurrence and reducing wound damage was cited by the authors as areas for future study [21].

S. aureus was effectively treated using PDT in an infected mouse bone model. This finding identified a potential role for PDT in the treatment of osteomyelitis [22].

Clinical Studies in Humans on the Antibacterial Effects of PDT

Erythrasma

Erythrasma is a superficial cutaneous infection caused by *Corynebacterium minutissimum*. *Corynebacterium* possesses significant levels of endogenous porphyrins which fluoresce coral red under Wood's light (UV) examination [23].

Using the photosensitizing properties of these endogenous porphyrins, a study assessing the efficacy of red light alone, without the addition of exogenous photosensitizers, was performed on 13 patients with erythrasma [24]. Lesions were irradiated with one treatment of red light (80 J/cm^2; broad band, peak 635 nm). Treated areas were assessed in 2 weeks, and if not completely resolved, a second treatment was conducted. Results showed that three patients had complete recovery and most other cases had reduction in the extent of the lesions (mean: 29% after one session).

The authors cited that while treatment parameters need to be further developed, using PDT to target endogenous photosensitizers presents an interesting approach with which to safely, inexpensively, and easily treating erythrasma.

PDT for Leg Ulcers

Clayton and Harrison [25] reported 72-year-old female patient with a chronic recalcitrant venous ulceration of the lower leg complicated by recurrent bouts of cellulites, allergic reactions to antibiotics, and colonized with MRSA who responded clinically to ALA PDT.

The patient had greater than 1-year history of lower leg ulceration measuring 19.6 cm. The lesion was refractory to management with compression bandaging, topical antiseptic therapies, and topical bacteriostatic dressings and resistant to larval therapy. Skin biopsies of the area showed no evidence of neoplasia.

PDT was initiated based on previously reported in vitro and animal model studies demonstrating its antimicrobial effects against various bacteria, including MRSA, and fungi using MB [26].

PDT using 5-ALA activated by red light (633 nm) was performed twice weekly for 4 weeks to 5 cm diameter areas. The patient tolerated the procedure well with minimal discomfort, despite no topical anesthesia being used. Wound cultures were negative and corresponded with significant clinical improvement of the ulcer.

The use of PDT as an antimicrobial strategy in treating localized cutaneous infections, particularly in the setting of antibiotic resistance and drug allergies, appears effective and well tolerated. ALA PDT, used as a primary or adjunctive therapy, has the potential to lessen dependence on antibiotic therapy. This promising clinical observation will require well-controlled clinical studies before PDT can be safely considered as a clinically viable therapeutic option in wound therapy.

Mycobacterium Infections

The treatment of mycobacterium infections usually involves prolonged antibiotic therapy, and in the case of tuberculosis, drug therapy has been complicated by multidrug resistance [27]. Alternatives to antibiotics as well as adjunctive therapy led to the study of PDT in a murine model for mycobacterium granulomas [28].

In the study, the photodynamic activity of two cationic photosensitizers (benzo[a]phenothiazinium chloride and benzo[a]phenoselenazinium chloride) against *Mycobacterium bovis* BCG was studied in vitro and in a murine model of a BCG-granuloma. BCG serves as a model for mycobacterium infections. Cell cultures of BCG were incubated with the two photosensitizers and illuminated with a 635-nm diode laser. In vivo studies involved the injection of the photosensitizers into the subcutaneous mycobacterium-induced granulomas followed by red light illumination. Both photosensitizers demonstrated good in vitro and in vivo antimycobacterium PDT activity with dose- and light-dependent toxicities. The study concluded that use of these cationic phenothiazine photosensitizers shows promise in antimycobacterium PDT for localized cutaneous and pulmonary granulomas.

Wiegell et al. reported a case of a patient with a biopsy-proven *Mycobacterium marinum* lesion on the hand, which failed therapy with doxycycline and was subsequently successfully treated with blue and red light alone followed by methyl ALA PDT [29]. *M. marinum* is the cause of "swimming pool" granulomas in individuals exposed to fish and fish tanks [30].

M. marinum contains porphyrins, most notably coproporphyrin III, which can be photoactivated to produce a cytotoxic effect. Because coproporphyrin III has a stronger absorption peak in the blue light region, the lesion was treated initially with 10 weekly doses of 7.8 J/cm^2 blue light (Lysta LC80 Dental Curing Light; Lysta A/S, Farum, Denmark). The thin part of the lesion resolved, but the thicker part remained unresponsive. This observation was attributed to the more shallow tissue penetration of blue light. Red light, because of its deeper tissue penetration, was then used to treat the thicker part of the lesion. Seven weekly 75 J/cm^2 doses of red light (Aktilite; Photocure ASA, Oslo, Norway) were performed with improvement of the lesion, but not resolution, and a new lesion developed at the border of the older lesion.

An in vitro incubation of ALA with *M. marinum* showed the accumulation of PpIX after 3 h. Based on these findings, the lesions were treated weekly for a total of 3 weeks with methyl ALA PDT using a 3-h incubation period and red light (Aktilite) 37 J/cm^2. Fluorescence photographs demonstrated the accumulation of PpIX in the active part of the lesion, but no accumulation in the previously resolved areas during the first two PDT sessions. The third and final session showed no accumulation of PpIX within the lesion which remained clinically resolved at 7 months posttreatment.

These findings suggest that in cases of *M. marinum*, particularly for antibiotic-resistant strains, PDT may be a reasonable therapeutic alternative.

PDT for Fungi

Superficial fungal infections of the skin, hair, and nails are one of the most prevalent infectious diseases worldwide. Therapy in most cases involves prolonged treatment with either topical or oral medications and patients are prone to relapse. The search for a safe, effective, convenient, and economically practical therapeutic alternative therapy led to the investigation of PDT as a treatment option. Until recently, little research in the area of PDT and its effect on fungi has been reported. Blood disinfection, a commercial use for PDT, has focused research efforts in the direction of eradication of bacteria and viruses from blood, whereas fungi are regarded as low-risk blood pathogens. However, recent reports demonstrate that both dermatophytes and yeast can be sensitized in vitro by the administration of photosensitizing agents [31]. These findings have in turn led to small clinical trials in humans.

Fungi, unlike mammalian cells, are surrounded by a fairly rigid cell wall composed of polysaccharides. The uptake of photosensitizers through the cell wall is increased by hydrophilic properties and electric charges and decreased by lipophilic properties. Once taken up into the cell, their intracellular distribution is almost exclusively located in the cytoplasm due to the restrictive nature of the nuclear membrane to penetration. This exclusion of the photosensitizer from the nucleus restricts its mutagenic potential. The observed peroxidation of lipids, inactivation of enzymes, and lysis of cell membranes, lysosomes, and mitochondria minimize the chance of resistance due to these multitargeting properties of PDT [32].

Four major groups of chemicals have been investigated for the treatment of fungi: phenothiazine dyes, phthalocyanines, porphyrins, and ALA. This group of photosensitizers is ideally suited because of their lack of toxicity when not photoactivated and lack of mutagenicity and genotoxicity. They also have a relative selectivity as the fungi tested were killed at doses of drug and light dosimetry at much lower doses than keratinocytes. Lastly, drug-resistant strains were never identified.

Phenothiazines in the oxidized state are cationic and possess a tricyclic planar structure unlike the larger conjugated structures of porphyrins. MB and toluidine blue (TBO) are the most widely used phenothiazines. Their maximum wavelength of absorption in water is 656 nm for MB and 625 nm for TBO [33].

In yeasts, specifically Candida species, TB and MB localize in the plasma membrane. However, the susceptibility of Candida to PDT is much less than that observed for prokaryotic bacteria such as *S. epidermidis*, *S. aureus,* and *Streptococcus pyogenes* [34].

Two plausible explanations for the difference in susceptibilities were offered by the authors of the study. First, yeasts are roughly 25–50 times larger than bacteria and therefore contain a proportionally larger number of potential molecular targets. Second, it is postulated that prokaryotic cells such as bacteria require damage to one of many equally susceptible molecular targets to result in cell death compared to eukaryotic cells (fungi) and require the damage to multiple sites for cell death to occur. In the same study, PDT using MB demonstrated an 18–200-fold higher selectivity for fungi compared to keratinocytes. Using MB and the same light dosimetry, no genotoxic or mutagenic effects were detected in either fungi or keratinocytes [35].

Candida has demonstrated PDT sensitivity to the clinically approved photosensitizer Photofrin. Possible mechanisms commonly used by microbes to avoid antimicrobial oxidative defenses or antimicrobial therapy, including the development of biofilms, were examined [36].

No adaptive response by *Candida albicans* to singlet oxygen-mediated stress due to Photofrin PDT was observed. Additionally, *C. albicans* biofilms were sensitive to Photofrin PDT in a dose-dependent manner and their metabolic activity following PDT was significantly lower than amphotericin B-treated biofilms.

The response of azole-resistant candidiasis was studied in an immunodeficient murine model using MB and 100 J/cm^2 of laser light (peak 664 nm) [37].

Therapeutic effects were light- and dose-dependent. Extrapolation of the findings to HIV+ patients who present with drug-resistant oral candidiasis suggests that PDT may provide an effective, nontoxic, relatively inexpensive therapy for oral infections. However, therapy in HIV+ patients may have limitations as there is often concomitant esophageal candidiasis which can be not only debilitating, but a reservoir of Candida to reinfect the oral cavity.

In vitro studies demonstrate that the fungal pathogen *Cryptococcus neoformans* is susceptible to photodynamic inactivation by use of a polycationic conjugate of polyethyleneimine and the photosensitizer chlorin (e6). A strain of the *C. neoformans* was identified and found to have a compromised cell wall, thereby permitting increased penetration of the photosensitizer when assessed by fluorescent uptake and confocal microscopy. The strain was found to be hypersusceptible to inactivation by PDT. This finding illustrates the significance of cell wall integrity in microbial susceptibility to PDT [38].

PDT using a UVA light source with two thiophenes (2,20:50,200-terthienyl and 5-(4-OH-1-butinyl) 2,20-bithienyl) was tested in vitro on eight strains of dermatophytes (*Trichophyton mentagrophytes*, *Trichophyton rubrum*, *Trichophyton tonsurans*, *Microsporum cookei*, *Microsporum canis*, *Microsporum gypseum*, *Epidermophyton floccosum*, *Nannizia cajetani*). Although complete inactivation was never achieved, there was a strong response to the PDT which was dose-dependent [39].

In vitro studies using *T. rubrum* in a liquid culture demonstrated that the addition of ALA to the medium resulted in the fungal production of PpIX. The generation of PpIX, which was measured by its red fluorescence, occurred in the range of 10–14 days following the addition of ALA to the medium of the slow-growing *T. rubrum*. The generation of PpIX was restricted to certain parts of the fungal mycelium. Irradiation with unfiltered halogen light in the range of 128 J/cm^2 resulted in a 50% inhibition of fungal growth. The slow cellular uptake of hydrophilic ALA prompted investigators to recommend esterification of the molecule to enhance cellular penetration [40].

Onychomycosis

Treatment failures for onychomycosis using combinations of topical and oral antifungals are very common. Combined with lengthy treatment courses and the possibility of drug–drug interactions, alternative treatments for onychomycosis have been sought. Studies have shown that fungi could be sensitized and killed using 5-ALA and light dosimetry at much lower levels than those used to kill keratinocytes. These findings prompted clinical trials using topical PDT to treat onychomycosis [41].

T. rubrum, which is responsible for approximately 90% of onychomycosis, underwent a 50% growth inhibition in vitro following ALA PDT [42].

This finding led to the clinical investigation of the treatment of onychomycosis by topical 5-ALA PDT. Two patients with dermatophyte onychomycosis of the big toe nails underwent 6 and 7 cycles of PDT using a 20% solution of methyl ALA in an aqueous cream followed by irradiation with an excimer-dye laser (630 nm; 100 J/cm^2). This resulted in a complete cure [43].

Piraccini et al. reported using PDT to treat onychomycosis in a single patient. The two large toe nails, one involved with total nail onychomycosis and the other with subungual proximal onychomycosis, were pretreated with 40% urea under occlusion followed by removal of the nail plate. This was followed by removal of the nail bed hyperkeratosis. Methyl-ALA cream (Metvix cream;160 mg/g; PhotoCure, Oslo, Norway) was applied under occlusion for 3 h followed by 37 J/cm^2 of red light (Aklilite CL128, PhotoCure, Oslo, Norway). After three treatment sessions 15 days apart, both KOH and culture were negative for dermatophytes and remained negative until the 24-month examination. The authors pointed out that removal of the nail plate and removal of hyperkeratotic debris in the nail bed are necessary for the maximizing PDT's effectiveness. The optimal number of treatments, light source, and dosimetry remain to be defined [44].

Cutaneous Leishmaniasis

In the early 1900s, the photosensitizing effect of acridine dyes was studied on protozoa. Recently, PDT has been reported in several studies to be effective in the treatment of cutaneous leishmaniasis, caused by the protozoa Leishmania major. The goal in treating this superficial protozoa infection is to eradicate the amastigotes and minimize the effect of potentially scarring cutaneous lesions.

Several studies have examined the efficacy and safety of PDT in treating leishmaniasis. Eleven patients (32 lesions) were treated with 1 or 2 weekly topical ALA PDT treatments using broadband red light. Initially, all smears were negative for amastigotes and reexamination at 3–6 months showed 31 of 32 lesions remained amastigote negative with lesion sizes decreasing an average of 67%. A smaller series of five patients were treated with ALA PDT repeated weekly for 4 weeks. Amastigotes were eradicated in all lesions (culture and smear) with no relapse at 4 months and a good cosmetic outcome was reported. MAL PDT has also been reported to be an effective therapy for leishmaniasis.

MAL PDT using red light was compared to the conventional daily topical treatment using paromomycin. The study involved ten lesions on the same patient. Following a total 28 MAL PDT treatments, 5 of 5 PDT-treated lesions and 2 of 5 paromomycin-treated lesions were histologically clear. However, no cultures were performed.

The largest randomized investigator-blinded study involved 57 patients (95 lesions total) who were randomized to receive weekly ALA PDT with red light, twice daily topical paromomycin, or placebo over a 4-week period. Lesion clearance measured at 8 weeks was 94% in the PDT group, 41% in the paromomycin group, and 13% in the placebo group. Clearance measured by smear was demonstrated in 100, 65, and 20%, respectively.

There have been two proposed mechanisms for the efficacy of PDT in treating leishmaniasis. The first is that PDT results in a nonspecific tissue destruction in which macrophages containing the leishmania are destroyed in the process. The other relies on in vitro data that demonstrate direct antiparasitic effects of porphyrins on intracellular leishmania [45, 46].

It is clear that PDT is an effective treatment for cutaneous leishmaniasis. Additional studies involving histology and culture data would be of benefit.

Disseminated Actinic Porokeratosis

Disseminated actinic porokeratosis (DSAP) is an autosomal dominant inherited skin disorder generally presenting in the 3rd or 4th decade of life with reduced penetration at younger ages. It is characterized by the development of multiple 3–6 mm slightly raised hyperkeratotic rings with central atrophy. Lesions may be erythematous or hyperpigmented and appear on sun-exposed areas of the arms and legs. The lesions likely are the result of a clonal expansion of keratinizing cells [47].

Numerous therapies aimed at eradicating the lesions have been tried, but met with little success. These include cryosurgery, which can result in scarring, topical tacalcitol, 5-fluorouracil, and topical and oral retinoids in combination with PUVA [48–50].

Reports on the use of PDT for this disorder have been limited to a few published case studies. In one study of three patients, the protocol involved carefully curetting off the surface scale followed by the application of 20% ALA in an emulsifying ointment (Porhin, Crawfords Pharmaceuticals) applied to lesions with a 1-cm overlap onto the surrounding skin. The area was covered for 5 h using Tegaderm and an opaque dressing and then exposed to 100 J/cm^2 of broadband red light (Waldman 1200) at 75 mW/cm^2. PpIX fluorescence in lesions before treatment was assessed and found to be present. Treatment failures were observed in all three patients following two courses 4 weeks apart [51].

In a literature review of the role of PDT in treating DSAP, Taub (unpublished observations) reported success in three patients using ALA PDT (Levulan 20% ALA; DUSA; Wilmington, MA) [3].

Caveats to successful treatment were listed as: multiple treatment sessions, long incubation periods, maximal light exposure, and pretreatment with a variety of agents including 5-Fluorouracil, imiquimod, salicylic acid, and retinoids either alone or in combination. Recurrences were common and annual retreatments were necessary.

The use of methyl ALA and red light to successfully treat biopsy-proven DSAP has been reported in a single patient [52].

The patient underwent two PDT sessions 1 week apart using MAL cream (Metvix,160 mg/g concentration. Galderma Italia S.p.A.) activated by red light (Aktilite; 635 nm; 37 J/cm^2). The examination at 1 year showed no residual DSAP. The authors attributed the efficacy of MAL PDT over ALA PDT to the increased lipophilicity and enhanced cellular penetration in MAL compared to ALA. Controlled trials involving both ALA and MAL PDT in a large series of patients with DSAP are needed.

Barrett's Esophagus

BE is a premalignant condition in which the normal squamous epithelium is replaced by metaplastic columnar epithelium. This predisposes patients to a stepwise progression from metaplasia through dysplasia to adenocarcinoma of the esophagus [53].

Most adenocarcinomas of the esophagus are thought to arise from high-grade dysplasia (HGD) in Barrett's. The presence of HGD in BE confers a 59% risk of developing cancer within 5 years [54].

Adenocarcinoma of the esophagus has a 5-year survival rate of less than 10% and its incidence is increasing in the western hemisphere [54–56].

PDT is an endoscopic alternative to the major surgical alternative, esophagectomy, for the treatment of HGD in BE. PDT in this disorder uses porfimer sodium and is an approved treatment in the USA, Canada, Japan, and Europe. However, it is associated with a high incidence of esophageal strictures with rates as high as 22% after a single treatment and up to 50% after multiple treatments. Treatment is associated with prolonged (4–6 weeks) photosensitivity [57, 58]. 5-ALA PDT provides an alternative to porfimer sodium as it has been shown to avoid the serious side effects [59].

Until recently, consensus on the most effective usage of ALA PDT in BE has been lacking. Mackenzie et al. recently demonstrated that using ALA 60 mg/kg activated by 1,000 J/cm^2 red light (635 nm) was more effective than 30 mg/kg ALA, which showed a higher relapse rate of HGD [60].

Green laser light (512 nm) was not as effective as red light. The overall optimal regimen showed an eradication rate of HGD of 89% and a cancer-free proportion of 96% at 36-month follow-up examination.

PDT Uses in Ophthalmology: Age-Related Macular Degeneration

ARMD is an age-related deterioration of the central part of the retina. There are two forms of ARMD: the atrophic (dry) form and the neovascular (wet) form in which new blood vessels emanating from the choriocapillaris grow into the subretinal space. Approximately one half to two thirds of ARMD is the "wet form." ARMD is the leading cause of blindness in Americans over the age of 65 with approximately 200,000 new cases diagnosed annually [61].

In "wet" ARMD, leakage of serous and/or lipid exudates into the subretinal space from the neovascularizing blood vessels causes separation of the retina from the choriocapillaris resulting in accumulation of waste products. This limits nutrient supply as well as causing intraretinal edema similar to that seen in patients with diabetic retinopathy. Hemorrhage, when occurs, releases iron which is toxic to the retina and results in permanent visual loss. These side effects result in distortion and scarring of the retina eventually leading to blindness.

PDT using verteporfin, a benzoporphyrin derivative, was approved in 2000 for the treatment of ARMD [62]. It is administered intravenously to a total dose of 6 mg/m^2 and accumulates preferentially in the choroidal neovascular tissue where it is activated by red (689 nm) laser light delivered into the eye at an intensity of 600 mW/cm^2 over 83 s to provide the recommended light dose of 50 J/cm^2. PDT induces apoptosis of the neovascular endothelial cells resulting in their selective destruction leaving normal retina blood vessels intact [63].

PDT was subsequently approved for the treatment of choroidal neovascularization (CNV) in pathological myopia. The treatment regimen for both is based on two prospective, multicentre trials (TAP and VIP studies [64]).

In ARMD, patients are treated every 3 months until the neovascular membrane is shut down. In phase 3 trials, PDT reduced the chance of severe visual loss by 66% compared to placebo and by 90% in patients with the "classic" form of neovascularization. However, most patients expressed dissatisfaction as only 13% of patients gained vision compared to 7% of placebo-treated patients. In 2005, the combined use of intravitreal triamcinalone acetonide, a corticosteroid, with verteporfin PDT significantly improved visual prognosis and reduced the number of treatments [65].

The development of clinical use of antivascular endothelial growth factors (anti-VEGF) and their superiority in treating ARMD when compared to PDT has resulted in the rare use of PDT as the sole therapy for exudative "wet" ARMD. Currently, PDT is used as an adjunctive therapy in combination with anti-VEGF injections for more aggressive lesions or in efforts to reduce the number of frequent injections of anti-VEGF.

Additional uses for PDT currently being evaluated include: idiopathic CNV, secondary CNV in inflammatory diseases of the retina and choroid, choroidal hemangioma, vasoproliferative tumors, malignant melanoma of the choroid, and central serous chorioretinopathy [66].

Chronic X-Ray Dermatitis (Radiodermatitis)

Radiodermatitis is the result of chronic exposure of the skin to very small doses of ionizing radiation. In the majority of cases, the exposure is occupational. The development of radiodermatitis is a slow insidious process in which atrophy is the first sign. Associated findings include dryness, hyperkeratotic areas, and thickened areas secondary to fibrosis and ulcers which can be debilitating. AKs and superficial squamous cell carcinomas (sSCC), histologically indistinguishable from sun-induced AKs and sSCC, commonly develop and can be quite extensive.

Management of the disorder includes: topical antibiotics for ulcers; topical corticosteroids; topical 5-fluorouracil, cryosurgery, electrodessication, and curettage to reduce the AKs burden; surgical excision; and grafting of necrotic tissue or areas of carcinoma involvement.

Five retired physicians, who used radioscopy without lead glove protection and subsequently developed radiodermatitis, were successfully treated with ALA PDT [67]. The rationale for using ALA PDT was based on its efficacy in treating AKs and nonmelanoma skin cancer [4]. ALA 20% in an oil-in-water cream base containing aqua, petrolatum, and EDTA was applied for 3 h and activated for 20 min with red (720 nm; 140 mW cm^2) and near infrared (1,250–1,600 nm; 70 mW cm^2) for a total dose of 252 J/cm^2 (VersaLight, ESC Medical Systems). All patients underwent multiple courses (range: 2–8) 4–8 weeks apart and were followed clinically for up to 33 months (range: 9–33).

Complete remission occurred in two patients and partial clinical remission in three patients. No complications were reported and the procedure was well tolerated. Significant pain relief was reported in all patients. The authors concluded that ALA PDT is a safe and useful treatment for radiodermatitis. It eliminates pain and preserves finger function by reducing tumor burden, minimizing need for surgery and possibly amputation.

Cutaneous Sarcoidosis

Sarcoidosis is a systemic disease of unknown etiology and is characterized by multiorgan involvement of noncaseous epitheloid cell granulomas. The lung is the most frequently involved organ and is affected in 90% of reported cases. The skin is involved in 25% of patients and may be the only manifestation of the disease [68, 69].

A single case was reported involving a patient who had a 17-year history of persistent sarcoid skin lesions refractory to conventional and alternative therapies. Treatment with ALA PDT resulted in complete resolution of her skin lesions [70].

The patient had no evidence of extracutaneous sarcoidal involvement and laboratory analyses were within normal limits. Skin lesions were reported only on the arms and legs. PDT was performed using 3% ALA in a gel containing 40% DMSO applied under dark occlusion for 6 h, then irradiated with an incoherent light source (PDT 1200; Waldmann Medizintechnik, VS-Schwenningen, Germany) at a wavelength of 580–740 nm (40 mW/cm^2; energy density, 20 J/cm^2). PDT was performed twice weekly for the first 8 weeks, followed by once weekly treatments. A total of 22 treatments were performed over a 3-month period. The only adverse effect was a slight burning sensation during treatment followed by erythema and edema lasting for 2 days after PDT. Lesions resolved within 3 months with histological clearance of a typical lesion at 4 months. At 18 months, the patient remained free of any cutaneous or visceral evidence of sarcoidosis.

It remains to be determined by what mechanism ALA PDT affects cutaneous sarcoid. The authors speculated that ALA PDT may exert an anti-inflammatory effect via release of cytokines from affected keratinocytes leading to a disruption of the formation of sarcoid granulomas.

Pyogenic Granuloma-Like Lesions Associated with Goltz Syndrome

Focal dermal hypoplasia syndrome (Goltz syndrome) is a rare genetic disorder characterized by ectodermal, mesodermal, and cutaneous defects

[71, 72]. Pyogenic granuloma-like lesions, while previously unreported to be associated with Goltz syndrome, presented in a patient as numerous painful exophytic granulation tissue lesions over a 15-year period [73].

The lesions were poorly responsive to topical steroids, silver nitrate application, cryotherapy, curettage, excision, and pulsed dye laser. Lesions treated with the combination of curettage and excision often recurred in 3–4 weeks. However, PDT combined with curettage provided significant long-term benefit.

PDT was performed with methyl ALA (160 mg/g Metvix; Photocure, Oslo, Norway) under occlusion for 3 h. Woods light revealed localization of PpIX within the lesions. The lesions were anesthetized with 1% lidocaine and illuminated with red light (631 nm; 37 J/cm^2 70–100 mW/cm^2). Lesions remained clear for up to 8 months following a single treatment.

A possible mechanism for the efficacy of PDT in these proliferating vascular lesions may be due to the finding that proliferating neovascular endothelium demonstrates low-density lipoprotein (LDL) expression. This is felt to allow selective uptake of a porphyrin-based sensitizer by LDL receptor-dependent endocytosis. This mechanism has been ascribed to the successful treatment of neovascular proliferation in ARMD. The same mechanism may be attributed to the successful treatment by PDT of the proliferating vessels in this case [74].

PDT in Necrobiosis Lipoidica Diabeticorum

Necrobiosis lipoidica diabeticorum (NLD) is an idiopathic granulomatous cutaneous disorder resulting in collagen degeneration leading to atrophy of the skin [75]. NLD is usually seen on the lower legs in patients with diabetes mellitus. In efforts to limit the inflammatory granulomatous process, a wide variety of anti-inflammatory measures have been used. The most commonly used treatments, topical high potency corticosteroids and intralesional corticosteroids, have limited application because of their tendency to cause atrophy. Systemic corticosteroids exacerbate blood glucose levels in diabetic patients and skin atrophy in both diabetics and nondiabetics. Other therapies directed at decreasing microangiopathy and thrombosis in NLD include: PUVA, allopurinol, stanozolol, inositol niacinate, nicofuranose, ticlopidine hydrochloride, pentoxifylline, retinoids, cyclosporine, chloroquine, and fumaric esters. These treatments have been found to be marginally effective and have not been subject to randomized controlled trials to determine efficacy [76–79].

A single case was reported involving a 60-year-old diabetic female with a 10-year history of histologically proven NLD who responded to methyl ALA PDT after failing conventional therapies [80].

The patient had previously been treated with mid-to-high potency topical corticosteroids, cryotherapy, Grenz ray, and 3 months of allopurinol with no response. Because of reports in the literature regarding the anti-inflammatory properties of PDT, the patient underwent treatment with methyl ALA activated by red light [81].

Three treatments 1 week apart were performed using methyl aminolevulinate (160 mg/g) applied to the lesion and kept under occlusion for 3 h. This was followed by activation with red light (CureLight 2: Photocure ASA; 37 J/cm^2 [LED, 580–670 nm], peak wavelength at 631 nm) for 8 min. No topical anesthesia was used. A marked reduction in lesion size and color was noted during the three treatments prompting a second series of three treatments using the same parameters. After a total of six treatments, the lesion disappeared clinically and histologically and remained clear 24 months later. No scarring was noted.

The immunologic mechanism by which PDT played a role in the clearance of NLD has yet to be determined. Methyl ALA PDT appears to be a safe and effective treatment for NLD. Additional well-controlled studies are necessary to fully evaluate treatment parameters and outcomes.

Summary

Considerable progress has been made over the last two decades in understanding the dynamic interactions between the three components of PDT: light, photosensitizer, and oxygen. Advances in technology have accelerated the ability to optimize PDT and further its adoption as a viable treatment option in the spectrum of neoplastic, infectious, and inflammatory diseases.

References

1. Morton CA, McKenna KE, Rhodes LE. Guidelines for topical photodynamic therapy: update. Br J Dermatol. 2008;159:1245–66.
2. Marcus SL, McIntyre WR. Photodynamic therapy systems and applications. Expert Opin Emerg Drugs. 2002;7(2):318–31.
3. Taub AF. Photodynamic therapy: other uses. Dermatol Clin. 2007;25:101–9.
4. Mark S. Nestor MD PhD (chair), a Michael H. Gold MD (co-chair), b Arielle N. B. Kauvar MD, c Amy F. Taub MD, d Roy G. Geronemus MD, c Eva C. Ritvo MD, e Dore J. Gilbert MD, f Mitchel P. Goldman MD, g Donald F. Richey MD h (Consensus Panel). The use of photodynamic therapy in dermatology: results of a consensus conference. J Drugs Dermatol. 2006;5(2):140–54.
5. Alexiades-Armenakas M. Aminolevulinic acid photodynamic therapy for actinic keratoses/actinic cheilitis/acne: vascular lasers. Dermatol Clin. 2007;25:25–33.
6. Niedre MJ, Yu CS, Patterson MS, Wilson BC. Singlet oxygen luminescence as an in vivo photodynamic therapy dose metric: validation in normal mouse skin with topical produce singlet oxygen using 5-aminolaevulinic acid. Br J Cancer. 2005;92:298–304.
7. Fritsch C, Homey B, Stahl W, Lehmann P, Ruzicka T, Sies H. Preferential relative porphyrin enrichment in solar keratoses upon topical application of 6-aminolevulinic acid methylester. Photochem Photobiol. 1998;68(2):218–21.
8. Likier HM, Levine JG, Lightdale C. Photodynamic therapy for completely obstructing esophageal carcinoma. Gastrointest Endosc. 1991;37:75–8.
9. Locicero J, Metzdorff M, Almgren C. Photodynamic therapy in the palliation of late-stage obstructing nonsmall-cell lung cancer. Chest. 1990;98:97–100.
10. Photofrin® (porfimer sodium). "package insert" that accompanies an FDA approved drug. It often contains relevant information that is not published in the public domain. Axcan Scandipharm, Inc.; 2000.
11. Strasswimmer J, Grande DJ. Do pulsed lasers produce an effective photodynamic therapy response? Lasers Surg Med. 2006;38:22–5.
12. Daniel MD, Hill JS. A history of photodynamic therapy. Aust N Z J Surg. 1991;61:340–8.
13. Hamblin MR, Hasan T. Photodynamic therapy: a new antimicrobial approach to infectious disease? Photochem Photobiol Sci. 2004;3(5):436–50.
14. Demidova TN, Hamblin MR. Photodynamic therapy targeted to pathogens. Int J Immunopathol Pharmacol. 2004;17(3):245–54.
15. Jori G, Fabris C, Soncin M, Ferro S, Coppellotti O, Dei D, et al. Photodynamic therapy in the treatment of microbial infections: basic principles and perspective applications. Lasers Surg Med. 2006;38(5):468–81.
16. Sharma M, Visai L, Bragheri F, Cristiani I, Gupta PK, Speziale P. Toluidine blue-mediated photodynamic effects on staphylococcal biofilms. Antimicrob Agents Chemother. 2008;52(1):299–305.
17. Menezes S, Capella MA, Caldas LR. Photodynamic action of methylene blue: repair and mutation in *Escherichia coli*. J Photochem Photobiol B. 1990; 5(3–4):505–17.
18. Millson CE, Wilson M, MacRobert AJ, Bown SG Exvivo treatment of gastric Helicobacter infection by photodynamic therapy. J Photochem Photobiol. 1996;32(1–2):59–65.
19. Maisch T. Phototoxicity of a novel porphyrin photosensitizer against MRSA in an ex-vivo porcine skin model. In: Presented at the sixth annual euro-PDT meeting. Berne, Switzerland, March 31–April 1, 2006.
20. Wong TW, Wang YY, Sheu HM, Chuang YC Bactericidal effects of toluidine blue-mediated photodynamic action on *Vibrio vulnificus*. Antimicrob Agents Chemother. 2005;49(3):895–902.
21. Lambrechts SA, Demidova TN, Aalders MC, Hasan T, Hamblin MR. Photodynamic therapy for *Staphylococcus aureus* infected burn wounds in mice. Photochem Photobiol Sci. 2005;4(7):503–9.
22. Bisland SK, Chien C, Wilson BC, Burch S. Preclinicalin vitro and in vivo studies to examine the potential use of photodynamic therapy in the treatment of osteomyelitis. Photochem Photobiol Sci. 2006;5(1):31–8.
23. Burns RE, Greer JE, Mikhail G, Livingood CS. The significance of coral-red fluorescence of the skin. Arch Dermatol. 1967;96:436–40.
24. Darras-Vercambre S, Carpentier O, Vincent P, Bonnevalle A, Thomas P. Photodynamic action of red light for treatment of erythrasma: preliminary results. Photodermatol Photoimmunol Photomed. 2006;22: 153–6.
25. Clayton TH, Harrison PV. Photodynamic therapy for infected leg ulcers. Br J Dermatol. 2007;156: 384–5.
26. Zeina B, Greenman J, Purdell WM, Das B. Killing of cutaneous microbial species by photodynamic therapy. Br J Dermatol. 2001;144:274–8.
27. Ma Z, Lienhardt C. Toward an optimized therapy for tuberculosis? Drugs in clinical trials and in preclinical development. Clin Chest Med. 2009;30(4): 755–68, ix.
28. O'Riordan K, Akilov OE, Chang SK, Foley JW, Hasan T. Real-time fluorescence monitoring of

phenothiazinium photosensitizers and their anti-mycobacterial photodynamic activity against *Mycobacterium bovis* BCG in in vitro and in vivo models of localized infection. Photochem Photobiol Sci. 2007;6(10):1117–23.
29. Wiegell SR, Kongshoj B, Wulf HC. *Mycobacterium marinum* infection cured by photodynamic therapy. Arch Dermatol. 2006;142:1241–2.
30. Aubry A, Chosidow O, Caumes E, et al. Sixty-three cases of *Mycobacterium marinum* infection: clinical features, treatment, and antibiotic susceptibility of causative isolates. Arch Intern Med. 2002;162: 1746–52.
31. Calzavara-Pinton PG, Venturini M, Sala R. A comprehensive overview of photodynamic therapy in the treatment of superficial fungal infections of the skin. J Photochem Photobiol B. 2005;78(1):1–6.
32. Bertoloni G, Zambotto F, Conventi L, Reddi E, Jori G. Role of specific cellular targets in the hematoporphyrin-sensitized photoinactivation of microbial cells. Photochem Photobiol. 1987;46:695–8.
33. Ito T. Toluidine blue: the mode of photodynamic action in yeast cells. Photochem Photobiol. 1977;25: 47–53.
34. Zeina B, Greenman J, Corry D, Purcell WM. Cytotoxic effects of antimicrobial photodynamic therapy on keratinocytes in vitro. Br J Dermatol. 2002;146: 568–73.
35. Greenman J, Corry D, Purcell WM. Antimicrobial photodynamic therapy: assessment of genotoxic effects on keratinocytes in vitro. Br J Dermatol. 2003;148:229–32.
36. Chabrier-Roselló Y, Foster TH, Pérez-Nazario N, Mitra S, Haidaris CG. Sensitivity of *Candida albicans* germ tubes and biofilms to photofrin-mediated phototoxicity. Antimicrob Agents Chemother. 2005;49(10):4288–95.
37. Teichert MC, Jones JW, Usacheva MN, Biel MA. Treatment of oral candidiasis with methylene blue-mediated photodynamic therapy in an immunodeficient murine model. Oral Surg Oral Med Oral Pathol Oral Radiol Endod. 2002;93:155–60.
38. Fuchs BB, Tegos GP, Hamblin MR, Mylonakis E. Susceptibility of *Cryptococcus neoformans* to photodynamic inactivation is associated with cell wall integrity. Int J Artif Organs. 2009;32(9):574–83.
39. Romagnoli C, Mares D, Sacchetti G, Bruni A. The photodynamic effect of 5-(4-hydroxy-1-butinyl)-2, 2-bithienyl on dermatophytes. Mycol Res. 1998;102:1519–24.
40. Kamp H, Tietz HJ, Lutz M, Piazena H, Sowyrda P, Lademann J, Blume-Peytavi U. Antifungal effect of 5-aminolevulinic acid PDT in *Trichophyton rubrum*. Mycoses. 2005;48(2):101–7.
41. Smijs TG, Mulder AA, Pavel S, Onderwater JJ, Koerten HK, Bouwstra JA. Morphological changes of the dermatophytes *Trichophyton rubrum*, after photodynamic treatment: a scanning electron microscopy study. Med Mycol. 2008;46:315–25.
42. Kamp H, Tietz HJ, Lutz M, Piazena H, Sowyrda P, Lademann J, et al. Antifungal effect of 5-aminolevulinic acid PDT in *Trichophyton rubrum*. Mycoses. 2005; 48:101–7.
43. Watanabe D, Kawamura C, Masuda Y, Akita Y, Tamada Y, Matsumoto Y, et al. Successful treatment of toenail onychomycosis with photodynamic therapy. Arch Dermatol. 2008;144:19–21.
44. Piraccini BM, Rech G, Tosti A. Photodynamic therapy of onychomycosis caused by *Trichophyton rubrum*. J Am Acad Dermatol. 2008;59:S75–6.
45. Kosaka S, Akilov OE, O'Riordan K, Hasan T. A mechanistic study of delta-aminolevulinic acid-based photodynamic therapy for cutaneous leishmaniasis. J Invest Dermatol. 2007;127:1546–9.
46. Abok K, Cadelas E, Brunk U. An experimental model system for leishmaniasis. Effects of porphyrin-compounds and menadione on leishmania parasites engulfed by cultured macrophages. APMIS. 1998;96: 543–51.
47. Reed RJ, Leone P. Porokeratosis – a mutant clone keratosis of the epidermis. Arch Dermatol. 1970; 101:340–3.
48. Böhm M, Luger TA, Bonsmann G. Disseminated superficial actinic porokeratosis: treatment with topical tacalcitol. J Am Acad Dermatol. 1999;40:479–80.
49. Shelley WB, Shelley ED. Disseminated superficial porokeratosis: rapid therapeutic response to 5-fluorouracil. Cutis. 1983;32:139–40.
50. Schwartz T, Seiser A, Gschnait F. Disseminated superficial actinic keratosis. J Am Acad Dermatol. 1982;11:724–30.
51. Nayeemuddin FA, Wong M, Yell J, Rhodes LE. Topical photodynamic therapy in disseminated superficial actinic porokeratosis. Clin Exp Dermatol. 2002;27:703–6.
52. Cavicchini S, Tourlaki A. Successful treatment of disseminated superficial actinic porokeratosis with methyl aminolevulinate-photodynamic therapy. J Dermatolog Treat. 2006;17:190–1.
53. Phillips RW, Wong RK. Barrett's esophagus: natural history, incidence, etiology, and complications. Gastroenterol Clin North Am. 1991;20:791–816.
54. Reid BJ, Levine DS, Longton G, Blount PL, Rabinovitch PS. Predictors of progression to cancer in Barrett's esophagus: baseline histology and flow cytometry identify low- and highrisk patient subsets. Am J Gastroenterol. 2000; 95:1669–76.
55. Montgomery E, Goldblum JR, Greenson JK, Haber MM, Lamps LW, Lauwers GY, Lazenby AJ, Lewin DN, Robert ME, Washington K, Zahurak ML, Hart J. Dysplasia as a predictive marker for invasive carcinoma in Barrett esophagus: a follow-up study based on 138 cases from a diagnostic variability study. Hum Pathol. 2001;32:379–88.
56. Schnell TG, Sontag SJ, Chejfec C, Aranha G, Metz A, O'Connell S, Seidel UJ, Sonneberg A. Long-termnonsurgical management of Barrett's esophagus with high-grade dysplasia. Gastroenterology. 2001; 120:1607–19.
57. Overholt BF, Panjehpour M, Haydek JM. Photodynamic therapy for Barrett's esophagus: follow-up in 100 patients. Gastrointest Endosc. 1999;49:1–7.

58. Overholt BF, Panjehpour M, Halberg DL. Photodynamic therapy for Barrett's esophagus with dysplasia and/or early stage carcinoma: long-term results. Gastrointest Endosc. 2003;58:183–8.
59. Regula J, MacRobert AJ, Gorchein A, Buonaccorsi GA, Thorpe SM, Spencer GM, Hatfield AR, Bown SG. Photosensitisation and photodynamic therapy of oesophageal, duodenal, and colorectal tumours using 5-aminolaevulinic acid induced protoporphyrin IX – a pilot study. Gut. 1995;36:67–75.
60. Gary D. Mackenzie & Jason M. Dunn & C. R. Selvasekar & C. Alexander Mosse & Sally M. Thorpe & Marco R. Novelli & Stephen G. Bown & Laurence B. Lovat. Optimal conditions for successful ablation of high-grade dysplasia in Barrett's oesophagus using aminolaevulinic acid photodynamic therapy. Lasers Med Sci. 2009;24:729–34.
61. Kaufman SR. Developments in age-related macular degeneration: diagnosis and treatment. Geriatrics. 2009;64(3):16–9.
62. Bressler NM. Treatment of age-related macular degeneration with photodynamic therapy (TAP) Study Group. Photodynamic therapy of subfoveal choroidal neovascularization in age-related macular degeneration with verteporfin: two-year results of 2 randomized clinical trials – tap report 2. Arch Ophthalmol. 2001;119(2):198–207.
63. Potter MJ, Szabo SM. Verteporfin photodynamic therapy-induced apoptosis in choroidal neovascular membranes. Br J Ophthalmol. 2006;90:1034–9.
64. Verteporfin Roundtable 2000 and 2001 Participants, Treatment of Age-Related Macular Degeneration with Photodynamic Therapy (TAP) Study Group, Verteporfin in Photodynamic Therapy (VIP) Study Group Principal Investigators. Guidelines for using verteporfin (visudyne) in photodynamic therapy to treat choroidal neovascularization due to age-related macular degeneration and other causes. Retina. 2002;22(1):6–18.
65. Spaide RF, Sorenson J, Maranan L. Photodynamic therapy with verteporfin combined with intravitreal injection of triamcinolone acetonide for choroidal neovascularization. Ophthalmology. 2005;112(2):301–4.
66. Lang GE, Mennel S, Spital G, Wachtlin J, Jurklies B, Heimann H, et al. Different indications of photodynamic therapy in ophthalmology. Klin Monatsbl Augenheilkd. 2009;226(9):725–39. Epub 2009 Jul 14 [Article in German].
67. Escudero A, Nagore E, Sevila A, Sanmartin O, Botella R, Guillenx C. Chronic-ray dermatitis treated by topical 5-aminolaevulinic acid – photodynamic therapy 2002 British Association of Dermatologists. Br J Dermatol. 2002;147:385–410.
68. Lessana-Leibowitch M, Monsuez JJ, Noble JP, Sedel D, Cadot M, Hewitt J. Manifestations cutanees de la sarcoidose. Ann Med Interne (Paris). 1984;135: 97–101.
69. Kerdel FA, Moschella SL. Sarcoidosis: an updated review. J Am Acad Dermatol. 1984;11:1–19.
70. Karrer S, Abels C, Beatrix Wimmershoff M, Landthaler M, Szeimies RM. Successful treatment of cutaneous sarcoidosis using topical photodynamic therapy. Arch Dermatol. 2002;138:581–4.
71. Goltz RW, Peterson WC, Gorlin RJ, Ravits HG. Focal dermal hypoplasia. Arch Dermatol. 1962;86:708–17.
72. Goltz RW. Focal dermal hypoplasia syndrome. An update. Arch Dermatol. 1992;128:1108–11.
73. Mallipeddi R, Chaudhry SI, Darley CR, Kurwa HA. A case of focal dermal hypoplasia (Goltz) syndrome with exophytic granulation tissue treated by curettage and photodynamic therapy. Clin Exp Dermatol. 2006; 31:228–31.
74. Ufret-Vincenty RL, Miller JW, Gragoudas ES. Photosensitizers in photodynamic therapy of choroidal neovascularization. Int Ophthalmol Clin. 2004;44:63–80.
75. Perez MI, Kohn SR. Cutaneous manifestations of diabetes. J Am Acad Dermatol. 1994;30:519–31.
76. Meurer M, Szeimies RM. *Diabetes mellitus* and skin diseases. Curr Probl Dermatol. 1991;20:11–23.
77. Norman A. Dermal manifestations for diabetes. In: Norman R, editor. Geriatric dermatology. New York: Parthenon Publishing Group; 2001. p. 143–54.
78. Kreuter A, Knierim C, Stucker M, Pawlak F, Rotterdam S, Altmeyer P, Gambichler T. Fumaric acid esters in necrobiosis lipoidica: results of a prospective noncontrolled study. Br J Dermatol. 2005;153:802–7.
79. De Rie MA, Sommer A, Hoekzema R, Neumann HA. Treatment of necrobiosis lipoidica with topical psoralen plus ultraviolet A. Br J Dermatol. 2002;147: 743–7.
80. Heidenheim M, Jemec GBE. Successful treatment of necrobiosis lipoidica diabeticorum with photodynamic therapy. Arch Dermatol. 2006;142:1548–50.
81. Babilas P, Karrer S, Sidoroff A, Landthaler M, Szeimeies RM. Photodynamic therapy in dermatology: an update. Photodermatol Photoimmunol Photomed. 2005;21:142–9.

Chemoprevention of Skin Cancer with Photodynamic Therapy

13

Robert Bissonnette

Abstract

Photodynamic therapy with ALA or MAL is safe and effective for the treatment and prevention of actinic keratoses. This modality has several advantages over 5-FU and imiquimod and its use should expand in the coming years with the wider availability of both photosensitizers.

Over the past 10 years, there has been a rapidly growing interest in the use of photodynamic therapy (PDT) for skin cancer prevention. Chemoprevention of skin cancer by PDT usually refers to treatment of large sun-damaged areas without visible premalignant or malignant lesions with the aim of preventing the appearance of skin cancer. At the time of this writing, two photosensitizer precursors were approved for the treatment of actinic keratoses (AK) and/or skin cancer: aminolevulinic acid (ALA) and methylaminolevulinate (MAL). This chapter focuses on the use of topical ALA solution and MAL cream as chemopreventive PDT agents. A patch containing ALA has also been shown to be effective for AK treatment, but it is not discussed in this chapter [1]. Systemic administration of ALA and possibly other photosensitizers has the potential to delay skin cancer appearance. However, systemic photosensitizers are not discussed as their use is not currently approved for the treatment of skin diseases.

R. Bissonnette (✉)
Innovaderm Research, 1851 Sherbooke East, Suite 502, Montreal, Canada H2K 4L5
e-mail: rbissonnette@innovaderm.ca

Evaluation of Patients Who Need Skin Cancer Prevention Strategies

Prevention of nonmelanoma skin cancer (NMSC) is regularly performed by clinicians. In contrast to patients with solid internal cancers, it is fairly easy to assess the risks of developing NMSC and AKs. The major risks include phototype and total exposure to UV radiation [2]. This information can easily be obtained by examining the patient's face and asking a few questions. For internal cancers, physicians usually need to conduct a careful medical history and obtain information on genetic and environmental risks. This is not always easy as some patients may not tell the truth about their exposure to known carcinogens such as nicotine or alcohol, while others may not remember or know details about work-related exposure or about their parents. Evaluation of risk factors for AKs and NMSCs is easier. Patients with phototype I or II can be identified by clinical examination, which can be confirmed with one or two simple questions about how patients tend to burn or tan. Patients may be evasive about their previous amount of sun exposure, but the presence of extensive small wrinkles, sallowness, dyspigmentation,

M.H. Gold (ed.), *Photodynamic Therapy in Dermatology*,
DOI 10.1007/978-1-4419-1298-5_13, © Springer Science+Business Media, LLC 2011

and possibly the presence of several AKs will suggest to the physician that the patient is at higher risk. This evaluation can easily be performed in less than a minute.

Patients at higher risk of skin cancer should have a thorough skin examination to detect and eventually treat existing AKs and skin cancers. In addition, physicians want to prevent new lesions from arising from chronically UV-exposed skin. Patients with numerous AKs, who have had more than one basal cell carcinoma (BCC) or squamous cell carcinoma (SCC), and patients on systemic immunosuppressants are typical candidates for skin cancer prevention strategies. Patients with only a few AKs or only one BCC or one SCC but with extensive facial sun damage will also benefit from prevention strategies. In addition to prevention of new AKs and skin cancers, they will benefit from an improvement in photoaging [3].

Current Options for Skin Cancer Prevention

All patients should be counseled about sun protection, sun avoidance, and the use of sunscreen. Current options to prevent AKs and NMSCs include 5 fluorouracil (5-FU), imiquimod, laser, peeling, and PDT (Table 13.1). 5-FU is very effective at treating AKs [4] and has been prescribed by clinicians for several years to prevent AKs and skin cancer. Daily, 5-FU applications usually give rise to erythema often associated with crusting and a burning sensation lasting for several weeks. Many physicians are prescribing 5-FU 2–3 times a week for several months to decrease the intensity of the reaction associated with daily use of 5-FU [5]. The disadvantage of this approach is that patients exhibit facial erythema for a longer time. In addition to erythema present during treatment, patients may develop prolonged erythema lasting for several months following 5-FU treatments.

Table 13.1 Topical modalities available for skin cancer prevention

Photodynamic therapy
5-FU
Imiquimod
Chemical peels
Laser

Imiquimod can also be used to prevent AKs. When used for skin cancer prevention, imiquimod is also administered for several weeks often with a second cycle after a few weeks of rest. Patients usually exhibit facial erythema for many months while being treated. A comparator trial suggested that 1 or 2 four-week courses of imiquimod were superior to a single course of 5-FU in preventing AKs [6]. A potential problem associated with both 5-FU and imiquimod is the possibility of poor adherence to treatment. Patients may forget applications or may misunderstand treatment regimen. This is more likely to occur if complex treatment regimens (on/off cycles, applications once or twice a week, addition of a topical corticosteroid or topical antibiotics) are used in elderly patients.

Peels such as phenol peels have been shown to be effective for the treatment of AKs when phenol is applied directly on lesions [7]. However, in most countries peels are not used very often to treat or prevent AKs. In addition, the long-term efficacy of peels has not been extensively studied as compared to other modalities.

Mechanism of Action of PDT for Skin Cancer Prevention

The exact mechanisms by which PDT prevents skin cancer are not well known. Animal studies using mice exposed chronically to UV radiation and treated with PDT on one half of the body showed that both ALA and light are required to induce a delay in skin cancer appearance [8]. This suggests that PDT prevents skin cancer mostly by local mechanisms. In addition, immune-mediated mechanisms could also be involved. Preclinical studies have shown that PDT can induce a cancer cell-specific immune response [9]. Repeated ALA or MAL-PDT could theoretically induce such a response and a recent report showed that tumor-specific immune response to BCC was higher following PDT than following standard surgical excision [10].

Local mechanisms of skin cancer prevention by PDT probably involve both specific and nonspecific phototoxic effects. ALA and MAL are both photosensitizer precursors that are transformed into porphyrins by cellular enzymes. Application of ALA or MAL on large skin areas with or without AKs followed by subsequent light exposure will induce a nonspecific phototoxic reaction on the entire area where the photosensitizer precursor was applied. This creates the equivalent of a nonspecific superficial peel that can eradicate small AKs and possible nonvisible AKs thus preventing new lesions.

Following addition of ALA or MAL, malignant cells have been shown to accumulate more porphyrins than their normal counterpart, probably because of their higher metabolic state. Preferential accumulation of porphyrins in dyskeratotic cells or in nests of dyskeratotic cells following ALA or MAL application on large skin surfaces may induce a more specific phototoxic effect, thus delaying the appearance of skin cancer.

Clinical Efficacy of PDT for Skin Cancer Prevention

Preclinical Studies

Following the report that ALA can be used as a photosensitizer precursor for the treatment of skin cancer in the early 1990s by Kennedy and Pottier, a number of studies were published on the ability of PDT to prevent skin cancer using UV-induced tumors in mouse models. In one of the first published PDT prevention studies, hairless mice were exposed to UV radiation to test the ability of various ALA-PDT regimens to prevent skin cancer [11]. This study found that multiple topical ALA-PDT sessions were able to delay the appearance of AK, but not the appearance of SCC. Subsequent studies conducted by our group using MAL or ALA in the commercially available hydro alcoholic solution showed that weekly ALA-PDT was able to delay the appearance of AK and cutaneous SCC [8, 12].

UV induction of BCC in animal models is more difficult than induction of AKs or SCCs. Our group conducted the first study on the ability of PDT to prevent BCC using a transgenic mouse model heterozygous for the PATCH gene. These mice eventually develop microscopic BCC following chronic UV exposure [13]. This study showed complete prevention of BCCs in mice exposed chronically to UV and treated weekly with MAL-PDT as compared to mice exposed chronically to UV and not treated with PDT.

Many of the early preclinical studies were conducted with broadband light sources that were different from the sources that were eventually approved by regulatory agencies for use with ALA and MAL. However, a study of the ability of ALA-PDT to prevent skin cancer in hairless mice performed with ALA in the commercially available hydro alcoholic vehicle and the Blue-U™ light source confirmed that ALA-PDT was able to delay the appearance of AK and SCC [14].

Clinical Studies

The efficacy of MAL-PDT for prevention of skin cancer was evaluated in a large multicenter trial involving 81 transplant patients with 889 lesions [15]. To be eligible, patients had to have 2–10 AKs within two symmetrical areas of 50 cm^2 located on each side of the body. On one side, MAL cream was applied on the entire area with occlusion for 3 h followed by 37 J/cm^2 of red light. This was performed at baseline and repeated after 1 week, 3, 9, and 15 months. On the other side (control area), individual AK lesions were treated (mostly with cryotherapy) at baseline, 3, 9, and 15 months. The difference in the number of new AKs between the MAL-PDT-treated side and the control area was significantly lower at 3 months, was at the limit of significance at 15 months, and was not statistically significant at 27 months. In addition to confirming results of preclinical studies, this study provided important information on how to use MAL-PDT to prevent AKs in transplant patients. These results and the personal experience of the author suggest that large surface MAL-PDT for skin cancer prevention should be performed at least twice a year on the same areas for transplant patients. Some transplant patients will require treatments every 2–3 months.

Another study was performed with 27 transplant patients where one area was treated with

MAL-PDT, while a nontreated area served as a control. A total of 63% of the MAL-PDT-treated areas were devoid of AKs at 1 year as compared to 35% of the control areas [16]. There was also a significant difference in the time for appearance of a new AK between the MAL-PDT-treated area and the control area. De Graaf et al. conducted a study where forearms of transplant patients who had at least ten keratotic lesions on each side were randomized to be treated with ALA-PDT or were left untreated [17]. They studied the appearance of new AKs and SCCs over a period of 2 years. They did not see any significant difference between the side treated with MAL-PDT and the control side. The results from this study are different from other clinical prevention studies conducted with ALA or MAL. The interpretation of the data from this study is difficult as the authors did not differentiate between AKs and benign keratotic lesions such as seborrheic keratoses. In addition, the PDT protocol they followed was probably not aggressive enough as they failed to show a decrease in keratotic lesions 3 months after PDT. Several other factors could explain the absence of difference in the number of new keratotic lesions including the fact that about half the patients received only one PDT treatment, the absence of lesion preparation (curettage), and the use of blue light instead of red light.

Preventive properties of PDT were recently studied in nonimmunosuppressed patients [18]. Two symmetrical areas of 50 cm^2 containing AKs were treated in immunocompetent patients with either ALA-PDT or vehicle PDT. ALA 20% was applied under occlusion for 3–5 h followed by red light exposure and this treatment was repeated 1 week later. There was a statistically significant difference in the number of new lesions 1 year after treatment. This study confirmed the preventive properties of PDT previously published in transplant patients. As opposed to the multicenter trial performed with MAL-PDT, the difference between the control and the PDT-treated area was statistically significant at 12 months suggesting that immune-competent patients probably do not have to be treated with large surface PDT as frequently as immuno-suppressed patients. In the author's experience, most patients who are not immuno-suppressed and who undergo repeated PDT treatments for skin cancer prevention can be treated once a year.

Combination of PDT with Other Modalities for Skin Cancer Prevention

There is limited literature on the combination of PDT with other modalities to prevent skin cancer. The product monograph for MAL requires the use of lesions preparation (mild curettage) prior to MAL application. This can be construed as combination therapy. In practice, physicians will often combine cyrotherapy, electrodessication and curettage or surgical excision to PDT. Using this approach, the larger or more keratotic AKs are first treated with cryotherapy, electrodessication, or surgery. This is followed by PDT in order to prevent new lesions. These more keratotic lesions can either be treated immediately before PDT or in the weeks prior to PDT treatment. If keratotic lesions are treated with electrodessication and curettage or with cryotherapy during the same visit, the author usually will not apply ALA or MAL on the treated area and will prescribe a topical antibiotic to be applied on these areas in order to prevent infection. However, application of ALA or MAL on treated AKs or BCCs could theoretically increase the cure rate of surgery, electrodessication, or cryosurgery. Formal trials are needed to evaluate and compare these two approaches.

Some physicians are using 5-FU before PDT to enhance penetration and possibly to increase efficacy [19]. Others have used 5-FU or Aldara after PDT both to increase efficacy in the treatment of visible lesions and for the chemopreventive effects. A study was conducted on 26 patients treated with ALA-PDT on the entire face at baseline and week 4 followed by half face randomization to either imiquimod for 16 weeks or vehicle for 16 weeks [20]. Reduction in the number of lesions was 89.9 vs. 74.5% at 52 weeks ($p<0.0023$) in favor of imiquimod. Unfortunately, the number of new lesions was not reported in this study. An important unanswered question when reviewing these combination studies is what is the benefit of combining PDT to another skin cancer prevention modality vs. performing additional PDT treatments. One of the reasons for choosing PDT as opposed to treatments like imiquimod and 5 FU is the shorter downtime. With combination therapy, patients still have long-term facial erythema as they often use imiquimod or 5-FU for many weeks or even many months.

An interesting study conducted with a human SCC cell line showed that the addition of etretinate, the metabolite of acitretin, enhanced the cytotoxic response to PDT [21]. More porphyrins accumulated in the cancer cells incubated with etretinate. The author has successfully treated with ALA or MAL-PDT several patients who were also taking acitretin. The outcome has always been positive, but clinicians should be aware that these patients are more sensitive to PDT and will probably have more important phototoxic effects. Studies are needed to assess the safety and efficacy of combining oral acitretin and PDT in patients.

Special Concerns When Using PDT to Prevent Skin Cancer

Pain

Pain during light exposure is expected with PDT. If a patient feels no pain or burning during light exposure, it usually means that there is not enough prophyrin accumulation to eradicate AK. The efficacy of ALA or MAL-PDT to prevent skin cancer when patients feel no pain is probably very low or nonexistent, although this has not been thoroughly investigated. PDT-induced pain increases when larger areas are treated. Therefore, pain management becomes an important issue when ALA or MAL-PDT is used for prevention of skin cancer as these treatments are usually performed on large areas such as the entire face. Most patients can tolerate large surface PDT sessions when strategies to alleviate pain are used (Table 13.2). However, some patients very sensitive to pain, especially older patients, may not tolerate PDT and another treatment modality may have to be used. The author will usually make sure that a member of the healthcare team, knowledgeable about PDT, is in the treatment room with the patient during the entire light exposure. This is especially important for the first PDT treatment as patients are more anxious if they never had PDT before. Patients should be told that pain will increase after the start of light exposure to eventually reach a plateau followed by a gradual decrease towards the middle or the end of exposure.

Table 13.2 Available strategies to alleviate pain when using PDT for skin cancer prevention

Strategy
Local anesthesia
Regional anesthesia
Fan
Cool air (Zimmer or equivalent)
Pause in light exposure
Water spraying
Cold packs

Several strategies can be used to alleviate pain including local or regional anesthesia, using a fan, spraying water on the exposed area, and the use of cold air. A randomized controlled study showed that both water spraying and the use of cold packs were able to decrease pain intensity in patients treated with PDT [22]. This study showed that the percentage of porphyrin photobleaching was lower on the area cooled with cold packs, but unfortunately efficacy data on AK were not reported. Local anesthesia is very useful when a BCC or Bowen's disease is treated, but has limited application when the entire face is treated. Local anesthesia should be performed without epinephrine to allow for sufficient oxygen to reach the lesion during exposure. Regional anesthesia can offer benefits in patients who are more pain-sensitive or when the physician wants to perform a PDT treatment with a long time between MAL or ALA application and light exposure [23]. In the author's hands, the use of cold air generated by a Zimmer device (Zimmer Medizinsystems, Germany) has proven to be a very useful way of controlling pain. However, one must be aware that too much cooling will decrease porphyrin production and may alter efficacy.

Photosensitivity and Photoprotection

Following ALA or MAL application, patients are sensitive to sunlight for about 2 days. Sensitivity is usually higher on the day PDT is done, but still significant on the day following PDT. Following red or blue light exposure, most porphryins are transformed into nonphotoreactive derivatives (a phenomenon called photobleaching). Additional porphryin synthesis occurs after the end of light exposure as there is residual photosensitizer precursor present in the skin. To decrease de novo synthesis of porphyrin after light exposure, patients should be asked to wash their face before light exposure to remove excess ALA or MAL. The author will usually ask patients to repeat this procedure after light exposure.

Photoprotection is usually not a major issue when PDT is used to treat BCC or Bowen's disease. An opaque dressing can be applied to the treatment site and changed daily for the first few days. However, this approach is not very practical when the entire face is treated. Patients should be warned that most sunscreens, even those with very high SPF, offer no protection against visible light. Visible light protection afforded by sunscreens is very difficult to evaluate both for patients and physicians as SPF cannot be used as an indicator of visible light protection. The author's group studied the ability of 2 SPF 55 physical sunscreens to protect against blue light sensitivity [24]. This study showed the Avene Compact 55 offers a protection factor of 22 against visible blue light. The author currently applies this sunscreen to the face of patients who undergo large surface facial PDT at his office, but still advises them to stay out of the sun and wear a large brim hat. The author has found that this has helped reduce severe phototoxic reactions in patients who undergo large surface PDT for skin cancer prevention. Patients are also told to seek the shade and use physical protection (opaque clothing) if they start feeling the same sensation they felt during blue or red light exposure at the clinic.

Prevention of Skin Cancer Outside the Face

PDT often tends to be less effective for the treatment of AKs outside the face and scalp. The same phenomenon is seen when large surface PDT is used for skin cancer prevention. Increasing the time between ALA or MAL application and light exposure will increase efficacy when PDT is performed on trunk and/or limbs. Many patients will require incubation of 2–3 h sometimes more for trunk and limbs. Other methods can also be used to increase efficacy such as using ALA under occlusion and/or pretreatment with microdermabrasion or glycolic acid peels. When using ALA for skin cancer prevention outside the face, the author usually uses occlusion with Tegaderm (3M) or Opsite (Smith & Nephew) and waits 1.5–3 h, sometimes more, between ALA application and light exposure. As this can significantly increase the phototoxic reaction in sun-damaged skin, it is advised to first treat small areas with different incubation times (for example 1, 2, and 3 h) before treating a limb or the entire trunk in order to determine the optimal time between ALA or MAL application and light exposure.

Use on Very Large Skin Surfaces

Both ALA and MAL come in units that are not ideal to treat very large skin surfaces. With an ALA Kerastick™, one can easily cover the entire face of a large patient, but it is difficult to cover significantly more than that area. If both forearms and hands have to be treated, two Kerastiks will probably have to be used. MAL comes in 2 g tubes and one tube used with occlusion can cover the face of a small- to medium-sized person. A single tube can still be sufficient for a patient with a larger face if areas without AKs and photodamage are left untreated. The use of more than one ALA Kerastick or more than 1 g of MAL during the same session is considered off-label in most countries. In addition, this significantly increases the cost of treatment.

Realistic Expectations

Patients sometimes have expectations that a single ALA or MAL-PDT session will prevent skin cancer and AK forever. This type of expectation is seen more often when patients are referred to a PDT center by clinicians who do not perform PDT and have a more limited knowledge of the technique. Clinical studies and experience gained by clinicians in the past 10 years show that such expectations are not realistic. Cases of long-term cure rate without appearance of new lesions were reported in patients with Gorlin's syndrome treated for multiple BCCs [25]. However, when ALA or MAL-PDT is used in older patients with AKs, a single session is not enough for long-term prevention. A single session may be enough to adequately treat all the visible AKs, but reappear lesions will eventually appear. One of the best strategies in patients with multiple AKs and a significant amount of past sun exposure is to perform regular PDT sessions. The first 2–3 sessions are performed at 2–4 weeks interval to clear all visible lesions. Thereafter, whole face PDT sessions can be performed on a regular basis to prevent new lesions. For most patients, a session every 6–12 months is sufficient. Immunosuppressed patients and some patients with very important skin photodamage will usually require more frequent sessions (every 2–6 months). The frequency of treatment is influenced by the intensity of the phototoxic reaction that the patient can tolerate. Sessions will have to be repeated more frequently if the incubation time between ALA and MAL and light exposure is short because of pain intolerance.

Protocol for Prevention of Skin Cancer Using ALA-PDT

Proper discussion of the PDT technique with advantages, disadvantages, side effects, and alternative treatment options is necessary before initiating treatment. Most of the explanations can be delegated to another healthcare professional. The author will ask for written informed consent from patients. Patients should be informed that the use of ALA or MAL for skin cancer prevention is off-label. Patients are told to bring a large brim hat to their PDT appointment and to make sure they don't have to walk outside under the sun after treatment.

In assessing potential patients for chemoprevention with ALA or MAL-PDT, the first step is to try to rule out the presence of skin cancer in the treatment field. The surface to be treated needs to be examined for the presence of melanoma, SCC and BCC. All suspicious lesions should be biopsied and adequately treated before performing PDT. If a biopsy shows the presence of a superficial BCC and the physician decides to use PDT for treatment, care should be taken to use parameters that are sufficient to adequately treat the lesion. For example, it is not advisable to use ALA without occlusion for 60–90 min for the treatment of a BCC. Even if these parameters are adequate for skin cancer prevention or for treatment of AK, they may not be sufficient for treatment of BCC and may mask the superficial portion of the tumor while intradermal growth is taking place. If AKs are present, the author usually performs a mild curettage for all hyperkeratotic lesions. In his hands, this increases efficacy, but makes the application of ALA somewhat painful as the hydroalcoholic solution tends to sting when applied on erosions or ulcers. Both ALA and MAL can be used for skin cancer prevention. The advantages and disadvantages of both treatments are summarized in Table 13.3.

Before ALA application, the author rubs the skin with acetone-soaked gauze. Care must be taken not to use too much acetone in order to avoid dripping into the eyes. This is followed by ALA application. The author uses the commercially available ALA solution (Kerastick™). Excess ALA is first applied on all visible AKs. This is followed by ALA application on the forehead, the nose, the temples, and the upper cheek. For nonimmune-suppressed patients who have little photodamage and have never had AKs or skin cancer on the lower cheeks and the chin, ALA is often not applied or applied in lesser quantity on these areas. This is often done for patients who

Table 13.3 Main advantages of ALA with blue light and MAL with red light for skin cancer prevention

ALA + blue light	MAL + red light
Lower cost to cover the same area	Less pain when cream is applied to eroded lesions
No need for occlusion	Possibly less pain during light exposure (controversial)
Commercial blue light unit covers a larger area	Approved (in some countries) for treatment of BCCs and Bowen

undergo their first treatment with ALA in order to try to minimize the phototoxic reaction. The incubation time for skin cancer prevention when ALA is applied on the entire face is usually between 60 and 120 min. Sometimes a lower incubation time of 45 min will be used for the first treatment of patients with numerous AKs and severe photodamage or in patients who are more anxious about the phototoxic reaction. Incubation time for skin cancer prevention rarely needs to exceed 120 min. The first treatment is usually performed with an incubation time of 60–75 min. The author uses a high-power UVA lamp to visualize fluorescent (red–orange) porphyrins at 60 min after application. If no fluorescence is detected, the incubation is increased until fluorescence is seen (patients are usually never exposed more than 90 min for a first treatment). Physicians who decide to use a UVA lamp to see fluorescence must individualize this technique to their practice as UVA lamps have different spectral output and irradiance. Before blue light exposure, patients are asked to rinse their face with water. The skin is then exposed to 10 J/cm^2 of blue light from a Blue-U device which corresponds to 16 min 40 s. Based on the fact that pain is often minimal after 10 min, incubation for 16 min 40 s is probably not necessary to obtain optimal efficacy. Immediately after light exposure, Compact Avene SPF 55 is applied. A prescription of topical antibiotics is given to patients with written instructions on what to do and what to expect in the days after PDT. Patients are required to stay inside the day PDT is performed as well as the following day. Patients are told that the phototoxic reaction is usually worst at 1–2 days after exposure. If there in an increase in pain, erythema, or crusting after 2 days, patients should come back to the clinic for reassement as this could suggest the presence of a complication such as impetigo or eczema herpeticum. Patients are usually seen after 1 month when a decision to perform a second treatment is made. The incubation time of the second treatment is adjusted according to the response and the magnitude of the phototoxic reaction following the first treatment. If a second treatment is required, the incubation time of the second treatment is usually increased to increase efficacy.

In most studies for AK prevention performed with MAL, the photosensitizer precursor is applied under occlusion and with an incubation time of 3 h. This usually induces a severe phototoxic reaction often associated with extensive erosions in patients with multiple AKs and significant photodamage. For skin cancer prevention, the author will either use MAL without occlusion or will perform tests on small areas of skin with MAL under occlusion. The incubation time for patients treated on the entire face without occlusion is around 60–90 min for the first session. This time can be increased for other sessions if the response is not sufficient. When occlusion is used on large surfaces, the author will expose small areas of skin to MAL under occlusion for 1, 2, and 3 h in order to find the highest incubation time associated with a tolerable phototoxic reaction. If PDT is used for skin cancer prevention, patients are seen at 1 month and the procedure is repeated if necessary.

Conclusions

PDT with ALA or MAL is safe and effective for the treatment and prevention of AK. This modality has several advantages over 5-FU and imiquimod and its use should expand in the coming years with the wider availability of both photosensitizers.

References

1. Hauschild A, Stockfleth E, Popp G, et al. Optimization of photodynamic therapy with a novel self-adhesive 5-aminolaevulinic acid patch: results of two randomized controlled phase III studies. Br J Dermatol. 2009;160:1066–74.
2. Roewert-Huber J, Stockfleth E, Kerl H. Pathology and pathobiology of actinic (solar) keratosis – an update. Br J Dermatol. 2007;157 Suppl 2:18–20.
3. Touma D, Yaar M, Whitehead S, Konnikov N, Gilchrest BA. A trial of short incubation, broad-area photodynamic therapy for facial actinic keratoses and diffuse photodamage. Arch Dermatol. 2004;140:33–40.
4. Askew DA, Mickan SM, Soyer HP, Wilkinson D. Effectiveness of 5-fluorouracil treatment for actinic keratosis–a systematic review of randomized controlled trials. Int J Dermatol. 2009;48:453–63.

5. Pearlman DL. Weekly pulse dosing: effective and comfortable topical 5-fluorouracil treatment of multiple facial actinic keratoses. J Am Acad Dermatol. 1991; 25:665–7.
6. Krawtchenko N, Roewert-Huber J, Ulrich M, Mann I, Sterry W, Stockfleth E. A randomised study of topical 5% imiquimod vs. topical 5-fluorouracil vs. cryosurgery in immunocompetent patients with actinic keratoses: a comparison of clinical and histological outcomes including 1-year follow-up. Br J Dermatol. 2007;157 Suppl 2:34–40.
7. Kaminaka C, Yamamoto Y, Yonei N, Kishioka A, Kondo T, Furukawa F. Phenol peels as a novel therapeutic approach for actinic keratosis and Bowen disease: prospective pilot trial with assessment of clinical, histologic, and immunohistochemical correlations. J Am Acad Dermatol. 2009;60:615–25.
8. Sharfaei S, Juzenas P, Moan J, Bissonnette R. Weekly topical application of methyl aminolevulinate followed by light exposure delays the appearance of UV-induced skin tumours in mice. Arch Dermatol Res. 2002;294:237–42.
9. Korbelik M. PDT-associated host response and its role in the therapy outcome. Lasers Surg Med. 2006;38: 500–8.
10. Kabingu E, Oseroff AR, Wilding GE, Gollnick SO. Enhanced systemic immune reactivity to a Basal cell carcinoma associated antigen following photodynamic therapy. Clin Cancer Res. 2009;15:4460–6.
11. Stender IM, Bech-Thomsen N, Poulsen T, Wulf HC. Photodynamic therapy with topical delta-aminolevulinic acid delays UV photocarcinogenesis in hairless mice. Photochem Photobiol. 1997;66:493–6.
12. Liu Y, Viau G, Bissonnette R. Multiple large-surface photodynamic therapy sessions with topical or systemic aminolevulinic acid and blue light in UV-exposed hairless mice. J Cutan Med Surg. 2004;8:131–9.
13. Caty V, Liu Y, Viau G, Bissonnette R. Multiple large surface photodynamic therapy sessions with topical methylaminolaevulinate in PTCH heterozygous mice. Br J Dermatol. 2006;154:740–2.
14. Bissonette R, Bergeron A, Liu Y. Large surface photodynamic therapy with aminolevulinic acid: treatment of actinic keratoses and beyond. J Drugs Dermatol. 2004;3:S26–31.
15. Wennberg AM, Stenquist B, Stockfleth E, et al. Photodynamic therapy with methyl aminolevulinate for prevention of new skin lesions in transplant recipients: a randomized study. Transplantation. 2008; 86:423–9.
16. Wulf HC, Pavel S, Stender I, Bakker-Wensveen CA. Topical photodynamic therapy for prevention of new skin lesions in renal transplant recipients. Acta Derm Venereol. 2006;86:25–8.
17. de Graaf YG, Kennedy C, Wolterbeek R, Collen AF, Willemze R, Bouwes Bavinck JN. Photodynamic therapy does not prevent cutaneous squamous-cell carcinoma in organ-transplant recipients: results of a randomized-controlled trial. J Invest Dermatol. 2006;126:569–74.
18. Apalla Z, Sotiriou E, Chovarda E, Lefaki I, Devliotou-Panagiotidou D, Ioannides D. Skin cancer: preventive photodynamic therapy in patients with face and scalp cancerization. A randomized placebo-controlled study. Br J Dermatol. 2010;162(1):171–5.
19. Gilbert DJ. Treatment of actinic keratoses with sequential combination of 5-fluorouracil and photodynamic therapy. J Drugs Dermatol. 2005;4:161–3.
20. Shaffelburg M. Treatment of actinic keratoses with sequential use of photodynamic therapy; and imiquimod 5% cream. J Drugs Dermatol. 2009;8:35–9.
21. Ishida N, Watanabe D, Akita Y, et al. Etretinate enhances the susceptibility of human skin squamous cell carcinoma cells to 5-aminolaevulic acid-based photodynamic therapy. Clin Exp Dermatol. 2009;34: 385–9.
22. Wiegell SR, Haedersdal M, Wulf HC. Cold water and pauses in illumination reduces pain during photodynamic therapy: a randomized clinical study. Acta Derm Venereol. 2009;89:145–9.
23. Paoli J, Halldin C, Ericson MB, Wennberg AM. Nerve blocks provide effective pain relief during topical photodynamic therapy for extensive facial actinic keratoses. Clin Exp Dermatol. 2008;33:559–64.
24. Bissonnette R, Nigen S, Bolduc C, Mery S, Nocera T. Protection afforded by sunscreens containing inorganic sunscreening agents against blue light sensitivity induced by aminolevulinic acid. Dermatol Surg. 2008;34: 1469–76.
25. Oseroff AR, Shieh S, Frawley NP, et al. Treatment of diffuse basal cell carcinomas and basaloid follicular hamartomas in nevoid basal cell carcinoma syndrome by wide-area 5-aminolevulinic acid photodynamic therapy. Arch Dermatol. 2005;141:60–7.

Fluorescence-Guided Photodynamic Therapy

14

Peter Bjerring and Kaare Christiansen

Abstract

The use of fluorescence-guided PDT is thought to be a standard component in every PDT treatment, and in photorejuvenation to ensure treatment efficiency, and to reduce risk of post-treatment phototoxicity. As protoporphyrin IX, in contrast to ALA, fluoresces at 634 nm (at 407 nm excitation), the transformation of ALA can be monitored noninvasively by detecting the skin surface fluorescence. This method has in the past been used in experimental clinical studies to optimize mechanical skin preparation, type of precursor, incubation time, topical delivery mechanism (vehicle) as well as the concentration of ALA.

The mechanism of ALA used in PDT is based on intracellular transformation of ALA to protoporphyrin IX (PpIX), followed by light exposure, which induces phototoxicity. The efficacy of this treatment modality is primarily dependent on efficient transformation of ALA into PpIX, which then provides the necessary phototoxicity upon the subsequent light exposure. As protoporphyrin IX, in contrast to ALA, fluoresces at 634 nm (at 407 nm excitation), the transformation of ALA can be monitored noninvasively by detecting the skin surface fluorescence. This method has in the past been used in experimental clinical studies to optimize mechanical skin preparation, type of precursor, incubation time, topical delivery mechanism (vehicle), as well as the concentration of ALA.

P. Bjerring (✉)
Department of Dermatology, Molholm Research, Molholm Hospital, Vejle, Denmark
e-mail: email@peterbjerring.dk

Recently a handheld fluorescence photometer (FluoDerm, Dia-Medico, FluoDerm Dia-Medico, Denmark [1], (Fig. 14.1) was introduced in the market. The FluoDerm was developed especially for the measurement of PpIX skin fluorescence independent of ambient light – thereby enabling easy routine monitoring of ALA transformation for individually optimized PDT treatment procedures.

Skin Preparation Prior to PDT Treatment

Standard guideline for skin preparation prior to PDT treatment for cosmetic purposes is degreasing of the skin surface by tape stripping, or more efficiently by wiping with gauze moistened with alcohol or/and acetone. For treatment of actinic keratoses (AK), basal cell carcinoma (BCC), and Bowen's disease (BD) curettage is normally performed to reduce tumor thickness and to improve penetration of ALA. As variation in

M.H. Gold (ed.), *Photodynamic Therapy in Dermatology*,
DOI 10.1007/978-1-4419-1298-5_14, © Springer Science+Business Media, LLC 2011

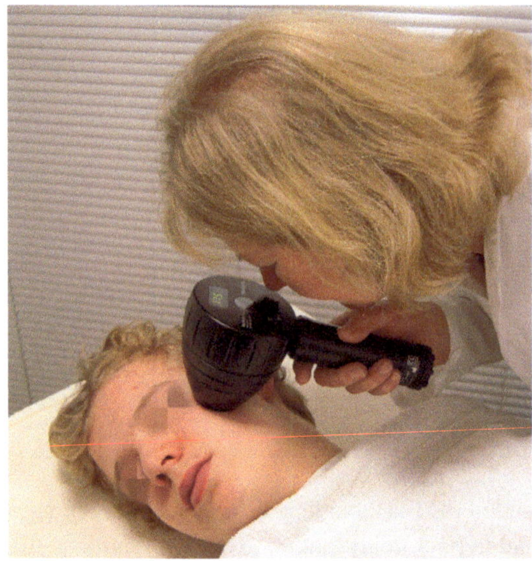

Fig. 14.1 Fluorescence monitoring with a hand held fluorescence photometer (FluoDerm, Dia-Medico, Denmark)

surface preparation of the lesions seem to vary from center to center, Moseley et al. [2] in 2008 decided to investigate the effect of either gentle curettage or abrasion with a spatula. ALA was left for 4 h (BCC) or 6 h (BD). The PpIX fluorescence was measured before and after surface preparation, and again immediately before and after light exposure. Only nonsignificant fluorescence difference between prepared (6.8 ± 1.8) and nonprepared controls (6.1 ± 1.2) were registered. The clinical assessment agreed with the fluorescence data as no significant different clinical outcome between prepared and unprepared halves of the lesion at 12 months was registered. This result is surprising and could indicate that beside the effect of degreasing of the skin, the thickness of stratum corneum may play a major role compared to partly removal of the epidermis.

Topical Precusors for PpIX Based PDT

Photodynamic treatment is based on accumulation of the photosensitive PpIX in the tissues. This is normally achieved by bypassing the limiting step of the haem biosynthesis cycle by exogenous administration of a precursor for PpIX in the form of 5-aminolaevulinic acid (5-ALA), or as an ester derivate of ALA such as methyl 5-aminolaevulinate (MAL), or hexyl 5-aminolaevulinate (HAL). ALA ester derivatives are more lipophilic [3] than 5-ALA, and the derivates are therefore expected to penetrate deeper into the skin than ALA.

In vitro investigations have shown up to 100 times higher transformation rate to PpIX for the ester derivative than for native 5-ALA [4, 5]. However, animal dosimetry models based on fluorescence spectroscopy in rat- and mouse skin performed by Casas et al. [6] and Juzeniene et al.,[7] showed only slightly higher PpIX levels for ALA esters than for 5-ALA. Identical results were found by Juzeniene et al. [8] in normal human skin (upper arm). Based on fluorescence emission spectra after 5-ALA applications less than 5 h resulted in higher PpIX levels than were obtained after MAL and HAL applications. For all three precursors, large inter-individual variations in PpIX fluorescence were registered. Measurements after 12 h application time showed that 5-ALA induced the highest average fluorescence intensity, and the average fluorescence from the MAL and HAL areas were 10 and 25% lower, respectively.

This corresponds well with investigations of human skin performed by Fritsch et al. [9] (biopsy based) and Wiegell et al. [10] (fluorescence based), where higher doses of MAL than 5-ALA were needed to achieve the same effect. The large inter-individual variation in PpIX fluorescence strongly indicates that PpIX fluorescence monitored treatment could increase cure rate as well as optimize treatment time and session numbers needed.

Fluorescence as Function of ALA Concentration

The most commonly used concentrations of pro-drugs for PDT treatments of AK and BBC are, according to a recent review covering 38 PDT investigations [11], 20% 5-ALA (Levulan® Kerastick®, Dusa, Wilmington, USA) and 16%

MAL(Metvix®,Galderma,Lausanne,Switzerland). Until now these concentrations have been more or less the golden standard and no efforts have been made to optimize the concentration for individual PDT treatments. However, Juzeniene et al. [8] published an investigation of PpIX fluorescence in different concentrations and application times in human skin.

Creams containing 0.2, 2 and 20% (w/w) of 5-ALA, MAL and HAL were applied on normal human skin of six volunteers for a 24-h test period. The amount of PpIX fluorescence in the skin was investigated by means of fluorescence spectroscopy. The correlation between PpIX fluorescence and amount of pro-drug concentration were nonlinear functions for all three products. After 4 h application time of 0.2, 2 and 20% 5-ALA, the registered fluorescence intensities were 7.5, 30 and 55 arbitrary units, respectively. The corresponding figures for MAL and HAL are seen in Table 14.1 and Fig. 14.2.

Table 14.1 PpIX fluorescence as function of used concentration after 4 h application time on normal human skin

Concentration	0.2%	2%	20%
ALA	7.5	30	55
MAL	1	7.5	40
HAL	5	30	40

Data from Juzeniene et al. [8], with permission

Low concentrations (0.2 and 2%) of MAL induced considerably less PpIX in normal human skin, than similar concentrations of ALA and HAL (Fig. 14.2). This corresponds very well to the findings that the necessary concentration to reach half of the maximum obtained fluorescence was 8.0±3.5% for MAL, but only 1.5±0.2% for 5-ALA, and 0.8±0.3% for HAL.

Recently, clinical use of lower concentration have been reported by Wiegell et al. [12] who obtained equivalent results after treatment of AKs with 8 and 16% MAL. Same MAL concentrations were tested by Braathen et al. [13] for PDT treatment of facial AKs, but here the lesion recurrence rate at 12 months follow-up after two treatments, increased from 19 to 44% by reduction of the MAL concentration from 16 to 8%. The registered difference in treatment efficacy again indicates that individual PpIX fluorescence monitoring might allow for standardizing the fluorescence before irradiation, and hence perhaps increase the cure rate and optimize irradiation dose and treatment time.

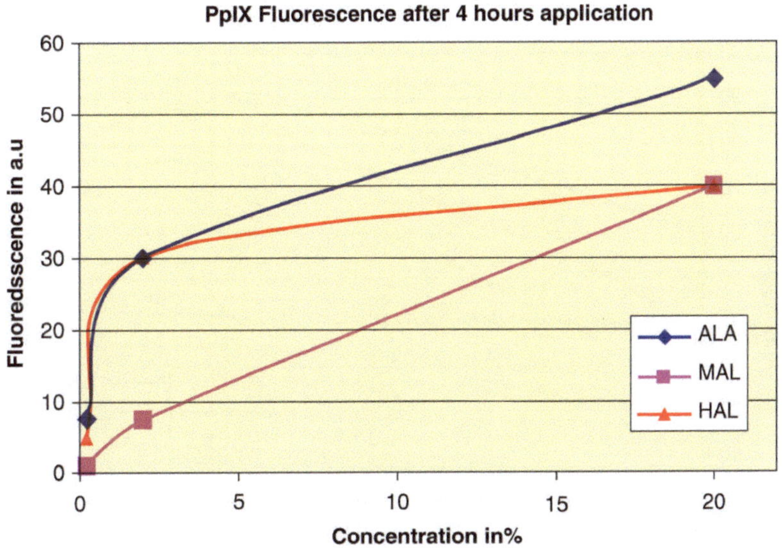

Fig. 14.2 PpIX Fluorescence as function of photosensitizer concentration after 4 h application time on normal human skin (data from Juzeniene et al. [8])

Fluorescence as Function of Incubation Time

In an in vivo dose study [8] on human skin of 0.2, 2 and 20% (w/w) of 5-ALA, MAL and HAL, a close correlation was found between application time and obtained fluorescence, as an indicator of the endogenously produced PpIX. In all three cases, the 0.2% concentration of the PpIX fluorescence level saturated after 8 h application time, while the fluorescence level continued to rise for the 2 and 20% concentration up to 14 h. For all three concentrations a linear correlation between application time and PpIX fluorescence was found for the first 6–8 h of application.

In 2007 we published a PpIX-fluorescence study of short time application of 20% 5-ALA [14]. Ten volunteers had 16 test sites designated on their backs. Twenty percent 5-ALA in a moisturizing cream base was applied under occlusion on four test sites, for 0.5, 1, 2 or 3 h. In eight other test sites, 1 or 0.5% liposome-encapsulated 5-ALA was sprayed every 15 min during the same time periods. Four additional test fields were used as controls, and each volunteer acted as their own control.

The skin surface PpIX fluorescence from each test field was measured before the 5-ALA application and again immediately after termination of the incubation time. During the following 3.5 h, fluorescence measurements were performed every 30 min, and for the subsequent 7 h, the time interval between measurements was extended to 1 h. In total, 2,240 skin fluorescence measurements were collected.

A strong linear correlation ($r^2=0.998$) between application time and skin fluorescence for 20% 5-ALA in cream was found in this study, which was in accordance with Juzeniene's observations [9, 14]. However, even more interesting was that the PpIX fluorescence continued to increase after the end of cream incubation and after washing of the skin surface. Figure 14.3 shows that independent of incubation time, the maximum PpIX fluorescence occurred approximately 8 h delayed (Average: 8:13 h, SD: 0:49 h).

The fluorescence obtained at that time varied from 1.6 to 9 times the fluorescence measured at the end of the 5-ALA application. There was a statistically significant difference between the observed fluorescence after 0.5 and 1 h incubation times ($P=0.0002$), but not between 1 and

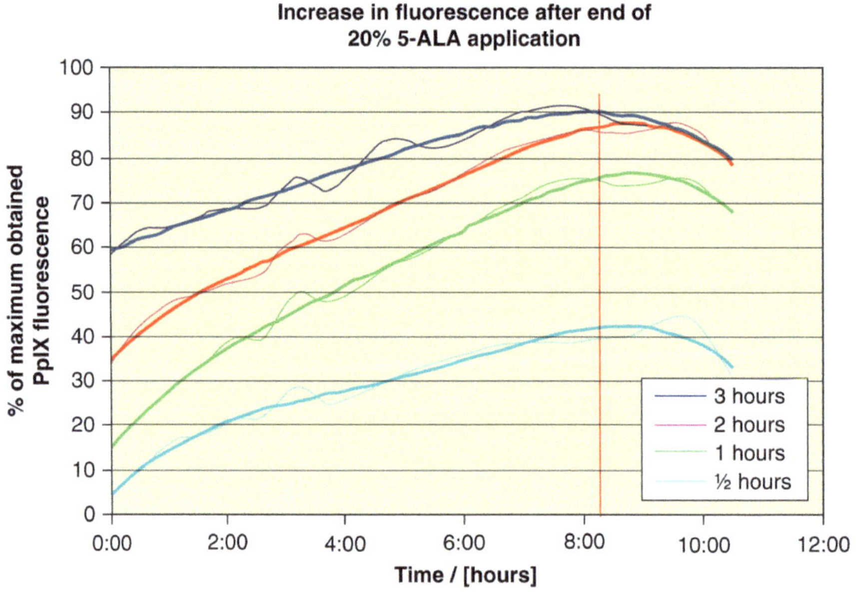

Fig. 14.3 PpIX fluorescence continues to increase up to 8 h after end of application of 20% 5-ALA in a moisturizing cream (time mark 0:00)

2 h, and not between 2 and 3 h incubation times ($P=0.069$, and $P=0.437$, respectively).

A comprehensive PpIX fluorescence investigation on normal human skin was performed by Lesar et al. [15] including both 20% 5ALA and 16% MAL. Application times of 1–6 h with steps of 1 h were used. As in a previous investigation [15] the maximum PpIX fluorescence occurred delayed. For 1–3 h application times the maximum PpIX fluorescence level for both 5-ALA and MAL occurred approximately 7 h after end of application, and the fluorescence increased by a factor 2.5–5 compared to the PpIX fluorescence measured immediately after end of ALA application. For 4–6 h application times the delay to maximum fluorescence was further extended to 24 h for 5-ALA, but unchanged 7 h for MAL (Table 14.2).

In general, if identical application time is used on normal human skin, MAL pretreatment results in approximately 50% of the PpIX fluorescence obtained with 5-ALA. Table 14.2 shows that the maximum PpIX fluorescence level, occurring 7 h after end of a 1-h application time, is approximate the half of the level obtained after the same application time with 5-ALA.

Table 14.2 PpIX fluorescence after 1 and 6 h application time measured 7 and 24 h post ended incubation of normal human skin

Application time/pro-drug	Measuring hours after end application (h)	One hour application time	Six hours application time
5-ALA	7	182 ± 113	220 ± 88
	24	52 ± 63	312 ± 88
MAL	7	97 ± 112	206 ± 99
	24	18 ± 14	68 ± 64

Data from Lesar et al. [15]

The 7–8 h delayed maximum PpIX fluorescence in normal human skin for both 20% 5-ALA and 16% MAL after application times of 1–3 h strongly indicates that light exposure immediately after end of cream application is not optimal. The efficacy of the light exposure is highly dependant on the formation of necessary amounts of PpIX, as well as the presence of oxygen in the skin during irradiation. The risk of normal skin phototoxicity due to exposure to ambient light after the therapeutic light treatment exists for as long as skin fluorescence is detectable. Therefore, the optimal light treatment after ALA application should start 7–8 h after end of ALA application when the maximum PpIX is fluorescence is reached.

A New Topical Delivery System

For cosmetic photodynamic photorejuvenation, reduced incubation time has been investigated in a series of split-face studies [16–19] with and without pretreatment with 20% 5-ALA. Significantly better clinical effect on fine lines and skin texture were reported for the 5-ALA-treated facial sides, with incubation times lasting between 30 and 60 min. Fluorescence measurements performed with FluoDerm after 30 and 60 min application of 20% 5-ALA in a moisturizing cream on nine volunteers [15] resulted in an increase in skin fluorescence of 4.0 FluoDerm Units, (FDU) and 15.4 FDU, respectively (Table 14.3).

Table 14.3 Increased skin fluorescence after short time application of 20% 5-ALA compared to spraying with 0.5% liposome encapsulated 5-ALA measured immediately after end of application ($N=9$ Caucasian volunteers)

	Skin fluorescence 20% 5-ALA application		Skin fluorescence after 1 h spraying with 0.5% liposome encapsulated 5-ALA		Skin fluorescence after 2 h spraying with 0.5% liposome encapsulated 5-ALA	
Caucasian skin type	30 min intervals	60 min intervals	15 min intervals	5 min intervals	15 min intervals	5 min intervals
Range of increase in skin fluorescence (FDU)	0–10	3–33	0–11.5	3–18	3–34	8–40.5
Average increase in fluorescence (FDU)	4.0 (SD:3.8)	15.4 (SD: 7.9)	4.7 (SD:3.9)	7.7 (SD: 4.7)	10.0 (SD:9.3)	19.8 (SD:9.6)

Due to the 7–8 h delayed response time for occurrence of maximally PpIX levels, side effects such as erythema, oedema, and crusting are often seen as adverse effects even after photorejuvenation with short application time of 20% 5-ALA [16, 18].

Therefore we investigated the efficacy of reduced 5-ALA concentrations down to 0.5%. In order to maintain sufficient transport over the skin barrier, the 5-ALA was encapsulated in liposomes (Photo Spray, Ellipse A/S, Hoersholm, Denmark). Also, the effect of different spraying intervals was investigated in a split face study, where nine Caucasian volunteers were randomized to spray with either 5 or 15 min intervals.

The baseline skin surface fluorescence from each test area on the cheeks was registered and fluorescence measurements were taken during the entire spraying period with 5 min intervals and further continued up to 2 h after end of spraying. After 1 h of spraying the volunteers obtained an average increase in skin fluorescence of 4.7 and 7.7 FDU for 15 and 5 min spraying intervals, respectively. After 2 h of spraying, the average increase in skin fluorescence was further elevated to 10.0 and 19.8 FDU (Table 14.3). The difference in skin fluorescence between 5 and 15 min spraying intervals was in both cases statistically significant $P=0.029$ and $P<10^{-4}$.

One hour of spraying with 5 min intervals resulted in an increase in skin fluorescence level which was higher than the fluorescence obtained after 30 min application of 20% 5-ALA in cream base (7.7 vs. 4.0 FDU).

For the treatment with 15 min spraying intervals, skin fluorescence continued to increase until approximately 40 min after the spraying was terminated, and reached a maximum level which was 47% higher than the fluorescence registered immediately at the end of the 2 h spraying period. In contrast, the increase in fluorescence level for spraying with 5 min intervals stopped shortly after termination of the spraying period and stays steady for 1 h before starting decreasing again (Fig. 14.4).

This short duration of post-treatment fluorescence after use of 0.5% liposome-encapsulated 5-ALA compared to the use of the standard 20% 5-ALA in a cream base may reduce the risk of unwanted clinical phototoxic reactions. Clinically equivalent outcomes with fewer side effects can be expected by changing from the standard 30–60 min application time of 20% 5-ALA cream to a new paradigm of 60 min spraying with 0.5% liposome encapsulated 5-ALA with 5 min intervals.

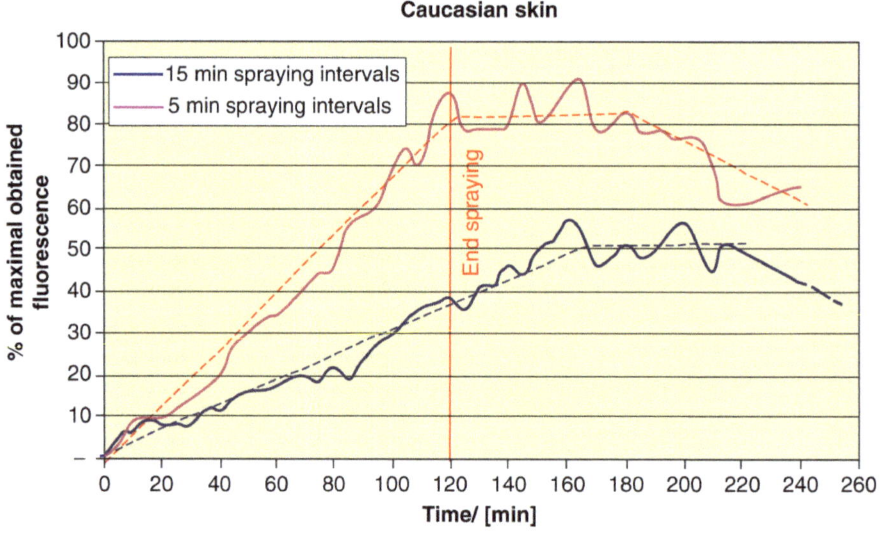

Fig. 14.4 Increase in skin fluorescence after 2 h of spraying with 0.5% liposomal-encapsulated 5-ALA with 5 min intervals and 15 min intervals

Effect on Different Skin Types

Also, skin type contribute to differences in transformation rate of 5-ALA into PpIX. In Asian skin the average increase in facial skin fluorescence was only 25–45% of that registered for Caucasian skin. After 1 h of spraying with 0.5% liposome encapsulated 5-ALA with either 15 or 5 min intervals, the increase in skin fluorescence was 0.94 and 3.9 FDU, respectively. The corresponding figures after 2 h of spraying were 2.3 vs. 8.7 FDU. These differences were statistically significantly different ($P<4\times10^{-5}$ and $P<6\times10^{-5}$) (Table 14.4).

A skin fluorescence level identical to 30 min application of 20% 5-ALA was obtained in Asian skin after spraying with 0.5% liposome-encapsulated 5-ALA with 5 min intervals for 50–90 min (average: 59.5 min, SD: 10.9 min). In Asian skin, a reduction in spraying intervals from 15 to 5 min resulted in an increase in skin fluorescence by a factor of approximate 4.0 (Table 14.4) after 2 h of spraying.

In contrast to Caucasian skin, Asian skin continues to build up skin fluorescence after 2 h of spraying independent of the spraying interval used (Fig. 14.5). The maximum skin fluorescence occurred approximately 45 min after end of spraying.

The average absolute increase in fluorescence after spraying of facial skin with 0.5% liposome encapsulated 5-ALA developed twice as quickly for Caucasian skin as for Asian skin (Fig. 14.6). The fluorescence level corresponding to 30–60 min application time of the standard 20% 5-ALA in a cream base was reached in Caucasian skin types after 40–90 min of spraying (5 min intervals). For Asian skin, the onset was delayed

Table 14.4 Increase in skin fluorescence in Asian skin after spraying with 0.5% liposome encapsulated 5-ALA measured immediately after termination of 2 h of spraying and again when the maximum skin fluorescence occurred ($N=9$)

	Skin fluorescence after 1 h spraying		Skin fluorescence after 2 h spraying	
Asian skin type	15 min intervals	5 min intervals	15 min intervals	5 min intervals
Range of increase in skin fluorescence (FDU)	0–3	1–6.5	0–5	4–11
Average increase in skin fluorescence (FDU)	0.94 (SD: 1.0)	3.9 (SD: 1.8)	2.3 (SD: 1.6)	8.7 (SD: 3.0)

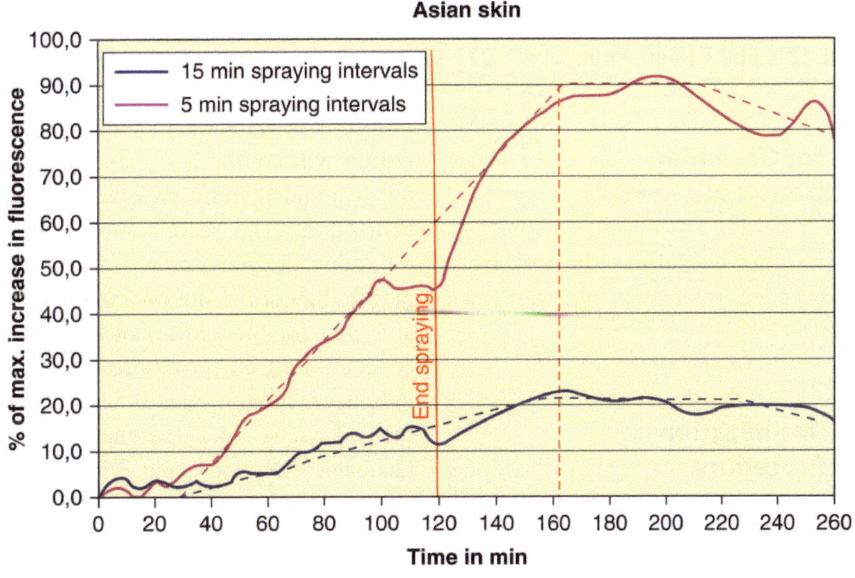

Fig. 14.5 Asian skin continues to build up skin fluorescence after termination of a 2-h spraying period independent of the spraying interval used (5 or 15 min)

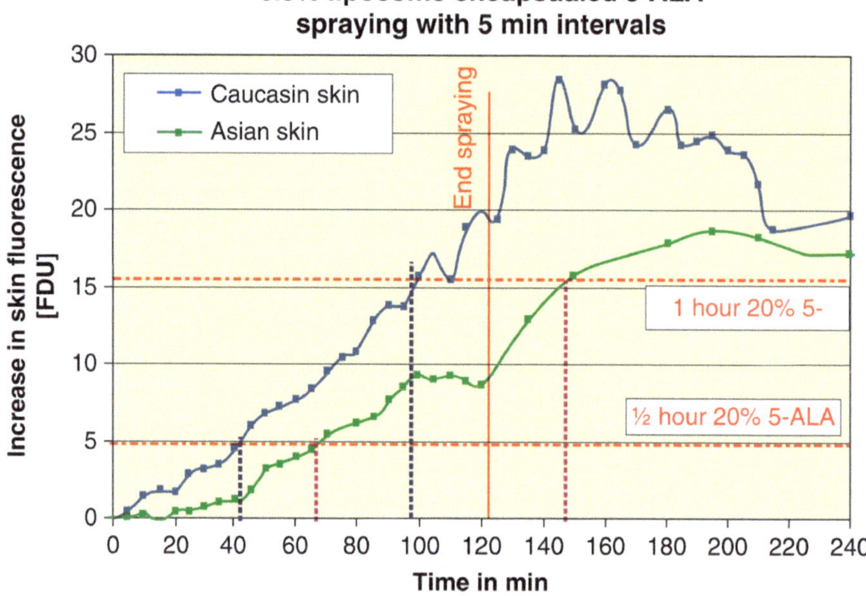

Fig. 14.6 The average increase in skin fluorescence after spraying of facial skin with 0.5% liposome-encapsulated 5-ALA developed twice as quickly in Caucasian skin as in Asian skin

and the same levels were first obtained after 65–145 min of spraying. This delayed onset may be due to the fact that Asian skin in general is thicker [20], with a corresponding longer diffusion distance and a larger distribution volume. This corresponds well to the negative correlation between skin fluorescence and thickness of stratum corneum, which has earlier been registered by Smits et al. [21] and Kleinpenning et al. [22].

Guidelines for Obtaining a Standardized Result in PDT

Table 14.5 presents guidelines derived from the previously cited references and our own experiments.

Individual Optimization of the PDT Procedure

As the inter-individual variation in transformation of ALA into PpIX is more than 10 times, and as differences in skin type as well as the used PpIX precursor both contribute with a factor of least 2, it is obvious, that no standard, fixed application time can be optimal for all patients.

There are at least two modalities for optimizing the treatment procedure, – both based on monitoring of the skin fluorescence development in each individual patient. In the first modality, the light exposure is performed as soon as the fluorescence has reached a level that is efficient for the actual type of PDT treatment. This procedure is the fastest, but does not take into consideration the fact that the PpIX concentration will continue to increase for the following 8 h and thereby pose a significant risk for skin burns. The second modality is based on removing the remaining 5-ALA from the skin before the correct fluorescence level is reached, and wait for the additional increase in fluorescence. Based on the fluorescence study of ten volunteers monitored at 0.5 h intervals for more than 11 h (Fig. 14.7) the final fluorescence level has been shown to occur 8 h after end application of 5-ALA. Even with the demonstrated large inter-individual difference in final transformation of ALA into PpIX (upper and lower limit marked with dotted lines in Fig 14.7), there is a clear correlation between the resulting added

Table 14.5 General guidelines for PDT treatment

Skin preparation	Degrease the skin prior to applying a topical PpIX precursor Gentle curettage to reduce tumor thickness seem not to improve the efficacy
Topical precursor	Use of 5-ALA results in higher PpIX level than MAL and HAL in human skin for application times less than 5 h
Precursor concentration	There is an nonlinear correlation between precursor concentration (5-ALA, MAL, HAL) and resulting PpIX concentration 5-ALA and HAL are less sensitive for variation in concentration as long as the concentration is higher than 2%
Incubation time	There is a close and linear correlation between incubation time and resulting PpIX level for application time less than 4 h The PpIX production continue to increase independently of application time for 7–8 h after end of application
Safety	Safety can be increased by reducing application time to 1–2 h and by postponing light exposure 7–8 h, enabling the skin to reach the maximum PpIX level For PDT-assisted photorejuvenation the use of low concentration, liposome encapsulated 5-ALA reduces the risk of post-treatment phototoxic reactions significantly [23]
Skin type	Asian skin need twice the application time compared to Caucasian skin to transform 5-ALA into PpIX
Inter-individual variations	The inter-individual variation in transformation rate of 5-ALA into PpIX can vary with more than a factor 10 Individualized treatment with fluorescence control is highly recommended

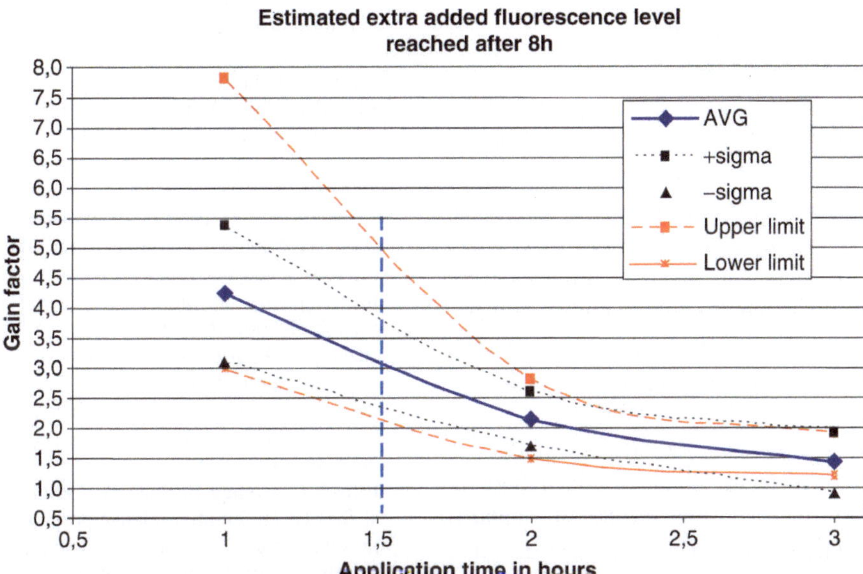

Fig. 14.7 Maximum fluorescence obtained 8 h after end of 5-ALA application. The *red line* is the average gain factor. The added fluorescence measured at the time when the 5-ALA application is stopped predicts the maximum fluorescence occurring 8 h later. +Sigma and – sigma are standard derivations (10 Caucasian patients)

fluorescence level at any given time, and the corresponding fluorescence level, which will be reached 8 h later.

For example: If a patient has a baseline skin fluorescence before ALA application of 20 FDU, and that this has reached a level of 60 FDU 1.5 h later, then the added fluorescence is 60–20 FDU = 40 FDU. According to Fig. 14.7 this patient will reach a maximal added fluorescence level of 40 FDU × 3.1 = 124 FDU 8 h later.

Taking the inter-individual difference in transformation rate into account, we can predict the lowest expected added fluorescence to be 40 FDU × 2.3 = 92 FDU. An added fluorescence level of 92 FDU will normally result in an efficient treatment in this body area, and therefore the 5-ALA application can be terminated, and the patient can be asked to return 8 h later for irradiation.

Skin Fluorescence in Aesthetic PDT (Photodynamic Photorejuvenation)

The added fluorescence needs to reach a certain level to ensure that the subsequent light exposure will result in an efficient treatment. Data from more than 100 PDT enhanced photorejuvenation procedures show that an added fluorescence of least 2 FDU has to be reached prior to light exposure.

Skin Fluorescence in PDT for Actinic Keratoses

In a study on AK 22 patients were treated on the cheeks, foreheads and scalps. The average added fluorescence level for treatment with no recurrence was 114 FDU (SD.: 51 FDU) vs. 76 FDU (SD.: 34 FDU) for treatment where recurrences were registered within 6 months after a single treatment. This difference is statistically significant ($P = 0.031$). No recurrence was seen in AK patients who had an added fluorescence higher than 90 FDU.

This study shows that the efficacy of PDT is highly correlated to the obtained added fluorescence before light exposure, and that a standardized efficient treatment can be ensured by a simple fluorescence measurement. Therefore we recommend not starting light exposure before a fluorescence level of at least 90 FDU has been reached.

Conclusion

The use of fluorescence guided PDT is suggested to be a standard component in every PDT treatment and in photorejuvenation, to ensure treatment efficiency and to reduce risk of post-treatment phototoxicity.

References

1. FluoDerm is a handheld device for objective real-time in vivo measuring of fluorescence. 2010. www.Dia-Medico.com. Accessed Feb 2010.
2. Moseley H, Brancaleon L, Lesar AE, Ferguson J, Ibbotson SH. Does surface preparation alter ALA uptake in superficial non-melanoma skin cancer in vivo? Photodermatol Photoimmunol Photomed. 2008;24(2):72–5.
3. Uehlinger P, Zellweger M, Wagnières G, Juillerat-Jeanneret L, van den Bergh H, Lange N. 5-Aminolevulinic acid and its derivatives: physical chemical properties and protoporphyrin IX formation in cultured cells. J Photochem Photobiol B. 2000;54:72–80.
4. Gaullier JM, Berg K, Peng Q, Anholt H, Selbo PK, Ma LW, Moan J. Use of 5-aminolevulinic acid esters to improve photodynamic therapy on cells in culture. Cancer Res. 1997;57:1481–6.
5. Kloek J, Akkermans W, Beijersbergen van Henegouwen GM. Derivatives of 5-aminolevulinic acid for photodynamic therapy: enzymatic conversion into protoporphyrin. Photochem Photobiol. 1998;67:150–4.
6. Casas A, Batlle AM, Butler AR, Robertson D, Brown EH, MacRobert A, Riley PA. Comparative effect of ALA derivatives on protoporphyrin IX production in human and rat skin organ cultures. Br J Cancer. 1999;80:1525–32.
7. Juzeniene A, Juzenas P, Iani V, Moan J. Topical application of 5-aminolevulinic acid and its methylester, hexylester and octylester derivatives: considerations for dosimetry in mouse skin model. Photochem Photobiol. 2002;76:329–34.
8. Juzeniene A, Juzenas P, Ma LW, Iani V, Moan J. Topical application of 5-aminolaevulinic acid, methyl 5-aminolaevulinate and hexyl 5-aminolaevulinate on normal human skin. Br J Dermatol. 2006;155(4):791–9.
9. Fritsch C, Homey B, Stahl W, Lehmann P, Ruzicka T, Sies H. Preferential relative porphyrin enrichment in solar keratoses upon topical application of deltaaminolevulinic acid methylester. Photochem Photobiol. 1998;68:218–21.
10. Wiegell SR, Stender IM, Na R, Wulf HC. Pain associated with photodynamic therapy using 5-aminolevulinic acid or 5-aminolevulinic acid methylester on tape-stripped normal skin. Arch Dermatol. 2003;139:1173–7.
11. Choudhary S, Nouri K, Elsaie ML. Photodynamic therapy in dermatology: a review. Lasers Med Sci. 2009;24(6):971–80.
12. Wiegell SR, Hædersdal M, Eriksen P, Wulf HC. Photodynamic therapy of actinic keratoses with 8% and 16% methyl aminolaevulinate and home-based

daylight exposure: a doubleblinded randomized clinical trial. Br J Dermatol. 2009;160:1308–14.

13. Braathen LR, Paredes BE, Saksela O, Fritsch C, Gardlo K, Morken T, et al. Short incubation with methyl aminolevulinate for photodynamic therapy of actinic keratoses. J Eur Acad Dermatol Venereol. 2009;23(5):550–5.
14. Christiansen K, Bjerring P, Troilius A. 5-ALA for photodynamic photorejuvenation –optimization of treatment regime based on normal-skin fluorescence measurements. Lasers Surg Med. 2007;39(4):302–10.
15. Lesar A, Ferguson J, Moseley H. A time course investigation of the fluorescence induced by topical application of 5-aminolevulinic acid and methyl aminolevulinate on normal human skin. Photodermatol Photoimmunol Photomed. 2009;25(4):191–5.
16. Alster TS, Tanzi EL, Welsh CW. Photorejuvenation of Facial skin with 20% 5-Amninolevulinic Acid and Intense Pulsed Light. J Drug Derm. 2005;4:35–8.
17. Dover JS, Bhatia AC, Stewart B, Arndt KA. Topical 5-aminolevulinic acid combined with intense pulsed light in the treatment of photoaging. Arch Dermatol 2005;141(10):1247–52.
18. Dover JS, Bhatia AC, Stewart B, Arndt KA. Topical 5-aminolevulinic acid combined with intense pulsed light in the treatment of photoaging. Arch Dermatol. 2005;141(10):1247–52.
19. Gold MH, Bradshaw VL, Boring MM, Bridges TM, Biron JA. Split-face comparison of photodynamic therapy with 5-aminolevulinic acid and intense pulsed light versus intense pulsed light alone for photodamage. Dermatol Surg. 2006;32(6):795–801; discussion 801–3.
20. Laurent A, Mistretta F, Bottigioli D, Dahel K, Goujon C, Nicolas JF, Hennino A, Laurent PE. Echographic measurement of skin thickness in adults by high frequency ultrasound to assess the appropriate microneedle length for intradermal delivery of Vaccine 2007;21:25(34):6423–30.
21. Smits T, Robles CA, van Erp PE, van de Kerkhof PC, Gerritsen MJ. Correlation between macroscopic fluorescence and protoporphyrin IX content in psoriasis and actinic keratosis following application of aminolevulinic acid. J Invest Dermatol. 2005;125(4):833–9.
22. Kleinpenning MM, Smits T, Ewalds E, van Erp PE, van de Kerkhof PC, Gerritsen MJ. Heterogeneity of fluorescence in psoriasis after application of 5-aminolaevulinic acid: an immunohistochemical study. Br J Dermatol. 2006;155(3):539–45.
23. Bjerring P, Christiansen K, Troilius A, Bekhor P, de Leeuw J. Skin fluorescence controlled photodynamic photorejuvenation (wrinkle reduction). Lasers Surg Med. 2009;41(5):327–36.

How I Perform ALA-Photodynamic Therapy in My Practice

15

Dore J. Gilbert

Abstract

ALA-PDT is a safe and efficacious therapy for the treatment and rejuvenation of sun-damaged skin, AKs and actinic porokeratoses, and acne. Clearance rates are typically very high with only several treatments. ALA-PDT does not require prolonged application and contact time compared with chemotherapeutic agents, resulting in reduced adverse events. Further, compared with other topical or systemic therapies, ALA-PDT is cost effective when applied to multiple lesions or broad areas. There may be some disadvantages associated with ALA-PDT including the downtime involved due to sun avoidance following a treatment, and the small-to-moderate risk of postinflammatory hyperpigmentation that directly relates to your skin type. In addition, many patients require multiple treatments to produce the desired results. Overall, ALA-PDT therapy provides a suitable alternative for treating sun-damaged skin, AKs, and acne.

Photodynamic therapy (PDT) is a fairly new and evolving treatment that uses a photosensitizing agent (that is activated by light exposure) and a light source to treat superficial skin cancers such as basal cell carcinoma (BCC), squamous cell carcinoma (SCC), and actinic keratosis [1–3]. This therapy is also used as a diagnostic aid for skin cancers. PDT is used for skin rejuvenation resulting from photoaging, and has proven to be an efficacious alternative therapy for the treatment of acne and rosacea [4–6]. Treatment is based on the application of light to activate the applied drug and release an activated oxygen molecule that can destroy targeted cells. The procedure is routinely performed in a physician's office or in outpatient settings.

The procedure for using PDT consists of three primary steps that include application of the photosensitizer, the incubation period with the photosensitizer, and light activation. The physician must determine if the patient is a reasonable candidate for PDT. For many patients, PDT side effects and recovery are usually milder with less downtime than alternative therapies such as freezing, chemotherapy creams (i.e., fluorouracil), or surgical procedures. The role of the physician also encompasses the evaluation of treatment, the expectations of the physician and patient for outcomes, the discussion of precautions regarding the use of PDT and possible adverse effects, as well as follow-up consultation and planning for additional treatment sessions or alternative treatment options.

D.J. Gilbert (✉)
Associate Professor of Dermatology,
University of California, Irvine, CA. Medical Director,
Newport Dermatology and Laser Associates,
Newport Beach, CA, USA
e-mail: lazrdoc@pacbell.net

M.H. Gold (ed.), *Photodynamic Therapy in Dermatology*,
DOI 10.1007/978-1-4419-1298-5_15, © Springer Science+Business Media, LLC 2011

This chapter focuses on three specific indications for PDT, utilizing the photosensitizer Levulan (5-aminolevulinic acid, or ALA). The three conditions that are covered include the treatment of sun-damaged skin, actinic keratosis, and recalcitrant acne (off label usage). This overview follows a patient from initial presentation, details the technical aspects of the PDT procedure, and discusses the expectations and outcomes of the physician and patient, and next steps for therapy.

PDT for Treatment of Sun-Damaged Skin

PDT improves the appearance of sun-damaged skin by increasing collagen production [7]. By comparison, most skin resurfacing treatments achieve results by removing layers of skin, resulting in healthier skin emerging as a result of the healing process. Orringer et al. indicate that protein Ki67, a marker of keratinocyte proliferation is significantly increased following PDT [7]. In addition, levels of both type I procollagen mRNA and type III procollagen mRNA (precursors to structural proteins in the skin) were increased following PDT and the effect lasted up to a month. Levels of the proteins procollagen I were increased 2.65 times compared with pretreatment levels and procollagen III was increased approximately 3.32 times compared with pre-treatment levels. Other molecular protein levels markers were also increased. The study utilized the photosensitizer ALA to increase the skin's sensitivity to light and improve overall outcomes.

The advantage of using PDT for sun-damaged skin compared with other therapies is the ability to selectively treat an entire area of skin damage, as well as precancers (blanket or field treatment). PDT also decreases the likelihood of lighter or darker skin areas that usually occur with other therapies due to postinflammatory hyper- or hypopigmentation (commonly observed with freezing procedures using liquid nitrogen). In addition, PDT facilitates an overall improved appearance due to balancing of skin color and tone and enhanced texture with smoother feel.

Initial Consultation: Selecting Appropriate Therapy

Following the initial consultation with the patient, the physician must determine if the patient is a reasonable candidate for PDT. Candidates that often exhibit the highest degree of success include those with lighter or fair skin and moderate degrees of sun damage. Patients with darker skin that easily discolors may not obtain the most desirable outcomes using PDT therapy. Patients who are sensitive to light, burn extremely easily, taking medications that may make them more photosensitive, or that are unable to stay out of sunlight for 48 h following the procedure, are also not good candidates for PDT. In addition, the physician must assess the location and type of skin lesions, the extent of damage, the success or adverse effects with past treatments, and overall level of health and degree of discomfort and cosmetic acceptability tolerated by the individual patient.

In the initial consultation, the physician should establish if the patient has sensitivity to light. These include previous sensitivities to light-based therapies, drugs that may increase photo reactions, and medical conditions such as systemic lupus erythematosus or porphyria [8–10]. The physician should also establish if other medical conditions exist that may affect overall wound healing. These conditions may include a history of staph or other skin infections in the recent past, frequent cold sores, as well as drug allergies to topical anesthetics or other photosensitizers. Further, the physician should be aware if the patient has a history of bruising tendencies, hepatitis, HIV/AIDS, or pregnancy.

At the initial consultation, I usually take photographs of the area to be treated as well as the surrounding area. The photograph documents the extent of the area to be treated, and is helpful upon subsequent visits as a comparison for the patient to visualize the degree of improvement. I also thoroughly discuss the procedure including the purpose, procedural aspects regarding cleansing and pretreatment with sensitizer, incubation period, as well as duration and type of light therapy. In addition I advise patients on continued use of their medications, discourage smoking for 1–2 days before and perhaps 1–2 weeks after the procedure, and refraining from heavy alcohol use before the procedure. I also advise patients on light exposure following the procedure, and the use of protective clothing and sunscreen and levels of physical activity they may incur.

Sensitizers Used for PDT

Photosensitizers are agents that have a stable electron configuration that at ground state is a singlet state. With exposure to light, absorbed photons of light convert the agent to a higher energy state. An ideal photosensitizer has low toxicity, is more rapidly accumulated by target tissue than surrounding tissue, is quickly cleared from normal tissue, activated at wavelengths of light that penetrate the tissue, and importantly, capable of producing a significant cytotoxic effect in targeted cells. Although many different sensitizers have been utilized for PDT, the current FDA approved photosensitizers include Levulan (ALA), Metvix (methyl-aminolevulinate), and Photofrin (porfimer sodium). Levulan and Metvix are applied topically for skin therapy, whereas Photofrin is used intravenously for internal cancers. Topically applied ALA and ester derivatives take advantage of the intrinsic cellular heme biosynthetic pathway to produce photoactive porphyrins. Through a series of enzymatic reactions between the mitochondria and cytosol, ALA is converted to protophorphyrin IX [11, 12]. This fluorescent molecule is essential to the transference of singlet oxygen species and the formation of free radicals, that ultimately damage various organelles as well as the plasma membrane [13]. The rate of porphyrin synthesis through this pathway is higher in malignant or premalignant cells, and is estimated to be from two- to tenfold greater, with a ratio of approximately 10:1 for porphyrin induction in skin tumor cells relative to surrounding tissue [14].

Light Sources for PDT

Light sources currently used for PDT include laser, intense pulsed light (IPL), light-emitting diodes (LEDs), red light, blue light, as well as other visible light. Photosensitizing agents can be activated by one or more types of light, and are excited by light in the ultraviolet and visible part of the spectrum [15]. The optimal wavelength is dependent upon the ideal wavelength for the particular drug used and the target tissue. Conventional light sources provide light covering the entire visible spectrum and include incandescent lamps, high-pressure arc lamps, low-pressure arc lamps, and light diodes. Incandescent lamps cover a wide range from 400 nm to infrared. High-pressure arc lamps contain mercury or xenon, while low-pressure arc lamps contain fluorescent material, whereas light diodes use narrow wavelength band of 20–50 nm, with no infrared emission. A disadvantage with these light sources is that they produce a large array of light, and it is difficult to focus the light on the target tissue. By comparison, lasers are a monochromatic light source, and have the ability to focus light on very small target areas with great precision due to the coherent nature of the light emitted. Diode lasers (632 and 670 nm) are used for PDT, as well as pulsed dye lasers (595 nm) [15]. Studies also show that pulsed laser light (on-off mode) is more effective than continuous illumination at the same power density, with the same photosensitizer [16].

PDT using Levulan and a proprietary blue light (BLU-U®; Dusa Pharmaceuticals, Inc.) is currently FDA approved for the treatment of minimally to moderately thick skin precancers termed actinic keratosis. This therapy is also designated as "super photo facial" when the photosensitizer is used with intense pulsed light. PDT aids in the removal of sun-damaged, precancerous skin cells. Sun damage, fine lines, and blotchy pigmentation is improved as a result of treatment with PDT. In my practice, I currently use ALA combined with IPL and/or Blu-U to treat sun-damaged or photo damaged skin, as the majority of patients respond extremely well to this treatment. Intense pulsed light therapy is a noninvasive and nonablative treatment that uses high intensity pulses of visible light for treating sun-damaged skin and for photo-rejuvenation. IPL systems work similar to lasers based on the principal that light energy is absorbed into particular target cells that contain color (chromophores) in the skin. The light energy is converted to heat energy, which causes damage to the specific target cells. IPL systems are different from lasers since they deliver many wavelengths in each pulse of light instead of just one wavelength. Filters are used to refine the energy output for the treatment of certain areas and to enhance penetration without using excessive energy levels. For patients with skin type I-light III, I prefer to utilize IPL with a 560-nm filter, 15–17 J, using a double pulse of 4.0 ms pulse duration incorporating a 20-ms pulse delay. For patients with darker skin type III and light IV, I utilize a 590 filter 17J, and a triple pulse of 4.0 ms pulse duration incorporating 30 ms pulse delays. In addition, following IPL treatment, the patient is placed under Blu-U for an additional 4–10 min, based on the severity of disease and what the patient can tolerate.

Alternatively, The BLU-U® offers effective, noninvasive and relatively pain-free (it may cause a burning sensation with ALA treatment) blue light in a narrow focused range at 417 nanometer (nm). The BLU-U delivers uniform narrow band blue visible light that efficiently activates porphyrins within targeted cells. When used in a series of brief exposure sessions (approximately 16 min), it provides a simple, noninvasive treatment regimen.

PDT Procedure

During the initial consultation, the patient is given a prescription for an antiviral as a precautionary measure to prevent the occurrence of cold sores that may erupt from latent virus as a result of light therapy. The patient will be placed on valacyclovir HCl (Valtrex®; GlaxoSmithKline) at a dosage of 1 g twice daily for 7 days starting the day before treatment. Although side effects with acute administration of Valtrex are infrequent, patients may occasionally experience headache or dizziness, nausea, or abdominal pain [17]. Photographs are taken of the patient either at the initial consultation or just prior to preparation for treatment.

The patient's face is cleansed to remove any make-up or moisturizers and then scrubbed with acetone to remove any surface oils that might interfere with the absorption of the Levulan (some offices use microdermabrasion to the tolerance level of the patient). The ALA ampules are gently crushed using the fingers, and the Kerastick is shaken for approximately 3 min keeping the sponge end up. Levulan is then applied in an even manner over the entire surface to be treated using gloved fingertips (we typically treat all sun exposed areas), with extra pressure applied to the target lesions. Care is taken to avoid the application of Levulan to mucous membranes. The Levulan is allowed to incubate for approximately 60 min (some patients may require up to 5 h of incubation) to enhance absorption. Following the incubation period, the patient rinses their face with water only (no soap). A numbing cream composed of benzocaine 20%, lidocaine 6% and tetracaine 4% is then applied and allowed to penetrate for approximately 15 min. The total incubation time for absorption of Levulan and numbing cream is approximately 75 min.

As noted earlier, based on the patient's skin type, for type I-light III, light therapy consists of IPL using a 560 filter, 15–17 J, with a double pulse of 4.0 ms pulse duration and a 20 ms pulse delay. For patients with darker skin types III to light IV, light therapy employing IPL with a 590-filter, 17 J, using triple pulse of 4.0 ms pulse durations and 30 ms pulse delays are used. During light therapy, there may be sensations of warmth, tingling, heat, or burning in some patients. A fan may be used to help cool off during light treatment. In addition, following IPL treatment, the patient is placed under Blu-U for an additional 4–10 min, based on the severity of disease and what the patient can tolerate.

Immediately following treatment, the patient's face is washed with mild soap and sunscreen is applied. Patients are advised to bring a hat with them to the office to wear after the treatment. The patient is then counseled on what to expect over the course of the next several days to weeks. Although for the majority of patients recovery is usually uneventful, some patients may experience mild dryness and a faint to mild sunburn of the treated area. A small percent of patients may have moderate or marked discomfort and experience a more eventful recovery resulting from increased skin dryness, redness, or burning. The majority of patients may experience some symptoms that include redness, scaling, crusting, and mild-to-moderate burning.

The patient is usually counseled regarding posttreatment home care on the day receiving ALA-PDT, and urged to apply ice packs to the treated areas and take pain medication as needed. Patients are counseled to stay indoors and avoid direct sunlight for 24 h immediately following ALA-PDT. PDT causes a temporary sensitivity to light, including natural sunlight and some indoor lights. The light sensitivity resolves with time, depending on both the photosensitizer used and dosage. It is recommended that patients be instructed to apply sunscreen to all exposed skin, not just the treated area and urged to wear a hat. Further, application of hydrocortisone 1% ointment to the treated area will help alleviate erythema, sensitivity, and reduce pain. The patient may take a shower if desired. For days 2–7 following the procedure, the patient should continue the use of ice packs and pain medication as needed. They should also continue to protect the treated area from sun exposure. If blisters develop on the treated area, patients are urged to use soaks consisting of white vinegar solution (1 tsp vinegar in 1 cup cold water). The patient should also apply ice over the vinegar-soaked areas for up to 20 min, and then pat dry. Petrolatum or hydrocortisone 1% ointment should then be applied. This procedure can be repeated every 4–6 h as needed. Petrolatum or hydrocortisone 1% ointment should be applied twice daily as needed during the week following the procedure. On day 7 following the treatment, if healing is complete patients may apply makeup if desired. Makeup should be applied over a moisturizer and the treated area should be protected from sun exposure using SPF 30 sun block for at least 2 weeks following treatment.

In general, many patients are able to resume normal indoor activities within 24 h of PDT. Most patients are able to resume normal activities such as work or school the 24–48 h following photodynamic therapy. However, for patients who must work outdoors, avoiding direct sunlight for the 48 h is crucial to avoiding a sensitivity response.

The patient is seen 1 week post treatment and then again 1 month later to determine whether second treatment is necessary. The patient is seen again at 3 months for follow-up and photographs (Fig. 15.1a and b).

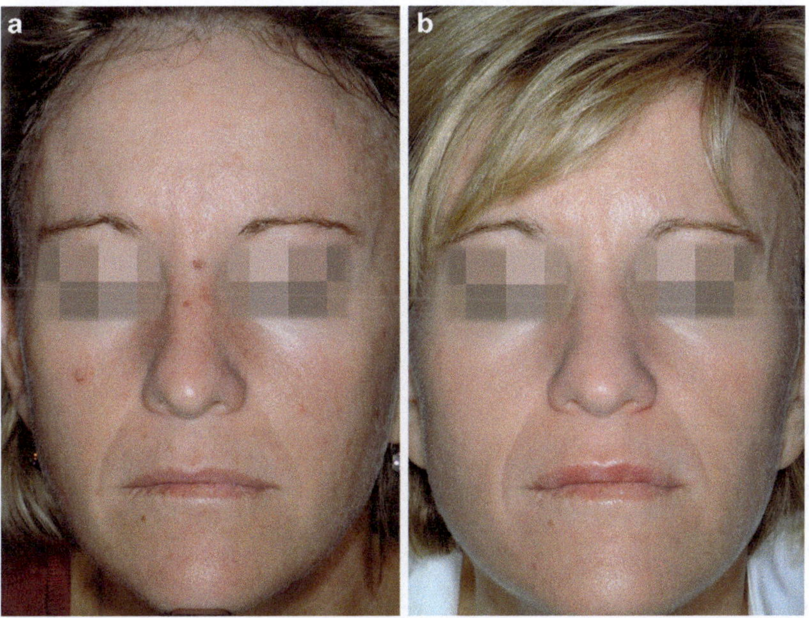

Fig. 15.1 PDT for sun-damaged skin. (**a**) The patient is seen pretreatment and then (**b**) posttreatment is necessary

Using PDT for Actinic Keratosis (AK) or Actinic Porokeratosis

Actinic keratosis is a UV light–induced lesion of the skin, that in some cases may progress to invasive squamous cell carcinoma (SCC) [18, 19]. AK is the most common lesion with the potential to develop into a malignant lesion on the skin and is commonly observed in fair-skinned persons in areas with long-term sun exposure, i.e., face, ears, bald scalp, forearms, and backs of the hands [20]. Frequency of actinic keratoses increase with age, proximity to the equator, and for persons employed in outdoor occupations, and is more common in men than in women; prevalence in the United States ranges from 11 to 26% [21].

Visual examination of AKs may range from barely perceptible rough spots on the skin to elevated, hyperkeratotic plaques that can extend to several centimeters in diameter. AKs may also contain an erythematous base covered by scale [22]. Lesions may gradually enlarge into broader, more elevated lesions. An actinic keratosis may follow one of three paths; it may regress, it may persist unchanged, or it may progress to invasive squamous cell carcinoma [21]. Although most actinic AKs do not progress to cancer, and as many as 26% usually regress spontaneously, up to 60% of cutaneous squamous cell carcinomas may arise from AKs [23]. Results of a recent study estimate that 1 in 25 clinically diagnosed AK lesions identified by histologic assessment were occult early-stage squamous cell carcinomas [24].

Patients with multiple, thin AKs on the face and scalp respond best to ALA-PDT. Patients that are suntanned should delay having ALA-PDT treatment until the suntan fades to avoid blistering, hypopigmentation, and reduced efficacy of treatment. A summary of patient selection and exclusion criteria is provided in Table 15.1.

Porokeratosis (PK) is a keratinization disorder characterized by one or more atrophic patches enclosed by a distinct ridgelike border termed the cornoid lamella [25]. The cornoid lamella is a histologic feature of all forms of porokeratosis and when stained, the keratinocytes beneath the cornoid lamella produce a pattern similar to that observed in squamous cell carcinomas. The PK lesion develops as a small, light brown, keratotic papule that slowly expands to form an irregularly shaped, annular plaque with a raised, ridgelike border. Lesions may be found anywhere, including the mucous membranes, although they most commonly occur on extremities. Risk factors for the development of porokeratosis include genetic inheritance, ultraviolet radiation, and immunosuppression [26]. Malignant degeneration is reported for all forms of PK, with estimated risks ranging from 7.5 to 11% [27, 28]. Treatment options for PK may include medical treatment (i.e., topical 5-fluorouracil, vitamin D3 analogs, imiquimod cream, oral isotretinoin, and acitretin), surgical removal of lesions, cryotherapy, and photodynamic therapy [29–32].

PDT Procedure for AK and Actinic Porokeratosis

The patient is pretreated with 5-fluorouracil (5-FU; Efudex, ICN Pharmaceuticals, Inc.) for 5 nights prior to treatment [33]. Although 5-FU is usually applied to AK lesions for 3 weeks, this reduced regimen is used since patients are able to receive the benefit of 5-FU prior to the onset of

Table 15.1 Criteria for selecting or excluding patients for ALA-PDT

Selection criteria	Exclusion criteria
Patients with multiple AKs from chronic sun exposure, Immunosuppression or organ transplant, or xeroderma Pigmentosum	Patients with photosensitivity, porphyria, hypersensitivity to porphyrins, or current use of photosensitizing drugs
Thin lesions that respond better than hyperkeratotic lesions	Pregnant or lactating patients
Patients with large or multiple AKs that have failed other therapies, or intolerant to other topical chemotherapeutic agents	Patients recently suntanned until tan fades or type IV–V skin

any adverse events. As previously reported, patients with multiple diffuse AKs may benefit from the application of 5-FU followed by ALA-PDT with IPL activation [33]. The results of this study of 15 patients with multiple and diffuse facial AKs in which 5-FU was applied nightly for 5 days, and the sixth day were treated with ALA-PDT demonstrate that at 1 month and 1 year posttreatment, 90% of treated AKs had resolved. Erythema resolved within 7–10 days following treatment. The patient is also placed on Valtrex 1 g twice daily for 7 days, starting the day before treatment.

The treatment procedure is essentially the same as previously outlined for ALA-PDT treatment of sun damaged skin except that the incubation time with Levulan may be increased due to severe actinic damage. Incubation time with Levulan may range from 1 to 5 h. Prior to treatment with Levulan, the patient's face is cleansed to remove any make-up or moisturizers, and then scrubbed with acetone to remove any surface oils and enhance the absorption of Levulan. Levulan is then evenly applied over the entire surface to be treated. Following the incubation period, the patient will rinse their face with water only (no soap). The numbing cream composed of benzocaine 20%, lidocaine 6% and tetracaine 4% is applied and allowed to penetrate for approximately 15 min.

For patients with type I-light III skin type, light therapy consists of IPL using a 560-filter, 15–17 J, with a double pulse of 4.0 ms pulse duration and a 20-ms pulse delay (Table 15.2). For patients with darker skin types III to light IV, light therapy employing IPL with a 590 filter, 17 J, using triple pulse of 4.0 ms pulse durations and 30 ms pulse delays are used. In addition, following IPL treatment, the patient is placed under Blu-U for an additional 4–10 min, based on the severity of disease and what the patient can tolerate.

Post procedure follow-up is essentially the same as described in the sun-damaged skin section. Immediately following treatment, the patient will wash their face with mild soap and then sunscreen is applied. Patients are advised to use a hat to wear after the treatment. The patient is counseled on the use of ice packs, moisturizers and sunscreens over the course of the next 2 weeks. We recommended the use of ice packs to the treated areas and pain medication as necessary. Sunscreen should be applied to all exposed skin, not just the treated area and when going outdoors, patients are urged to wear a hat. Further, application of hydrocortisone 1% ointment to alleviate erythema, sensitivity, and reduce pain is also recommended. If blisters develop on the treated area, the use of white vinegar soaks followed by ice packs is useful. Following use of soaks and

Table 15.2 IPL settings for use of ALA-PDT in skin types I–IV

Skin type (hyperpig. color), treatment number,	Mode	Pulse duration (ms)	Pulse delay (ms)	Fluence (J/cm^2)	Cut-off filter (wavelength, nm)
I–III (mild)					
1	Double	4.0/4.0	20	15	560
2–4	Double	4.0/4.0	20	17	560
III (dark)					
1	Double	4.0/4.0	30	15	590–640
2–4	Double	4.0/4.0	30	16	590–640
3–5	Triple	4.0/4.0/4.0	30	19–20	590–640
IV (lighter)					
1	Triple	4.0/4.0/4.0	30	15	590–640
2–5	Triple	4.0/4.0/4.0	30	15	590–640
IV (darker)					
1	Triple	4.5/4.5/4.5	50	15	640
2	Triple	4.5/4.5/4.5	40	15	640
3–5	Triple	4.5/4.5/4.5	40	15	640

Adapted from Gilbert [52]. Copyright Elsevier 2008

ice, petrolatum or hydrocortisone 1% ointment should be used. Petrolatum or hydrocortisone 1% ointment should be applied twice daily during the week following the procedure. One week after treatment if the healing process is complete the patient may apply makeup over a moisturizer if desired. The patient should also continue to apply SPF 30 sun block for at least 2 weeks following treatment.

The patient is seen 1 week post treatment and then again 1 month later to determine if additional treatments are required (Fig. 15.2a and b). At a 3-month follow-up session, photographs and review of patient expectations and progress are discussed, along with the physician's expectation of outcomes. The efficacy of treatment is assessed by the number or percentage of lesions cleared. The response is in part determined by the thickness, size, and location of the lesion. Clearance rates are typically greater on the face and scalp compared with extremities. The larger and more keratotic the lesion, the less likely it will be cleared with a single session. Although more aggressive treatments may result in greater efficacy of clearing and outcomes, aggressive protocols may also result in increased incidence of adverse effects and downtime. Most patients require at least two or more treatments for complete resolution. The durability of the response (time that the area remains clear) is also a measure of efficacy. The more effective the treatment, the longer the area will stay clear. Piacquadio et al. report in 243 patients receiving ALA plus blue light therapy, 86% of lesions responded completely after a single treatment [34]. There was 94% clearance after two treatments compared with 32% clearance after two treatments with placebo and light. In another study of 36 patients, 88% of AKs cleared completely after a single PDT compared with 6% following treatment with vehicle and light [35]. Similar results, complete clearance in 93% of AK patients were also reported by Clark et al. [36].

Using PDT to Treat Acne

Acne is a prevalent skin disease that may affect up to 80% of the population at some time during their lifetime. While the majority of cases clear over time with the use of over the counter washes and topical therapies, many patients are recalcitrant to treatment and require more aggressive therapy. For these patients, conventional treatments

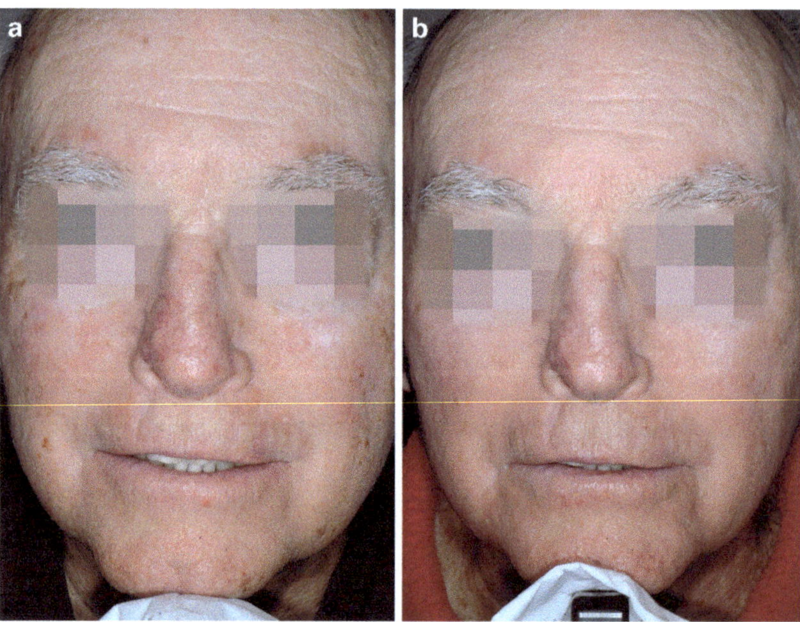

Fig. 15.2 PDT for actinic keratosis. The patient is seen (**a**) before and (**b**) after treatment

utilizing topical retinoids and antimicrobials, benzoyl peroxide, and oral antibiotics, contraceptives and antiandrogens often produce satisfactory outcomes. When patients fail to respond to these therapies, the use of oral isotretinoin may be required. Due to stringent Food and Drug Administration guidelines on the use and dispensing of oral isotretinoin, the use of light and laser therapies are often sought as alternatives for recalcitrant acne patients.

PDT combined with the use of ALA photosensitizing agent is an effective treatment (off-label indication) for mild to moderate acne [37, 38], intractable acne [39, 40], and moderate to severe acne [41]. The basis for PDT use in treating acne is that *Propionibacterium acnes* (*P. acnes*), the main bacteria that proliferates and initiates inflammation in sebaceous glands, produces porphyrins (specifically coprophoryphrin III) [42]. The prophorphyrins act as protophores that mediate a PDT response following exposure to blue light as a result of the generation of singlet oxygen that causes bacterial destruction. However, the use of blue light to treat acne only demonstrated mild to moderate effectiveness due to poor skin penetration by blue light. The combined use of ALA with PDT greatly enhances the efficacy of treatment for acne [43, 44]. ALA is known to accumulate in sun-damaged skin cells, nonmelanoma skin cancer cells, and in the pilosebaceous unit. Since exogenous ALA concentrates in sebaceous glands, combination therapy is more effective in reducing *P.acnes* since the bacteria concentrates in sebaceous follicles. Three possible modes of action for ALA-PDT in acne may result including the photodynamic killing of *P. acnes* that sterilizes the sebaceous follicle, direct photodynamic injury to sebaceous glands that significantly inhibits sebum production, and reducing follicular obstruction by enhancing keratinocyte shedding and hyperkeratosis [45]. In acne patients receiving PDT, high levels of light therapy may eradicate bacteria in a single treatment. However, high levels of light therapy may result in erythema, swelling, reactive acne, or pigmentation changes. As a result, lower light levels are used with repeated visits to prevent downtime for patients.

In one study, the use of blue light alone for 4 weeks resulted in a 21% clearing of lesions compared with 32% when ALA was used in combination; the authors indicated that ALA combined blue light is superior to the use of blue light alone [44]. When patients received two-to-four ALA-PDT treatments over 4–8 weeks, 11 of 12 patients in the study had a 50% improvement, and 5 of 12 experienced a 75% improvement in acne [46]. Goldman treated 22 patients with moderate-to-severe inflammatory acne vulgaris using blue light, with and without ALA. This study reported a greater response for the ALA-PDT blue light group than that achieved with the blue light group alone, with no adverse events reported [47]. In a recent study comparing IPL, radiofrequency (RF) and IPL, or blue light in combination with ALA, the results showed that at 1 month and 3 months median investigator-assessed improvements were greatest with IPL activation and less with blue light activation. The investigators concluded that ALA-PDT with activation by IPL appears to provide greater, longer-lasting, and more consistent improvement than either RF-IPL or blue light activation for the treatment of moderate to severe acne vulgaris [48]. The use of ALA combined with IPL is used to treat moderate to severe acne. When comparing patients treated on one side of the face with IPL alone vs. IPL plus ALA pretreatment, IPL decreased lesion counts by nearly 67% and IPL plus ALA reduced lesion counts by approximately 88% ($P<0.01$) at 12 weeks following three sessions [49]. These findings are similar to those reported in other studies, and suggest that ALA-PDT using IPL is an efficacious treatment option for patients with moderate to severe inflammatory acne [41, 50].

PDT for Acne: Initial Consultation and Treatment

At the initial consultation, it is important to question the patient regarding the history and prior treatment of their acne. Questions often include how long has the patient been suffering from acne; the use of antibiotics, dosage, and the duration of therapy; does the patient have a history of herpes simplex; does the patient have any photosensitivity; and, has the patient had any photo-induced drug reactions or dermatitis. The condition of the patient's skin is also evaluated to determine if it is seborrheic, normal, or dry.

Care must be taken during the procedure to protect the eyes, conjunctiva, lips, and mucosa during light therapy. During light therapy, most patients feel a burning sensation. If there is no sensation, the dose of light therapy may be too low; conversely, if the burning sensation is excessive, the dosing of light therapy may be too high. A series of three or more treatments is usually performed at monthly intervals. This protocol is consistent with others and in a study by Alexiades-Armenakas an average drug incubation time of 45 min and three PDL treatment sessions produced clearance in all 14 patients [51]. The number of treatments recommended depends on the severity of acne. Some patients may notice improvement following the first treatment. Unfortunately, more challenging problems often result from downtime following treatment, especially in adolescents. For adolescent patients, incubation times are usually cut in half and the patient is treated with either the IPL or Blu-U but not both. The advantages of PDT are the rapid treatment of acne lesions over the entire face with no scarring, no surgical excisions, and no systemic side effects. The skin appears refreshed and younger following these treatments. ALA-PDT is effective for decreasing pore size, shrinking oil glands, and reducing oily skin. The disadvantage of using ALA-PDT is that the patient's skin may redden and there may be some skin peeling for several days following treatment. Usually, the first 1–2 days present the most uncomfortable symptoms. As noted with discussion of other disorders, the patient is recommended to remain indoors the day following treatment to avoid sun exposure, and may be photosensitive for approximately 24 h after PDT. Topical acne lotions can be used in between Levulan treatments once the sensitivity and redness has subsided over a period of a several days. Unlike the use of Accutane, ALA/PDT does not result in the same serious side effects that result from the use of a systemic medication since ALA stays confined within the sebaceous glands, associated adverse effects are greatly reduced.

Most PDT treated patients should plan to stay indoors and avoid sunlight for at least the first 24 if not 48 h. In general, most patients will be able to resume all normal indoor activities the first day and are able to return to work or school the 24–48 h following PDT therapy. Again, avoiding direct sunlight for the first 1–2 days is paramount to avoiding an exuberant (red) response.

Typically, there is minimal to moderate pain or discomfort following PDT. Some patients report mild to moderate skin irritation that may include stinging and/or burning sensation and erythema or edema of the lesions, and mild to moderate dryness and tight feeling of their skin after PDT. This discomfort is usually improved with frequent application of topical emollients such as petrolatum or the use of hydrocortisone 1% ointment. Mild to moderate redness or swelling is not uncommon the first day or two after PDT and can be reduced by application of ice packs. For any blisters that develop on the treated area, patients can apply white vinegar soaks, alternating with ice packs. Following the use of the soaks and ice for blisters, petrolatum or hydrocortisone 1% ointment should be applied. This procedure can be repeated every 4–6 h as needed.

Follow-up appointments should be used to assess the efficacy of treatment and discuss outcomes of treatment from both the patient and physicians perspective. Three to four weeks between treatments should be allowed to provide adequate evaluation of the effectiveness of earlier treatments. The total number of treatments will depend on the degree of improvement with successive treatments coupled with the patient expectations. If after several treatments successful outcomes are not achieved, the option of continuing the present therapy or possible alternative therapies should be discussed.

Summary: Benefits, Comfort, Convenience

ALA-PDT is safe and efficacious therapy for the treatment and rejuvenation of sun-damaged skin, AKs and actinic porokeratoses, and acne.

Clearance rates are typically very high with only several treatments. ALA-PDT does not require prolonged application and contact time compared with chemotherapeutic agents, resulting in reduced adverse events. Any discomfort encountered with the procedure usually resolves within 24 h immediately following treatment. If erythema and desquamation occur, it generally resolves within the first week. Patients are usually able to resume normal duties at home and work activities within 3–7 days following therapy. Further, compared with other topical or systemic therapies, ALA-PDT is cost effective when applied to multiple lesions or broad areas. There may be some disadvantages associated with ALA-PDT including the downtime involved due to sun avoidance following a treatment, and the small to moderate risk of postinflammatory hyperpigmentation that directly relates to your skin type. In addition, many patients require multiple treatments to produce the desired results. Overall, ALA-PDT therapy provides a suitable alternative for treating sun-damaged skin, AKs, and acne.

References

1. Ericson MB, Wennberg AM, Larko O. Review of photodynamic therapy in actinic keratosis and basal cell carcinoma. Ther Clin Risk Manag. 2008;4:1–9.
2. Stritt A, Merk HF, Braathen LR, von Felbert V. Photodynamic therapy in the treatment of actinic keratosis. Photochem Photobiol. 2008;84:388–98.
3. Tierney E, Barker A, Ahdout J, Hanke CW, Roy RL, Kouba DJ. Photodynamic therapy for the treatment of cutaneous neoplasia, inflammatory disorders, and photoaging. Dermatol Surg. 2009;35:725–46.
4. Taylor MN, Gonzalez ML. The practicalities of photodynamic therapy in acne vulgaris. Br J Dermatol. 2009;160:1140–8.
5. Nybaek H, Jemec GB. Photodynamic therapy in the treatment of rosacea. Dermatology. 2005;211:135–8.
6. Katz B, Patel V. Photodynamic therapy for the treatment of erythema, papules, pustules, and severe flushing consistent with rosacea. J Drugs Dermatol. 2006;5:6–8.
7. Orringer JS, Hammerberg C, Hamilton T, et al. Molecular effects of photodynamic therapy for photoaging. Arch Dermatol. 2008;144:1296–302.
8. Poh-Fitzpatrick MB. Porphyrias, photosensitivity and phototherapy. Methods Enzymol. 2000;319:485–93.
9. Breuckmann F, Gambichler T, Altmeyer P, Kreuter A. UVA/UVA1 phototherapy and PUVA phtochemotherapy in connective tissue diseases and related disorders: a research based review. BMC Dermatol. 2004;4:1–11.
10. Abramson AL, Aivi A, Mullooly VM. Clinical exacerbation of systemic lupus erythematosus after photodynamic therapy of laryngotracheal papillomatosis. Lasers Surg Med. 2005;13:677–9.
11. Fuchs J, Weber S, Kaufmann R. Genotoxic potential of porphyrin type photosensitizers with particular emphasis on 5-aminolevulinic acid: implications for clinical photodynamic therapy. Free Radic Biol Med. 2000;28:537–48.
12. Taylor EL, Brown SB. The advantages of aminolevulinic acid photodynamic therapy in dermatology. J Dermatol Treat. 2002;13:S3–11.
13. Barr H, Kendall C, Reyes-Goddard J, Stone N. Clinical aspects of photodynamic therapy. Sci Prog. 2002;85:131–50.
14. Szeimies RM, Landthaler M. Photodynamic therapy and fluorescence diagnosis of skin cancers. Recent Results Cancer Res. 2002;160:240–5.
15. Szeimies RM, Calzavara-Pinton PG, Karrer S, et al. Topical photodynamic therapy in dermatology. J Photochem Photobiol. 1996;36:213–9.
16. Muller S, Walt H, Dobler-Girdziunaite D, et al. Enhanced photodynamic effects using fractionated laser light. J Photochem Photobiol B. 1998;42:67–70.
17. Dworkin RH, Johnson RW, Breuer J, et al. Recommendations for the management of herpes zoster. Clin Infect Dis. 2007;44 suppl 1:S1–26.
18. Glogau RG. The risk of progression to invasive disease. J Am Acad Dermatol. 2000;42:23–4.
19. Leffell DJ. The scientific basis of skin cancer. J Am Acad Dermatol. 2000;42:18–22.
20. Salasche SJ. Epidemiology of actinic keratoses and squamous cell carcinoma. J Am Acad Dermatol. 2000;42:4–7.
21. Anwar J, Wrone DA, Kimyai-Asadi A, Alam M. The development of actinic keratosis into invasive squamous cell carcinoma: evidence and evolving classification schemes. Clin Dermatol. 2004;22:189–96.
22. Roewert-Huber J, Stockfleth E, Kerl H. Pathology and pathobiology of actinic (solar) keratosis – an update. Br J Dermatol. 2007;157 suppl 2:18–20.
23. Marks R, Rennie G, Selwood TS. Malignant transformation of solar keratoses to squamous cell carcinoma. Lancet. 1988;1:795–7.
24. Ehriq T, Cockerell C, Piacquadio D, Dromgoole S. Actinic keratoses and the incidence of occult squamous cell carcinoma: a clinical-histopathologic correlation. Dermatol Surg. 2006;32:1261–5.
25. Kang BD, Kye YC, Kim SN. Disseminated superficial actinic porokeratosis with both typical and prurigo nodularis-like lesions. J Dermatol. 2001;28:81–5.
26. Herranz P, Pizarro A, De Lucas R, et al. High incidence of porokeratosis in renal transplant recipients. Br J Dermatol. 1997;136:176–9.
27. Guenova E, Hoetzenecker W, Metzler G, Rocken M, Schaller M. Multicentric Bowen disease in linear porokeratosis. Eur J Dermatol. 2007;17:430–9.
28. Sasson M, Krain AD. Porokeratosis and cutaneous malignancy. A review. Dermatol Surg. 1996;22:339–42.

29. Danby W. Treatment of porokeratosis with fluorouracil and salicylic acid under occlusion. Dermatol Online J. 2003;9:33.
30. Harrison PV, Stollery N. Disseminated superficial actinic porokeratosis responding to calcipotriol. Clin Exp Dermatol. 1994;19:95.
31. Jain S. Successful treatment of porokeratosis of Mibelli with imiquimod 5% cream. Clin Exp Dermatol. 2006;97:77–8.
32. Garcia-Navarro X, Garces JR, Baselga E, Alomar A. Linear porokeratosis: excellent response to photodynamic therapy. Arch Dermatol. 2009;145: 526–7.
33. Gilbert DJ. Treatment of actinic keratoses with sequential combination of 5-fluorouracil and photodynamic therapy. J Drugs Dermatol. 2005;4:161–3.
34. Piacquadio DJ, Chen DM, Farber HF, et al. Photodynamic therapy with aminolevulinic acid topical solution and visible blue light in the treatment of multiple actinic keratoses of the face and scalp: investigator-blinded, phase 3, multicenter trials. Arch Dermatol. 2004;140:41–6.
35. Jeffes EW, McCullough JL, Weinstein GD, Kaplan R, Glazer SD, Taylor JR. Photodynamic therapy of actinic keratoses with topical aminolevulinic acid hydrochloride and fluorescent blue light. J Am Acad Dermatol. 2001;45:96–104.
36. Clark C, Bryden A, Dawe R, Moseley H, Ferguson J, Ibbotson SH. Topical 5-aminolaevulinic acid photodynamic therapy for cutaneous lesions: outcome and comparison of light sources. Photodermatol Photoimmunol Photomed. 2003;19:134–41.
37. Goldman MP, Boyce S. A single-center study of aminolevulinic acid and 417 nm photodynamic therapy in the treatment of moderate to severe acne vulgaris. J Drugs Dermatol. 2003;2:393–6.
38. Pollock B, Turner D, Stringer MR, et al. Topical aminolaevulinic acid-photodynamic therapy for the treatment of acne vulgaris: a study of clinical efficacy and mechanism of action. Br J Dermatol. 2004;151: 616–22.
39. Itoh Y, Ninomiya Y, Tajima S, Ishibashi A. Photodynamic therapy for acne vulgaris with topical 5-aminolevulinic acid. Arch Dermatol. 2000;136: 1093–5.
40. Itoh Y, Ninomiya Y, Tajima S, Ishibashi A. Photodynamic therapy of acne vulgaris with topical delta aminolevulinic acid and incoherent light in Japanese patients. Br J Dermatol. 2001;144:575–9.
41. Gold MH, Bradshaw VL, Boring MM, Bridges TM, Biron JA, Carter LN. The use of a novel intense pulsed light and heat source and ALA-PDT in the treatment of moderate to severe inflammatory acne vulgaris. J Drugs Dermatol. 2004;3 suppl 6:S15–9.
42. Schaller M, Loewenstein M, Borelli C, et al. Induction of a chemoattractive proinflammatory cytokine response after stimulation of keratinocytes with Propionibacterium acnes and coproporphyrin III. Br J Dermatol. 2005;153:66–71.
43. Gold MH. Efficacy of lasers and PDT for the treatment of acne vulgaris. Skin Therapy Lett. 2007;12:1–6.
44. Akaraphanth R, Kanjanawanitchkul W, Gritiyarangsan P. Efficacy of ALA-PDT vs blue light in the treatment of acne. Photodermatol Photoimmunol Photomed. 2007;23:186–90.
45. Hongcharu W, Taylor CR, Chang Y, et al. Topical ALA-photodynamic therapy for the treatment of acne vulgaris. J Invest Dermatol. 2000;115:183–92.
46. Taub AF. Photodynamic therapy for the treatment of acne: a pilot study. J Drugs Dermatol. 2004;3:S10–4.
47. Goldman MP. Using 5-aminolevulinic acid to treat acne and sebaceous hyperplasia. Cosmetic Dermatol. 2003;16:57–8.
48. Taub AF. A comparison of intense pulsed light, combination radiofrequency and intense pulsed light, and blue light in photodynamic therapy for acne vulgaris. J Drugs Dermatol. 2007;6:1010–6.
49. Rojanamatin J, Choawawanich P. Treatment of inflammatory facial acne vulgaris with intense pulsed light and short contact of topical 5-aminolevulinic acid: a pilot study. Dermatol Surg. 2006;32:991–6.
50. Santos MA, Belo VG, Santos G. Effectiveness of photodynamic therapy with topical 5-aminolevulinic acid and intense pulsed light versus intense pulsed light alone in the treatment of acne vulgaris: comparative study. Dermatol Surg. 2005;31:910–5.
51. Alexiades-Armenakas MR. Long-pulsed dye laser-mediated photodynamic therapy combined with topical therapy for mild-to-severe comedonal, inflammatory, or cystic acne. J Drugs Dermatol. 2006;5:45–55.
52. Gilbert DJ. Treatment of sebaceous hyperplasia. In: Goldman MP, editor. Photodynamic therapy. 2nd ed. Philadelphia: Saunders; 2008.

How We Perform Photodynamic Therapy MAL in Clinical Practice

16

Hannah C. de Vijlder and H.A. Martino Neumann

Abstract

Many clinical trials have been reported on MAL-PDT for treating nonmelanoma skin cancer (NMSC), and acne vulgaris. Although response rates are high for NMSC, they do not match the response rates of (Mohs' micrographic) surgery, especially for deeper lesions. The delivery of sufficient (precursor of) PpIX and light to the full depth of the lesion and sufficient supply of oxygen are critical in topical PDT. Optimization of these factors to improve the response rates for the deeper lesions is an area under investigation. Beside this technical limitation, pain associated with PDT is an important patient-related limitation of PDT. Although a lot of research has been done into the efficiency of PDT, more work needs to be done on the effect of various treatment variables on the efficiency and adverse effects of PDT in order to develop an optimum treatment protocol for both NMSC and acne vulgaris.

Photodynamic therapy (PDT) has become very popular in the last decade, especially for treating (pre)malignant cutaneous lesions. In Europe, PDT plays an important role in everyday dermato-oncology care. Other good indications such as acne vulgaris and skin rejuvenation are not frequently treated with PDT in Europe.

Methyl-aminolevulinate (MAL) is the main photosensitizer that is used in Europe. It is commercially known as Metvix® or Metvixia® (PhotoCure ASA, Oslo, Norway) with marketing rights by Galderma (Europe/USA). Metvix® has European Union approval for the treatment of nonhyperkeratotic actinic keratoses (AKs) on the face and the scalp, and for the treatment of superficial (s) and/or nodular (n) basal cell carcinoma (BCC), which are "unsuitable" for conventional therapy. Moreover, it has approval for the treatment of Bowen's disease when excision is less suitable. MAL has not yet been registered in Europe for treating other indications such as acne vulgaris and skin rejuvenation. In the USA, MAL has FDA approval for the treatment of thin and moderately thick, nonhyperkeratotic, nonpigmented Aks on the face and the scalp in immunocompetent patients.

PDT is often repeated in the treatment of malignant cutaneous lesions because a single treatment yields poor long-term results. Therefore, MAL-PDT for the treatment of sBCCs and Bowen's disease, using the Galderma Metvix®

H.C. de Vijlder (✉)
Department of Dermatology, Erasmus Medical Center Rotterdam, Rotterdam, The Netherlands
e-mail: h.devijlder@erasmusmc.nl

M.H. Gold (ed.), *Photodynamic Therapy in Dermatology*,
DOI 10.1007/978-1-4419-1298-5_16, © Springer Science+Business Media, LLC 2011

protocol is repeated 7 days after the first treatment. Another strategy to improve the effectiveness of PDT is by splitting the illumination scheme into two light fractions separated by a dark interval on the same day. The effect of fractionated 5-aminolevulinic acid (ALA)-PDT was investigated in preclinical and clinical studies. It was reported in the preclinical studies that the response to ALA-PDT following a twofold illumination scheme in which the two light fractions were separated by a dark interval of 2 h was significantly increased, as compared with the response to a single illumination scheme [1]. The increase in efficacy using fractionated PDT was confirmed in randomized clinical trials (RCTs) [2, 3]. However, using this illumination scheme for MAL-PDT did not lead to an increased response [4]. Differences in the biophysical and the biochemical characteristics of ALA and MAL may be important for the differences in the response to fractionated PDT. Thus, although the basic principle of MAL- and ALA-PDT may be the same, it is impossible to translate MAL to ALA and vice versa because of the difference in their chemical structure.

This difference may also be responsible for the difference in adverse effects such as pain during illumination. A drawback of PDT is the stinging and burning pain that can accompany treatment. The severity of pain varies from a transient discomfort to severe pain. Fewer adverse effects with MAL-PDT than with ALA-PDT in the treatment of both acne vulgaris and nonmelanoma (pre)malignant skin lesions were reported in two studies [5, 6].

We discuss "How to use MAL" for treating nonmelanoma (pre) malignant skin lesions and acne vulgaris in this chapter. The proposed treatment schemes represent "best practice," and should be up-dated as and when the evidence supporting the improvements becomes available.

How the Authors Perform MAL PDT for Skin Cancers

There is no argument today as to whether MAL-PDT is an effective treatment for AKs and sBCCs [7]. Theoretically, carcinoma in situ-Bowen's disease is also an excellent indication for PDT, but good RCTs reporting long-term results are lacking. In our opinion, PDT is not the treatment of choice for nBCCs. Although topical MAL was reported to effectively penetrate into thick nodular BCC lesions [8], high efficacy in the treatment of nBCCs as compared with excision could not be clinically confirmed [9]. Our recommendation is that (Mohs' micrographic) surgery is the first choice of treatment for nBCCs.

The following protocol for the proper use of MAL applies to Metvix®. Metvix® contains 160 mg/g MAL (Figs. 16.1–16.9). One treatment session is recommended for the treatment of AKs. The treatment session should be repeated at 7 days for the treatment of sBCCs and Bowen's disease.

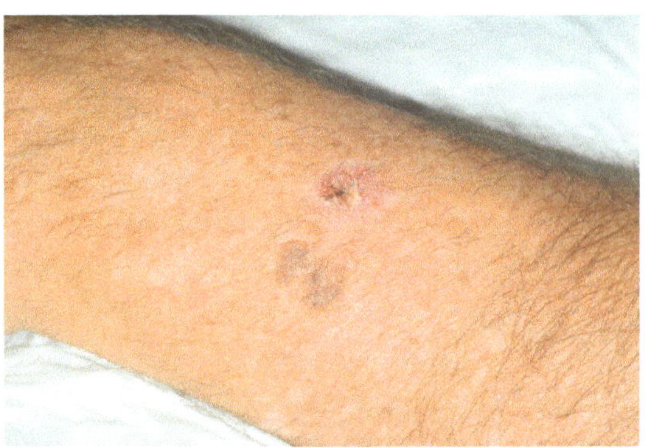

Fig. 16.1 Documentation: pretreatment photograph of lesion (Bowen's disease)

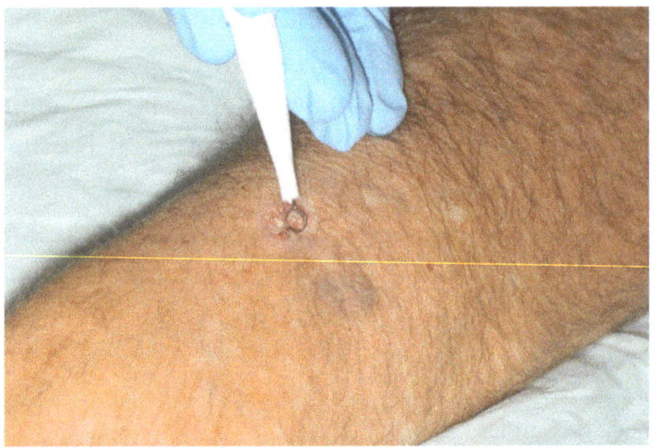

Fig. 16.2 Lesion preparation: gently remove the scales and the crusts and roughen the surface of the lesion before applying MAL

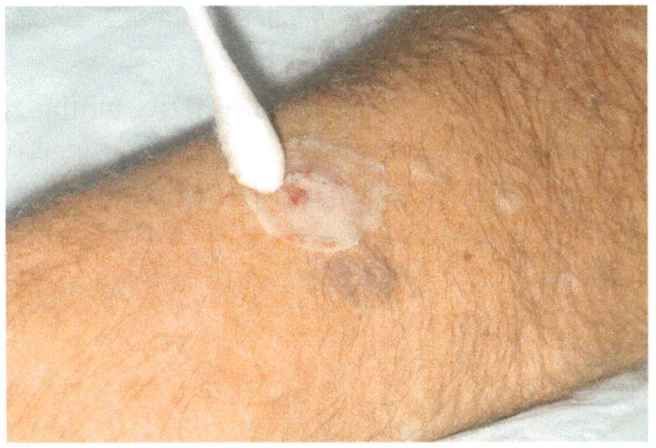

Fig. 16.3 Application of MAL cream in a 1-mm-thick layer with a margin of 10-mm around the lesion

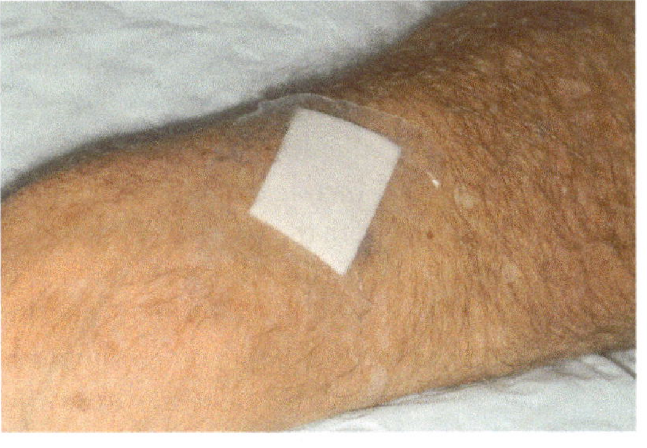

Fig. 16.4 Occlusion with an adhesive dressing (e.g., Opsite®) in order to retain the cream at the site

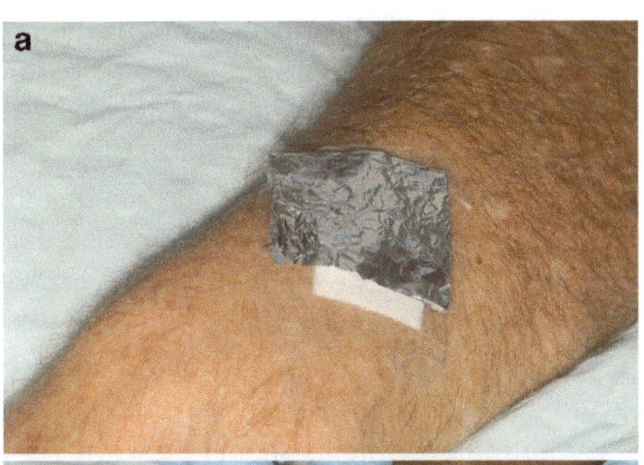

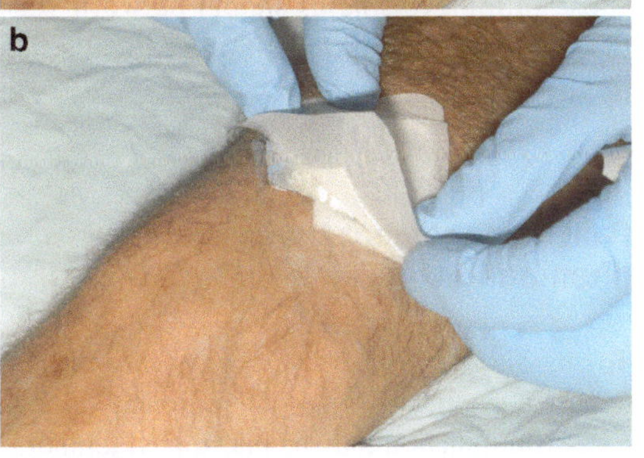

Fig. 16.5 Occlusion with a light protective dressing (e.g., tinfoil) to minimize ambient light exposure

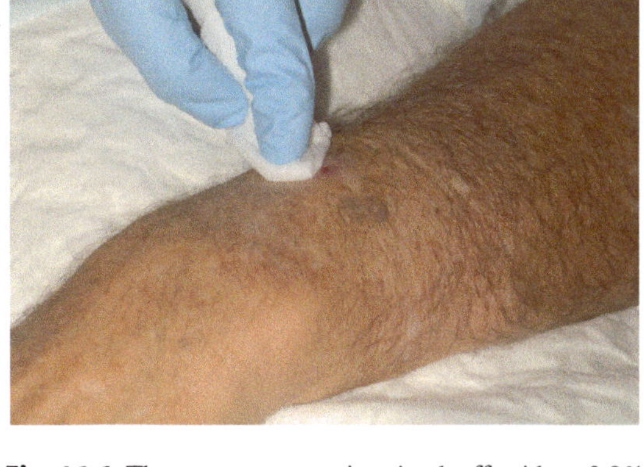

Fig. 16.6 The excess cream is wiped off with a 0.9% saline solution-wetted gauze after incubation for 3 h.

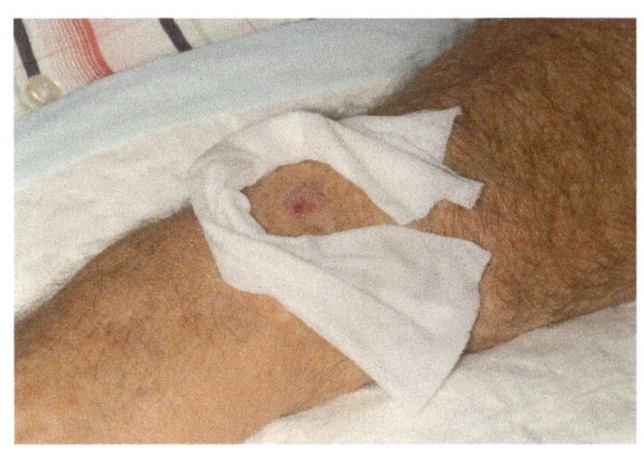

Fig. 16.7 Lesion ready for illumination

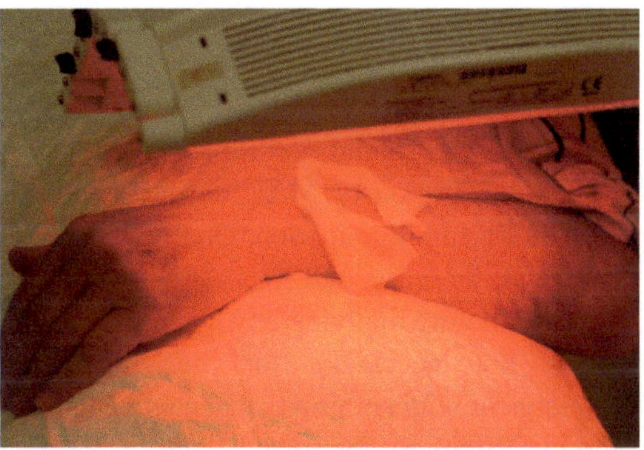

Fig. 16.8 Noncoherent red light with a continuous spectrum of 570–670 nm (e.g., Waldmann Omnilux®) is used for illumination. The total light dose should be 37.5 Jcm^{-2} at the surface of the lesion. Therefore, the light source should be positioned at a distance that ensures even illumination of the treatment area at the desired intensity

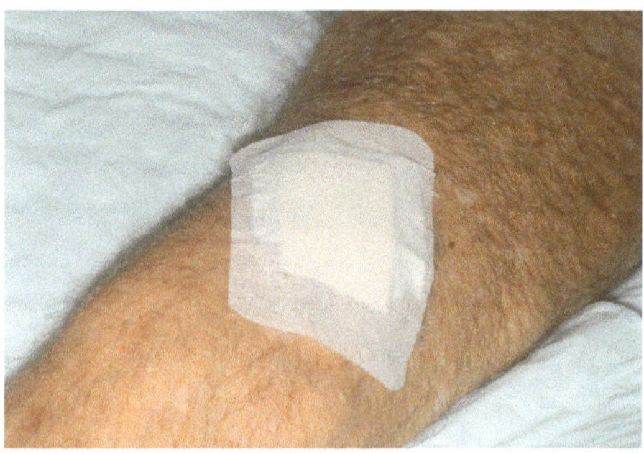

Fig. 16.9 Apply a nonadherent dressing to the treated area for 24–48 h after illumination

Documentation

The site, the size, the number, and diagnosis of the lesion(s) should be clearly documented before starting PDT treatment. Pretreatment photographs (overview and detail) may also be useful in the accurate identification of the lesion(s). A diagnostic biopsy to establish growth pattern and thickness of the BCC is mandatory.

Lesion Preparation

Hyperkeratosis should be removed to permit optimal penetration of MAL during incubation and light during illumination. Gently remove the scales and the crusts and roughen the surface of the lesion before applying MAL. Local anesthesia is not necessary for this procedure. Pretreatment with keratolytic agents may be considered particularly for crusted areas.

Application of MAL

MAL cream should be applied evenly in a 1-mm-thick layer on the lesion, as well as on a minimum margin of 5-mm around each lesion after curettage. Many dermatologists, including ourselves, have increased this margin to 10-mm. Thereafter, the lesion should be occluded with an adhesive dressing (e.g., Tegaderm®,Opsite®) in order to retain the cream at site and a light protective dressing (e.g., tinfoil) to minimize the ambient light exposure and thus wastage of protoporhyrin IX. The bandages are removed and the excess cream is wiped off with 0.9% saline solution-wetted gauze after 3 h of incubation, just before illumination.

Light Source and Illumination Scheme

Noncoherent red light with continuous spectrum of 570–670 nm (e.g., Aktilite® or Waldmann Omnilux®) is used for illumination. A light dose of 37.5 Jcm^{-2} should be delivered at the surface of the lesion. The light dose depends on several factors such as the distance of the light source from the surface of the lesion, the size and the shape (flat, concave, convex) of the treatment area, and the duration of the illumination. Therefore, the light source should be positioned at a distance that ensures even illumination of the treatment area at the desired intensity. The total light dose received and the intensity of illumination must be mentioned in the patient's record. In principal, strictly defined doses and parameters are preferred to ensure that the treatment results are comparable with those in already published RCTs. There is no need to protect the healthy skin surrounding the lesion(s) during illumination. Patients and doctor/nurse should wear suitable filter spectacles to limit the transmission of the high intensity light, and to avoid discomfort and temporary disturbance in color perception during PDT. Close-fitting eye shields should be worn when the area of illumination is in the patient's field of vision.

Pain Management During Light Illumination

To monitor pain levels during illumination, dynamic cooling devices is sufficient in most cases. Illumination may be interrupted temporarily to anesthetize the treated area if necessary. Lidocaine 1% may be administered subcutaneously (field block or nerve block). The toxic dose of 4.5 mg/kg ,or a total dose of 300 mg will not be reached under normal circumstances.

End of Treatment and Aftercare

Immediately after treatment, the treated area may appear erythematousand there may be swelling with some exudation. This will settle down within a day. Apply a nonadherent dressing. The patient may remove the dressing after 24–48 h. The areas where MAL had been applied must be protected from sunlight for 48 h. The treated area heals over a period of 3–6 weeks.

Follow-Up

Evaluation of the response of the treated area should be performed 3 months after the treatment. If (pre)malignant lesions are visible in the treated area, then we regard this treatment failure as recurrence and will act according to the guidelines (Table 16.1).

How the Authors Perform MAL PDT for Acne Vulgaris

Although acne vulgaris is a good indication for MAL-PDT, it is not widely used in Europe. Effectiveness of MAL-PDT was reported in several clinical trials. An improvement of acne vulgaris of 59–70% was reported after 1–4 PDT sessions using Metvix® [5, 10–13].

However, PDT was also associated with moderate-to-severe pain during treatment, and mild-to-moderate adverse events such as erythema, skin swelling, pustular eruption, and epithelial exfoliation after treatment were noted. Optimization of the treatment regimen is necessary for a more patient friendly approach. The treatment schemes being used in the trials seem to be based on the Metvix® protocol for (pre) malignant cutaneous lesions:

1. Acne lesions are counted and pretreatment photographs (overview) are taken before starting PDT-treatment for comparison after the treatment.
2. A 1-mm-thick layer of Metvix® cream is applied evenly on the face avoiding the eye area, the nose and the lips (≈ 2 g of Metvix® for half face). The face is then occluded with a dressing for light protection. The dressing and the remaining cream are removed after 3 h of incubation, just before illumination. The incubation time for Metvix® was 30 min in the study reported by Yeung et al. [13].
3. The illumination in three RCTs was with noncoherent red light with continuous spectrum with an average wavelength of 635 nm and a light dose of 37.5 J cm^{-2} (Aktilite®). In one study the illumination was with nonpurpuric LPDL using parameters of 7.5 Jcm^{-2}, 10 ms, 10-mm spot size [12]. In another study the illumination was with intense pulsed light (530–750 nm, 7–9 Jcm^{-2}) [13].
4. In the RCTs pain was managed with dynamic cooling devices or cool water sprays. All patients treated with MAL-PDT described

Table 16.1 How the authors use MAL-PDT for skin cancers

Documentation	Site, size, number, clinical diagnosis, (in case of BCC) histological examination for growth pattern, depth of lesion, pretreatment photographs
Lesion preparation	Crust removal, cream application (MAL, 160 mg/g), 10-mm border, dressings (occlusive and light-protective) for 3 h
Lesion treatment	Rinse off excess of cream, position light source (noncoherent red light with continuous spectrum of 570–670 nm (Waldmann Omnilux®), light dose of 37.5 Jcm^{-2} at surface of lesion, irradiance 50–100 m W cm^{-2}), monitor pain level during illumination, interrupt treatment temporarily for local anesthesia if necessary
Lesion aftercare	Apply nonadherent dressing. Protection from sunlight for 48 h
Follow-up	AKs: one treatment session, sBCCs and Bowen's disease: repeat treatment at 7 days. Response evaluation at 3 months

Table 16.2 How the authors use MAL-PDT for acne vulgaris

Documentation	Pretreatment photographs of the area to be treated
Lesion preparation	Short-contact (90 min or less) application of MAL (160 mg/g), light-protective dressing during this period
Lesion treatment	Rinse off excess cream, position noncoherent light source (blue light, light dose of 37.5 Jcm^{-2} at the surface of the lesion, irradiance of 25–50 mW cm^{-2})
Regimen	Treatment interval of 2–4 weeks, frequency of treatments: up to satisfaction (2–4 treatments)

moderate to severe pain during illumination. In at least two RCTs a few patients did not receive a second treatment because of pain during and after the first treatment [10, 11]. The fluence rate was halved in one RCT in order to reduce pain during the treatment [11]. However, the effect of the halved fluence rate on pain during treatment was not compared with the fluence rate that was used in the Metvix® protocol.

5. After illumination the majority of patients in the RCTs experienced mild to moderate adverse events such as erythema, skin swelling, pustular eruption, and epithelial exfoliation. The treatment schemes were repeated at 2 or 3 weeks in the majority of the trials.

Optimization of the treatment regimen minimizing the adverse events, and maintaining the efficacy is necessary before a consensus protocol for the treatment of acne vulgaris can be compiled. In a literature review by Taylor et al. which focused on the treatment-specific queries on the photosensitizer, the route of administration, the treatment intervals, the light sources, and the patient selection, the following conclusions were drawn regarding the efficacy and the adverse events: topical short-contact (90 min or less) of MAL (or ALA) using a noncoherent light source at 2–4 weeks intervals for a total of two to four treatments produced the highest clinical effect [14]. Wiegell et al. reported that the low fluence- compared with the high fluence MAL-PDT was associated with less pain in the treatment of acne vulgaris [15]. The optimum photosensitizer concentration, the wavelength of the noncoherent light source and its settings are still areas needing more research. Lower MAL concentrations penetrate to shallower depths [8]. Therefore, lower concentrations may not be absorbed sufficiently to have sustained effect on the pilosebaceous units. A reduction in MAL concentration is possible without losing effect on the pilosebaceous unit by using MAL encapsulated in liposomes, which have the capacity to transport the encapsulated drug more selectively into the sebaceous gland. [16] The effect of low fluence (rate) and the influence of the wavelength on the pain are dealt with in more details in the discussion (Table 16.2).

Discussion

Many clinical trials have been reported on MAL-PDT for treating nonmelanoma skin cancer (NMSC) and acne vulgaris. Although response rates are high for NMSC, they do not match the response rates of (Mohs' micrographic) surgery, especially for deeper lesions. The delivery of sufficient (precursor of) PpIX and light to the full depth of the lesion and sufficient supply of oxygen are critical in topical PDT. Optimization of these three factors in order to improve the response rates for the deeper lesions is an area under investigation. Beside this technical limitation, pain associated with PDT is an important patient-related limitation of PDT. Pain associated with PDT is a burning, stinging pain, which usually resolves quickly but can persist for up to 24 h and rarely up to several days [17]. The severity of pain may be a decisive factor whether a treatment can be completed [18] or may be a decisive factor in a patient's choice for a next NMSC to be treated with PDT. Pain has been noted to depend on several factors, such as the PpIX precursor, the wavelength, the illumination settings, and the protoporphyrin IX fluorescence intensity. There are two studies reporting fewer adverse events with MAL-PDT than with ALA-PDT [5, 6]. The influence of the wavelength was investigated recently by Mikolajewsksa et al. [19]. They reported that ALA-PDT using red light (632 nm) induced pain earlier than ALA-PDT using violet light (405 nm). However, there was no significant difference in the pain perception between MAL-PDT using red light and MAL-PDT using purple light. Based on these results they concluded that the choice of blue/violet light for ALA-PDT induced less pain in the patients than red light when deep light penetration was not required. The choice of light for MAL-PDT should be determined by the area and the thickness of the lesions only since there was no statistically significant difference between the induction times for pain with red and violet light irradiation. High irradiance may also increase pain during treatment. Cottrell et al. did a systematic clinical investigation on the effect of irradiance on ALA-PDT efficiency and pain and they observed that lowering the irradiance reduced the pain during PDT, while maintaining the efficacy in the treatment of sBBCs [20]. Wiegell et al. reported that low fluence- compared with high fluence MAL-PDT was associated with less pain in the treatment of acne vulgaris [14]. In conclusion, although a lot of research has been done into the efficiency of PDT, more work needs to be done on the effect of various treatment variables on the efficiency and adverse effects of PDT, in order to develop an optimum treatment protocol for both NMSC and acne vulgaris. One should realize that the optimum treatment variables for MAL-PDT will not be automatically the optimum treatment variables for ALA-PDT, and vice versa, because of the differences in their biophysical and biochemical characteristics. The standardized Galderma Metvix® protocol that is used for MAL-PDT may not be the optimum protocol, but has the main advantage that treatment results are comparable with those in published RCTs.

References

1. Robinson DJ, de Bruijn HS, Star WM. Dose and timing of the first light fraction in two-fold illumination schemes for topical ALA-mediated photodynamic therapy of hairless mouse skin. Photochem Photobiol. 2003;77:319–23.
2. De Haas ERM, Kruijt BM Sterenborg HJ. Fractionated illumination significantly improves the response of superficial basal cell carcinoma to aminolevulinic acid photodynamic therapy. J Invest Dermatol. 2006;126:2679–86.
3. De Haas ERM, de Vijlder HC, Sterenborg HJ. Fractionated aminolevulinic acid-photodynamic therapy provides additional evidence for the use of PDT for non-melanoma skin cancer. J Eur Acad Dermatol Venereol. 2008;22:426–30.
4. De Bruijn HS, de Haas ERM, Hebeda KM. Light fractionation does not enhance the efficacy of methyl 5-aminolevulinate mediated photodynamic therapy in normal Mouse skin. Photochem Photobiol Sc. 2007;6:1325–31.
5. Wiegell SR, Wulf HC. Photodynamic therapy of acne vulgaris using 5-aminolevulinic acid versus methyl aminolevulinate. J Am Acad Dermatol. 2006;54:647–51.
6. Moloney FJ, Collins P. Randomized, double-blind, prospective study to compare topical 5-aminolevulinic acid photodynamic therapy for extensive scalp actinic keratosis. Br J Dermatol. 2007;157:87–91.
7. Braathen LR, Szeimeis R, Basset-Seguin N. Guidelines on the use of photodynamic therapy for nonmelanoma skin cancer: An international consensus. J Am Acad Dermatol. 2007;56:125–43.
8. Peng Q, Soler AM, Warloe T. Selective distribution of porphyrins in skin thick basal cell carcinoma after topical application of methyl 5-aminolevulinate. J Photochem Photobiol B. 2001;62:140–5.
9. Rhodes LE, de Rie MA, Leifsdottir R. Five-year follow-up of a randomized, prospective trial of topical methyl aminolevulinate photodynamic therapy versus surgery for nodular basal cell carcinoma. Arch Dermatol. 2007;143:1131–6.
10. Horfelt C, Funk J, Frohm-Nilson M. Topical methyl aminolevulinate photodynamic therapy for treatment of facial acne vulgaris of a randomized, controlled trial. Br J Dermatol. 2006;142:973–8.
11. Wiegell SR, Wulf HC. Photodynamic therapy of acne vulgaris using methyl aminolaevulinate: a blinded, randomized, controlled trial. Br J Dermatol. 2006;154:969–76.
12. Haedersdal M, Togsverd-Bo K, Wiegell SR. Long-pulsed dye laser versus long-pulsed dye laser-assisted photodynamic therapy for acne vulgaris: a randomized controlled trial. J Am Acad Dermatol. 2008;58:387–94.
13. Yeung CK, Shek SY, Bjerring P. A comparative study of intense pulsed light alone and its combination with photodynamic therapy for the treatment of facial acne in asian skin. Lasers Surg Med. 2007;39:1–6.
14. Taylor MN, Gonzalez ML. Practicalities of photodynamic therapy in acne vulgaris. Br J Dermatol. 2009;160:1140–8.
15. Wiegell SR, Skiveren J, Philipsen PA, Wulf HA. Pain during photodynamic therapy is associated with protoporhyrin IX fluorescence and fluence rate. Br J Dermatol. 2008;158:727–33.

16. de Leeuw J, de Vijlder HC, Bjerring P. Liposomes in dermatology today. J Eur Acad Dermatol Venereol. 2009;23:505–16.
17. Wennberg AM. Pain relief and other practical issues in photodynamic therapy. Australas J Dermatol. 2005;46:S3–4.
18. Morton CA, McKenna KE, Rhodes LE. Guidelines for topical photodynamic therapy: update. Br J Dermatol. 2008;159:1245–66.
19. Mikolajewsksa P, Lani V, Juzeniene A, et al. Topical aminolaevulinic acid- and aminolaevulinic acid methyl ester-based photodynamic therapy with red and violet light: influence of wavelength on pain and erythema. Br J Dermatol. 2009;161:1173–9.
20. Cottrell WJ, Paquette AD, Keymel KR, et al. Irradiance-dependent photobleaching and pain in d-Aminolevulinic acid-photodynamic therapy of superficial basal cell carcinomas. Clin Cancer Res. 2008;14:4475–83.

The Future of Photodynamic Therapy

17

Macrene Alexiades-Armenakas

Abstract

The field of PDT is increasing its accuracy at targeting specific tissues, organisms, and other matter for ever-advancing applications in therapeutics. Of importance is the broadening of the classes of photosensitizers that are being developed for use in PDT, along with the development of novel wavelengths and light sources. Technologically advanced, microtargeted delivery systems are being developed that will enable photosensitizers to penetrate to desired targets with increasing specificity and efficiency. Finally, the applications of PDT to various clinical conditions are advancing, with the advent of its use for the treatment of acne, light hair removal, and infections.

Photodynamic therapy has evolved extensively since its inception over a century ago and holds more promise than ever as a therapeutic modality as it progresses in the centuries to come. The stimulation of photosensitizing compounds by specific wavelengths is a scientific method with innumerable permutations and applications. This approach will continue to be developed for diagnostics and research, in addition to therapeutic interventions, though the latter is the focus of this chapter. The number and variety of photosensitizers have only begun to be studied and designed. A classification system is put forth to chemically classify the new and emerging photosensitizers, as well as existing ones. Secondly, novel delivery systems are rapidly being developed to improve targeting and uptake of photosensitizers, thus improving specificity and therapeutic efficacy. In addition, only a fraction of wavelengths have been explored thus far. The range and types of light sources being developed for PDT are discussed. In this chapter, we take an overview of the current and new directions in which the field of PDT is progressing.

M. Alexiades-Armenakas (✉)
Department of Dermatology,
Yale University School of Medicine,
New York, NY, USA
and
Dermatology and Laser Surgery Center,
New York, NY, USA
e-mail: dralexiades@nyderm.org

Photosensitizer Development

Current Porphyrin Photosensitizers

Numerous photosensitizers have been studied over the past century, overwhelmingly of the porphyrin variety [1]. Initially, systemic photosensitizers

M.H. Gold (ed.), *Photodynamic Therapy in Dermatology*,
DOI 10.1007/978-1-4419-1298-5_17,

were employed, with the more recent advent of topical photosensitizers over the past three decades [2]. While systemic photosensitizers continue to be used for internal tumors, the transition from systemic to topical photosensitizers occurred in an effort to mitigate untoward systemic photosensitivity when treating skin lesions, and has been highly successful in achieving this goal [1]. Currently, the four FDA-approved photosensitizers in the United States are porphyrins of the heme variety: porfimer sodium (Photofrin®, 1995, Axcan Pharma Inc.), verteporfin (Visudyne®, 2000, Novartis/QLT Phototherapeutics, Inc.), aminolevulinic acid (20% aminolevulinic acid solution, Levulan Kerastick®, 1999, DUSA Pharmaceuticals, Wilmington, Massachusetts), and methyl aminolevulinic acid (16.8% methyl aminolevulinate cream, Metvixia Cream®, 2004 PhotoCure ASA, Oslo, Norway, Galderma, Fort Worth, Texas). Photofin is approved to treat esophageal carcinoma, Barrett's esophagus, and non-small-cell lung cancer (see Chap. 12). Verteporfirin is approved for the treatment of subfoveal choroidal neovascularization. ALA and MAL are FDA-approved for the treatment of actinic keratoses.

Future Classes of Photosensitizers

What trends and future progress can we predict in the field of photosensitizers? Firstly, additional classes of photosensitizers, in addition to the heme porphyrins, are under study; among these are the chlorophyll porphyrins, fullerenes, phthalocyanins, and phenothiazines. In this chapter, a classification of current and new photosensitizers based on their basic molecular structure is presented (Table 17.1).

Pyrroles

The first class of photosensitizers based on chemical structure is the pyrrole class, which includes porphine, heme and chlorophyll (Table 17.1) [3–5]. Pyrroles are heterocyclic (containing at least one atom of carbon, and at least one element other than carbon, such as sulfur, oxygen or nitrogen within a ring structure) aromatic organic compounds, characterized by a five-membered ring with the formula C_4H_4NH [3–5]. Porphine contains four pyrrole molecules, joined to form a larger aromatic ring system, which is highly stable. Porphine is the parent compound of the class of molecules termed porphyrins, in which hydrogen atoms on the outside of the porphine ring are replaced by various substituents [3–5]. As many of these substances form purple crystalline solids, their name is derived from the Greek word for "purple" which is "porphyros." Porphyrins are ubiquitous in nature, and characteristic of systems involving respiration, as in the cases of heme and chlorophyll. Porphine compounds include Porforin Sodium, Verteporfin, and tetra-substituted N-methyl-pyridyl-porphine (TMP).

Heme protoporphyrin IX (PPIX) is a porphyrin derivative in which an iron(II) ion is held rigidly by the nitrogen atoms in the center of its macrocycle. Both ALA and MAL are precursors

Table 17.1 Classes of photosensitizers under development

Class	I. Pyrroles			II. Fullerenes	III. Phthalocyanines	IV. Phenothiazines
Types	a. Porphine	b. Heme	c. Chlorophylls			
	Porfimer sodium	ALA	Phaeophytin	Buckminister fullerene C(60) C(60) fullerene Huang et al. 2009	Zinc (II)-Phthalocyanine (ZnPc)	Methylene blue
	Verteporfirin	MAL	Phaeophorbide	C (70)	Phthalocyanine 4 (Pc4)	Toluidene blue
	Tetra-substituted N-methyl-pyridyl-porphine (TMP)			Nanotubes		

of PPIX. PPIX has its strongest absorptive peak in the Soret band 360–400 nm, and smaller peaks in the Q bands spanning the red region of the spectrum between 500 and 635 nm [1].

Chlorophyll, which is named from the Greek *chloros* "green" and *phyllon* "leaf," is a porphyrin derivative found in green plants and *Cyanobacteria*, which enables these organisms to perform photosynthesis. The chlorophylls hold a magnesium ion in the center of their porphyrin macrocycles. Chlorophyll absorbs visible light in the violet (~420 nm) and red (~680 nm) regions of the spectrum; hence, the light that is reflected off this pigment is green [6]. The energy from the sunlight absorbed by chlorophyll in the chloroplasts of green plants is used to drive the synthesis of carbohydrates such as glucose ($C_6H_{12}O_6$) from carbon dioxide and water. The potential use of chlorophyll in PDT has been proposed [7].

Phaeophytin and phaeophorbide are chlorophyll derivatives lacking the magnesium ion [8]. They are porphyrin molecules currently being studied as future photosensitizing compounds for use in PDT [8]. For example, sodium-pheophorbide has been studied in combination with a variety of light sources for treating methicillin-resistant *Staphylococcus* with PDT [9]. The pheophorbide photosensitizer was mixed with the bacteria and successful bactericidal activity was measured following irradiation [9]. Chlorin e6 and pheophorbide a were tested for potential use as topical PDT agents [10]. The phaeophorbide accumulated with a much higher rate in keratinocytes in vitro, and both resulted in apoptosis upon illumination [10].

Fullerenes

Buckminsterfullerene, or C_{60}, is a 60 carbon atom with a molecular shape resembling a soccer-ball [11]. The molecule was discovered by H.W. Kroto, R.E. Smalley, and R.F. Curl in the 1980s in experiments involving graphite vaporized with lasers for which they were awarded the Nobel Prize in Chemistry in 1996 [11]. The icosahedron, with its 12 pentagons and 20 hexagons, reminded them of the shape of the geodesic dome designed by the architect R. Buckminster Fuller, and they named the molecule in his honor [11]. Similar spherical- or oval-shaped carbon-only molecules, such as C_{70}, are often referred to as *fullerenes* or "buckyballs." *Nanotubes* are cylindrical versions of the fullerenes and have been described as resembling a chain link fence rolled into a cylinder, with a dome-shaped cap on the end [12].

The fullerenes are currently being explored for their potential future use in PDT for the treatment of neoplasms [13]. Early studies of fullerenes have also demonstrated their broad-spectrum antimicrobial activity as PDT photosensitizers [14, 15].

Phthalocyanines

A phthalocyanine is a macrocyclic compound with an alternating nitrogen atom-carbon atom ring structure [16, 17]. The structure of a phthalocyanine molecule is closely related to that of the naturally occurring porphyrin systems [18]. It contains a copper ion instead of iron. Phthalocyanines are being extensively tested and studied as potential photosensitizers for PDT [19]. Examples of potential photosensitizers in this class that have been studied for use in PDT include zinc (II)-phthalocyanine (ZnPc) and phthalocyanine 4 (Pc4) [20, 21].

Phenothiazines

Phenothiazine is an organic tricyclic compound that occurs in anti-psychotic and anti-histamine drugs [22]. It is a yellow compound with the formula $S(C_6H_4)_2NH$ and related to thiazines [22]. Phenothiazine was introduced in 1935 as a pesticide and still in some use to treat parasites in livestock. The synthetic dye methylene blue, first described in 1876, is a phenothiazine derivative and has very recently been used as a photosensitizer for PDT of plaque psoriasis [23]. Methylene blue is also being studied as a potential photosensitizer for PDT application as an anti-microbial [24]. Toluidene blue is also a phenothiazine being explored for use in PDT [25–27].

Novel Photosensitizer Delivery Systems

In addition to new photosensitizer molecule classes, the future of PDT involves manipulating the mode of delivery of photosensitizers (Table 17.2).

Silica Nanoparticles

Mesoporous silica has been coated onto NaYF(4) upconversion nanocrystals to form a core-shell structure and then loaded with the photosensitizer zinc (II)-phthalocyanine (ZnPc) into its porous silica [20]. The nanoparticles displayed a uniform spherical shape with an average diameter of about 50 nm and were then applied to murine bladder cancer cells. Subsequent irradiation with 980 nm demonstrated photodynamic effect, with singlet-oxygen mediated apoptosis of the cells [20].

This approach is being applied experimentally to melanoma cells, using silica nanoparticle encapsulated Pc4 [21]. Since Pc4 aggregates in aqueous solutions, which dramatically reduces its PDT efficacy and therefore limits its clinical application, an alternative delivery system has been developed. Pc4 has been encapsulated using silica nanoparticles (Pc4SNP), which not only improved the aqueous solubility, stability, and delivery of the photodynamic drug, but also increased its photodynamic efficacy compared to free Pc4 molecules. Cell viability measurements demonstrated that Pc4SNP was more phototoxic to A375 or B16-F10 melanoma cells than free Pc4 [21].

Micelle Delivery

Another novel photosensitizer delivery approach is the use of micelles to overcome the hydrophobicity of the photosensitizing molecules. A typical micelle is a nano-sized vesicular membrane which is soluble in water by virtue of having a hydrophilic (water-loving) "head" facing the outside, while the hydrophobic (water-hating) "tails" surround the fat soluble nutrient inside [28]. Such micelles formation is referred to as *emulsification*, a process that allows a compound normally insoluble (in the solvent being used) to dissolve, and this natural formation is referred to as a "nano-emulsion" [28].

This micelle formation enables the delivery of lipophilic photosensitizers into target structures. Recently, biocompatible PEG-PCL micelle nanoparticles have been developed which involve encapsulation of Pc4 within the micelle core by hydrophobic association with the PCL block [29]. In vitro PDT studies of the micelle-formulated Pc4 in MCF-7c3 human breast cancer cells studies demonstrated efficient encapsulation of Pc4 in the micelles, intracellular uptake of the micelle-formulated Pc4 in cells, and significant cytotoxic effect of the formulation upon photoirradiation [29].

Liposomal Delivery

Liposomal delivery is another novel delivery method for introducing photosensitizers into target tissues. Lipid spheres that contain an aqueous core are called *liposomes*, from the Greek for "fat body." Liposomes are different from micelles structurally in that they have a

Table 17.2 Novel photosensitizer delivery systems for PDT

Silica nanoparticles	Micelles	Liposomes	Peptide nanoparticles	Gold nanoconjugates
Guo et al. [20] and Zhao et al. [21]	Seddon and Templer [28] and Master et al. [29]	Torchilin [30], Oku and Ishii [31], Fadel et al. [32], and de Leeuw et al. [33]	van Hell et al. [34, 35]	Wieder et al. [36]

bilayer membrane [30]. In the human body, natural liposomes, like micelles, are composed of lecithin phospholipids. Liposomes differ from micelles also in that they are generally larger and have the advantage of being able to carry *both* fat-soluble *and* water-soluble contents [30].

Recently, benzoporphyrin derivative monoacid ring A (BPD-MA) photosensitizer was prepared in a clever liposomal formulation and tested for PDT activity in angiogenic target cells [31]. The investigators endowed the liposomes with an active-targeting probe, Ala-Pro-Arg-Pro-Gly (APRPG), a peptide specific for angiogenic endothelial cells. They then showed that APRPG-PEG-LipBPD-MA strongly suppressed tumor growth by PDT treatment [31].

Liposomal delivery of methylene blue photosensitizer is being applied to the treatment of acne vulgaris [32]. Liposomes loaded methylene blue (LMB) were prepared and studied for different pharmaceutical properties and formulated in hydrogel (MB 0.1%). Permeability and selective sebaceous gland targeting in mice skin was studied. Gel containing LMB was used for treating 13 patients complaining of mild-moderate acne vulgaris once a week for 2 weeks. After only two sessions, there was 83.3% reduction in the number of inflammatory acne lesions, and a 63.6% reduction in the number of noninflammatory acne lesions. At 12 weeks, 90% of patients had a moderate-to-marked improvement of their acne in the treated areas [32].

In another recent publication, assessment of the efficacy and the safety of PDT using 5-ALA 0.5% in liposomal spray and intense pulsed light (IPL) in combination with topical peeling agents (Li-PDT-PC) in acne vulgaris was conducted [33]. After a mean period of 7.8 months and a mean number of 5.7 treatments the mean total number of lesions dropped from 34.6 to 11.0 lesions, resulting in a mean improvement of 68.2% [33]. While the safety of this modality must be rigorously tested and the efficacy findings reproduced, this approach holds great future potential and interest in the field.

Peptide Nanocarriers

Peptide carriers are another method of nanoparticle delivery being employed. A group of scientists have shown that recombinantly produced amphiphilic oligopeptides with amino acid sequence Ac-Ala-Ala-Val-Val-Leu-Leu-Leu-Trp-Glu-Glu spontaneously assemble into nano-sized vesicles with an average diameter of 120 nm [34]. Moreover, peptide vesicles could be stabilized by introducing multiple cysteine residues within the hydrophobic domain of these amphiphilic oligopeptides, allowing the formation of intermolecular disulfide bridges. Water-insoluble phthalocyanines could be quantitatively entrapped within the hydrophobic domains of these peptide vesicles [35]. Upon illumination, the phthalocyanine-containing peptide vesicles showed an active photodynamic response towards the cells leading to effective cell killing. In contrast, the free phthalocyanine or empty peptide vesicles did not show any cytotoxicity [35]. Thus, these experiments demonstrate the critical importance of the mode of photosensitizer delivery in yielding efficacy in PDT.

Gold Nanoconjugates

Phthalocyanine-gold nanoparticle conjugates have been designed and synthesized for PDT [36]. The phthalocyanine photosensitizer stabilized gold nanoparticles have an average diameter of 2–4 nm. The synthetic strategy interdigitates a phase transfer reagent between phthalocyanine molecules on the particle surface that solubilizes the hydrophobic photosensitizer in polar solvents enabling delivery of the nanoparticle conjugates to cells. The phthalocyanine is present in the monomeric form on the nanoparticle surface, absorbs radiation maximally at 695 nm and catalytically produces the cytotoxic species singlet oxygen with high efficiency. Irradiation of the nanoparticle conjugates within the HeLa cells induced substantial cell mortality through the photodynamic production of singlet oxygen. The PDT efficiency of the nanoparticle conjugates, determined using colorimetric assay, was twice that obtained using the free phthalocyanine derivative [36].

Light Sources Under Development

The pyrrole class of photosensitizers exhibit a very typical absorption spectrum with the highest peak at approximately 405 nm with the Soret-band and the aforementioned lesser Q-bands, the last having an absorption peak at 635 nm. Although the latter red peak is much smaller than that at 405 nm, this wavelength is preferentially used for cutaneous PDT, since light in the red spectrum shows the best tissue penetration [1, 2, 37]. As the new photosensitizer classes continue to be developed, more wavelengths will be employed.

Prior PDT Light Sources

The initial light sources used for PDT included broadband, noncoherent lights, such as quartz, xenon, tungsten, or halogen lamps [1]. The wavelengths of light chosen spanned the 360–400 nm Soret band, and red around 650 nm because of the latter Q band [1]. Systemic photosensitizers caused prolonged photosensitivity and broadband light sources had limitations and side effects. The development of topical photosensitizers, such as ALA, and the advent of lasers in recent years advanced PDT for cutaneous use. In the 1990s, red lasers were applied due to their increased skin penetration despite lesser absorption by porphyrins. Broad-band blue light and red light were also studied extensively, the former achieving FDA-approval in combination with topical ALA for the treatment of AK in 1997. These lasers and light sources caused significant side effects, such as discomfort, erythema, crusting, blistering and dyspigmentation [1]. The two light sources FDA-approved in the United States for PDT are blue light in combination with ALA, and red light in combination with MAL for the treatment of actinic keratoses.

Novel PDT Light Sources

Two relatively recent light sources for PDT include pulsed dye lasers (PDL) and IPL devices.

LP PDL

Among the Q bands in the PPIX absorption spectrum, a peak at 575 nm had been shown to be amenable to activation through PDL [38]. It was subsequently shown that the application of the long-pulsed pulsed dye laser (LP PDL, 595 nm) following topical ALA greatly minimized side effects without compromising efficacy in treatment of AK, AC, sebaceous hyperplasia, lichen sclerosus, and most recently acne vulgaris [37, 39–42].

IPL

IPL sources have been shown to be effective in mediating PDT to treat photodamage and acne, offering advantages of versatility in wavelengths and applications. A split-face design study, comparing three treatments at 3-week intervals with topical ALA and IPL on one side of the face vs. IPL alone on the contralateral side, demonstrated greater improvement in rhytides, photoaging, and mottled pigmentation on the ALA IPL side [43]. In another randomized, split-design study, moderate to severe acne patients received three monthly sessions with ALA plus IPL on one side of the face vs. IPL alone on the other side. In that study, the mean reduction of inflammatory acne lesions was statistically different between the long incubation (90 min) ALA and IPL and the IPL-only [44].

Future PDT Light Sources

The future light sources for PDT will likely involve light-emitting diodes (LEDs) and portable light sources. These offer an inexpensive, convenient and practical method for mediating PDT, and are only now beginning to be explored. They also allow for lower-cost, facile, and versatile delivery of wavelengths.

LEDs

Several studies have published high efficacy and safety with LEDs combined with topical photosensitizers, such as ALA, for the treatment of cutaneous neoplasms. One study of a low-irradiance, potentially disposable, lightweight, organic light-emitting diode (OLED), with an area-emitting light source (2 cm diameter), for the treatment of Bowen's disease and superficial basal cell carcinoma demonstrated complete clearance in 7 of 12 cases following two treatments (45–60 J/cm^2 red light, 550–750 nm, peak 620 nm, irradiance 5 mW/cm^2) 1 month apart following topical ALA at 4 h incubation [45].

In another split-design study, subjects with actinic keratoses received topical MAL and subsequent irradiation with an LED system (120 mW/cm^2; 40 J/cm^2, LEDA, WaveLight AG, Erlangen, Germany) on one side of the face as compared to incoherent lamp (160 mW/cm^2; 100 J/cm^2, PDT 1200L, Waldmann Medizintechnik, Villingen-Schwenningen, Germany) to the other [46]. Six months following treatment there was no statistically significant difference between the keratosis scores between the two light sources. The remission rate was 78.5% (LED system) vs. 80.3% (incoherent lamp) [46].

The combination of topical photosensitizers with LEDs is also being explored for the treatment of inflammatory disorders. Plaque psoriasis was effectively treated with topical methylene blue and a 565 mW LED 670 nm. Complete clearance was reported in 16 patients [23]. The application of at-home phototherapy has been explored for psoriasis, yet the concept of topical PDT in combination with at-home UVA devices has yet to be published [47, 48].

Acne treatment with LED PDT offers many advantages. LEDs alone have been reported to demonstrate some efficacy in treating acne. In a recent study, combination of 415 nm and near-infrared (IR) LED therapy for moderate acne demonstrated mixed lesional improvements [49]. Potentially combining ALA with LEDs in the red potion of the spectrum may yield improvements, though side effects may still be encountered. Blue LEDs would also be potential candidates, provided that the UVA portion of the spectrum is blocked.

Portable/At-Home Light Sources

In addition to the hand-held or portable LEDs, various other at-home light sources are being developed to mediate PDT. One obvious choice is daylight. Thirty patients with mostly thin-grade AK of the face or scalp were treated with 16 and 8% MAL-PDT in two symmetrical areas after application of sunscreen. Immediately after, patients left the hospital with instructions to spend the remaining day outside the home in daylight. The complete response rate after 3 months was 76.9% for 16% MAL and 79.5% for 8% MAL ($P=0.37$). Patients spent a mean of 244 min outdoors and received a mean effective light dose of 30 J/cm2. Light doses of 8–70 J/cm2 induced similar response rates ($P=0.25$) [50]. Recently, the possibility of specific wavelengths to be programmed in hand-held devices has also been raised.

Novel PDT Applications Under Development

Major new applications for PDT include the treatment of acne, unwanted hair, and infections, including bacterial and fungal.

Acne

The treatment of acne with PDT is well underway, yet FDA-approval is lacking. The combination of topical ALA and MAL with various light sources has demonstrated safety and high efficacy rates for this modality. Twenty-one clinical trials and case series have been published to date, demonstrating the safety and efficacy of PDT for the treatment of acne [51]. One may categorize laser and light-based treatments of acne according to efficacy, and PDT ranks highest in terms of acne lesional clearance rates.

Topical ALA (1 h) followed by LP PDL (595 nm) demonstrated 77% lesional clearance rate per treatment, as compared to 32% with LP PDL alone, when combined with topical therapy, with sustained clearance [40].

Additional studies of ALA PDT employing blue and red light or lasers, or IPL demonstrated lesional clearance rates of 32–75% after multiple treatments [52]. Most recently, combination of

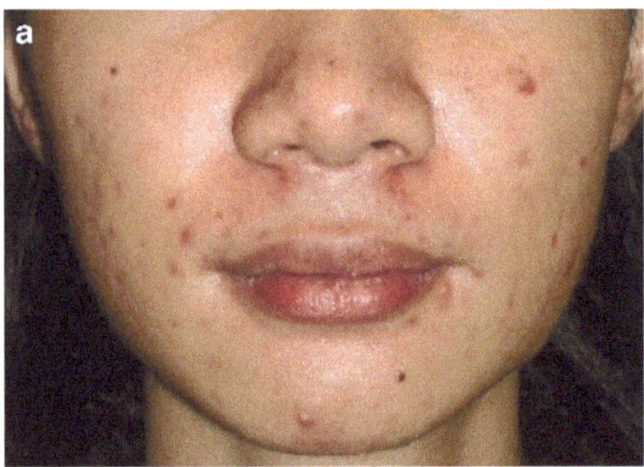

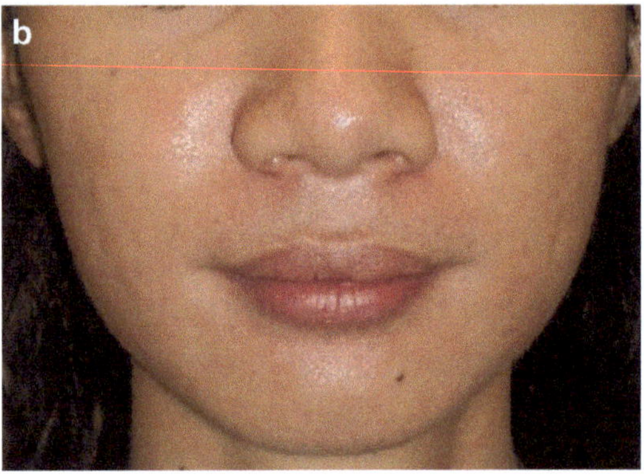

Fig. 17.1 Cystic acne treated with ALA LP PDL PDT combined with diode laser. A recalcitrant cystic acne patient is shown at baseline (**a**) and following two sessions of ALA PDT with long-pulsed dye laser combined with 1,450 nm diode laser (**b**) with sustained clearance to 1-year follow-up

ALA PDT with LP PDL with diode (1,450 nm) laser boosted clearance rates (MAA, manuscript in preparation), suggesting that combination therapy of PDT with other modalities may be a possible method to advance efficacy. In Fig. 17.1, a subject is shown with recalcitrant cystic acne (a), with sustained clearance to 1 year following two sessions of PDT with diode laser (b) (Fig. 17.1).

Unwanted Hair

The treatment of blonde or white hair with laser or light-based approaches has been unsuccessful. Some data suggest potential efficacy through the use of topical photosensitizers with irradiation with wavelengths to target the matrix cells of the hair follicle. Intraperitoneal ALA injection resulted in PPIX fluorescence in sebaceous glands and hair follicles of albino mice and allowing illumination, a persistent reduction in the number of hair follicles was observed [53]. PPIX fluorescence was also reported in mice following topical ALA application [54]. Recently, PDT-induced damage to not only sebaceous glands, but also hair follicles in a rat model following application of liposomal ALA and irradiation with a red filtered halogen lamp was demonstrated [55]. Liposomal delivery of topical ALA to intact or depilated rat skin demonstrated PPIX expression in pilosebaceous units, with maximal expression in anagen hairs. Inhibition of hair induction after depilation was observed [55].

The only published clinical study regarding the use of PDT for hair disorders in humans aimed at treating the hair loss disease alopecia areata with topical ALA followed by red light. This study demonstrated no increase in hair growth following treatment, which would be expected should PDT to hair follicles result in their destruction [56]. Clearly, clinical studies are needed in order to evaluate this potential modality as a mode of hair removal.

The author has conducted an experimental protocol to evaluate topical 5-ALA and IPL (580–980 nm) for the removal of blonde and gray hair [52]. A photographic example of a patient with excessive vellus hairs on the face prior to (a) and following ALA PDT with IPL (b) is shown in Fig. 17.2. Regrowth following treatment increased from an estimated 30% at 1 month to 40% at 2 months, and 50% at 3 months follow up (Fig. 17.2b). It will be necessary to follow patients long term to 6 months and 1 year follow up in order to make an assessment regarding long-term reduction.

Anti-Microbial

PDT using various photosensitizers and light sources is under study to treat infections, including bacterial, fungal, and protozoal. Such studies have been experimental, and not yet tested clinically in humans.

Anti-Bacterial

One approach has been to introduce bioluminescent tags to bacteria as a model system for studying

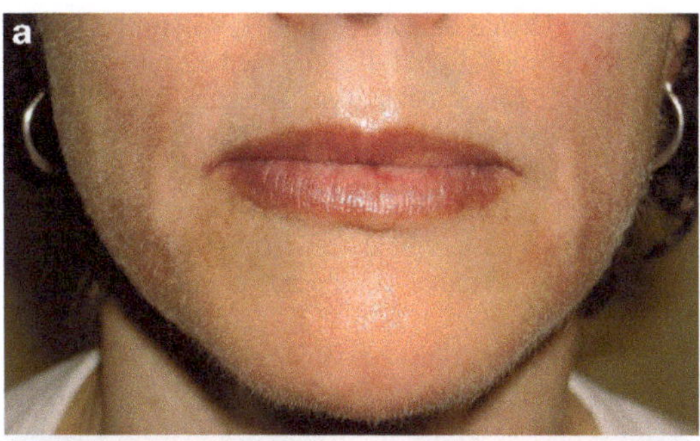

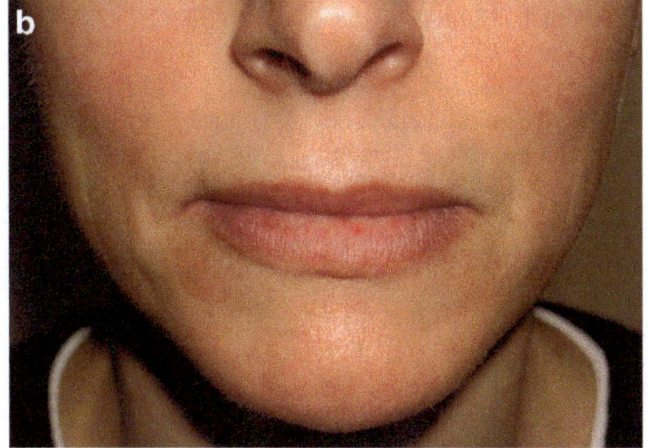

Fig. 17.2 Blonde vellus hairs treated with ALA PDT. A subject with excessive blonde vellus facial hair at baseline (**a**) is shown following a single treatment with ALA PDT using IPL at 3 months follow-up (**b**), with approximately 50% regrowth

the efficacy of PDT in skin infections in the murine system [57]. As discussed in detail in Chap. 12, differences in PDT efficacy and photosensitizer penetration have been noted between gram+ and gram– bacteria.

Staphylococcus

PDT is being tested to clear staphylococcal biofilms, which play an important role in nosocomial infections, as well as methicillin-resistant *Staphylococcus aureus* (MRSA), a major cause of morbidity and mortality in our hospital and now ambulatory population [26, 58]. PDT has shown some promise in treating *S. aureus* colonized wounds in a murine model [59, 60].

Other Bacteria

PDT is also being applied to less common bacteria, including *Vibrio vulnificus* which causes opportunistic infections and cellulitis, with promise for decreasing mortality rates in a mouse model [61]. As discussed earlier, the combination of methylene blue and white light has demonstrated bactericidal activity against *Escherichia coli* in vitro [24]. Toluidene and methylene blue followed by copper vapor-pumped dye laser demonstrated bactericidal activity against *Heliobacter* using an ex vivo ferret gastric mucosa model without damage to the mucosa [62].

Erythrasma, a skin infection in the skin folds, is caused by *Corynebacterium minutissimum*, a bacterium that fluoresces under Wood's light. Endogenous PDT shows promise in clinical studies of patients in a study using red (635 nm) light [63].

Mycobacteria

The application of PDT to treat mycobacteria infections is an attractive option, however limited by the location of the granulomas and the accessibility to light activation. Thus far, in vitro and murine models of subcutaneous granulomas have demonstrated the potential efficacy of this approach [64, 65].

Anti-Fungal

Several studies have investigated the future role of PDT in treating *Candida albicans* infections. The FDA-approved Photofrin has been studied in murine and in vitro models [66, 67]. The treatment of dermatophytes with PDT has been more rigorously studied. Its application has been reported in several in vitro studies, which demonstrated both fungicidal and fungistatic effects of PDT on dermatophytes, most notably *Trichophyton rubrum* [68, 69].

Of tremendous interest is its future use as a potentially approved treatment for onychomycosis. Several case reports in humans have shown early evidence of clinical efficacy using both topical ALA and MAL, combined with red light [70, 71]. Large-scale clinical studies will determine its ultimate future role [72].

Summary

In sum, the field of PDT is increasing its accuracy at targeting specific tissues, organisms, and other matter for ever-advancing applications in therapeutics. Of importance is the broadening of the classes of photosensitizers that are being developed for use in PDT, along with the development of novel wavelengths and light sources. Technologically advanced, microtargeted delivery systems are being developed, that will enable photosensitizers to penetrate to desired targets with increasing specificity and efficiency. Finally, the applications of PDT to various clinical conditions are advancing, with the advent of its use for the treatment of acne, light hair removal, and infections.

References

1. Alexiades-Armenakas MR. Laser-mediated photodynamic therapy. Clin Dermatol. 2006;24(1):16–25.
2. Marcus SL, McIntyre WR. Photodynamic therapy systems and applications. Expert Opin Emerg Drugs. 2002;7(2):318–31.
3. Atkins PW. Molecules. 2nd ed. Cambridge: Cambridge University Press; 2003. p. 46–8, 143, 144–51, 168–9.
4. Bruice PY. Organic chemistry. 4th ed. Upper Saddle River: Prentice-Hall; 2004. p. 594–9.
5. Fox MA, Whitesell JK. Organic chemistry. 3rd ed. Sudbury: Jones and Bartlett Publishers; 2004. p. 64–74.
6. Buschmann C. Variability and application of the chlorophyll fluorescence emission ratio red/far-red of leaves. Photosynth Res. 2007;92(2):261–71.
7. Nyman ES, Hynninen PH. Research advances in the use of tetrapyrrolic photosensitizers for photodynamic therapy. J Photochem Photobiol B. 2004;73(1-2): 1–28.
8. Krasnovsky Jr AA, Neverov KV, Egorov SYu, Roeder B, Levald T. Photophysical studies of pheophorbide a and pheophytin a. Phosphorescence and photosensitized singlet oxygen luminescence. J Photochem Photobiol B. 1990;5(2):245–54.
9. Yamamoto T, Iriuchishima T, Aizawa S, Okano T, Goto B, Nagai Y, et al. Bactericidal effect of photodynamic therapy using Na-pheophorbide a: evaluation of adequate light source. Photomed Laser Surg. 2009;27(6):849–53.
10. Radestock A, Elsner P, Gitter B, Hipler UC. Induction of apoptosis in HaCaT cells by photodynamic therapy with chlorin e6 or pheophorbide a. Skin Pharmacol Physiol. 2007;20(1):3–9.
11. Kroto HW, Heath JR, O'Brien SC, Curl RF, Smalley RE. C60: buckminsterfullerene. Nature. 1985;318: 162–3.
12. Mitchel DR, Brown Jr RM, Spires TL, Romanovicz DK, Lagow RJ. The synthesis of megatubes: new dimensions in carbon. Materials. 2001;40(12):2751–5.
13. Mroz P, Pawlak A, Satti M, Lee H, Wharton T, Gali H, et al. Functionalized fullerenes mediate photodynamic killing of cancer cells: Type I versus Type II photochemical mechanism. Free Radic Biol Med. 2007;43(5):711–9.
14. Tegos G, Demidova T, Arcila-Lopez D, Lee H, Wharton T, Gali H, et al. Cationic fullerenes are effective and selective antimicrobial photosensitizers. Chem Biol. 2005;12(10):1127–35.
15. Huang L, Terakawa M, Zhiyentayev T, Huang YY, Sawayama Y, Jahnke A, et al. Innovative cationic fullerenes as broad-spectrum light-activated antimicrobials. Nanomedicine. 2010;6:442–52.
16. Leznoff CC, Lever ABP, editors. The phthalocyanines, Vols. 1–4. New York: Wiley; 1986–1993.
17. McKeown NB. Phthalocyanine materials – synthesis, structure and function. Cambridge: Cambridge University Press; 1998.
18. Kadish K, Smith KM, Guilard R, editors. The porphyrin handbook, Vols. 15–20. New York: Academic Press; 2003.
19. Leznoff CC, Vigh S, Svirskaya PI, Greenberg S, Drew DM, Ben-Hur E, et al. Synthesis and photocytotoxicity of some new substituted phthalocyanines. Photochem Photobiol. 1989;49(3):279–84.
20. Guo H, Qian H, Idris NM, Zhang Y. Singlet-oxygen induced apoptosis of cancer cells using upconversion fluorescent nanoparticles as a carrier of photosensitizer. Nanomedicine. 2010;6:486–95.
21. Zhao B, Yin JJ, Bilski PJ, Chignell CF, Roberts JE, He YY. Enhanced photodynamic efficacy towards melanoma cells by encapsulation of Pc4 in silica nanoparticles. Toxicol Appl Pharmacol. 2009;241(2):163–72.
22. Taurand G. Phenothiazine and derivatives. In: Ullmann's encyclopedia of industrial chemistry. Weinheim: Wiley; 2005.
23. Salah M, Samy N, Fadel M. Methylene blue mediated photodynamic therapy for resistant plaque psoriasis. J Drugs Dermatol. 2009;8(1):42–9.
24. Menezes S, Capella MA, Caldas LR. Photodynamic action of methylene blue: repair and mutation in *Escherichia coli*. J Photochem Photobiol B. 1990; 5(3–4):505–17.
25. Sharma M, Bansal H, Gupta PK. Virulence of *Pseudomonas aeruginosa* cells surviving photodynamic treatment with toluidine blue. Curr Microbiol. 2005;50(5):277–80.
26. Sharma M, Visai L, Bragheri F, Cristiani I, Gupta PK. Speziale P toluidine blue-mediated photodynamic effects on staphylococcal biofilms. Antimicrob Agents Chemother. 2008;52(1):299–305.
27. Lin J, Bi LJ, Zhang ZG, Fu YM, Dong TT. Toluidine blue-mediated photodynamic therapy of oral wound infections in rats. Lasers Med Sci. 2010;25:233–8.
28. Seddon JM, Templer RH. Polymorphism of lipid-water systems. In: Lipowsky R, Sackmann E, editors. Handbook of biological physics, vol.1. Elsevier: Amsterdam; 1995.
29. Master AM, Rodriguez ME, Kenney ME, Oleinick NL, Gupta AS. Delivery of the photosensitizer Pc 4 in

PEG-PCL micelles for in vitro PDT studies. J Pharm Sci. 2010;99:2386–98.

30. Torchilin VP. Multifunctional nanocarriers. Adv Drug Deliv Rev. 2006;58(14):1532–55.
31. Oku N, Ishii T. Antiangiogenic photodynamic therapy with targeted liposomes. Methods Enzymol. 2009;465:313–30.
32. Fadel M, Salah M, Samy N, Mona S. Liposomal methylene blue hydrogel for selective photodynamic therapy of acne vulgaris. J Drugs Dermatol. 2009;8(11):983–90.
33. de Leeuw J, van der Beek N, Bjerring P, Martino Neumann HA. Photodynamic therapy of acne vulgaris using 5-aminolevulinic acid 0.5% liposomal spray and intense pulsed light in combination with topical keratolytic agents. J Eur Acad Dermatol Venereol. 2010;24:460–9.
34. van Hell AJ, Costa CI, Flesch FM, Sutter M, Jiskoot W, Crommelin DJ, et al. Self-assembly of recombinant amphiphilic oligopeptides into vesicles. Biomacromolecules. 2007;8(9):2753–61.
35. van Hell AJ, Fretz MM, Crommelin DJ, Hennink WE, Mastrobattista E. Peptide nanocarriers for intracellular delivery of photosensitizers. J Control Release. 2010;141:347–53.
36. Wieder ME, Hone DC, Cook MJ, Handsley MM, Gavrilovic J, Russell DA. Intracellular photodynamic therapy with photosensitizer-nanoparticle conjugates: cancer therapy using a "Trojan horse". Photochem Photobiol Sci. 2006;5(8):727–34.
37. Alexiades-Armenakas MR. Aminolevulinic acid photodynamic therapy for actinic keratoses/actinic cheilitis/acne: vascular lasers. Dermatol Clin. 2007;25: 25–33.
38. Karrer S, Bäumler W, Abels C, Hohenleutner U, Landthaler M, Szeimies RM. Long-pulse dye laser for photodynamic therapy: investigations in vitro and in vivo. Lasers Surg Med. 1999;25(1):51–9.
39. Alexiades-Armenakas MR, Geronemus RG. Laser-mediated photodynamic therapy of actinic keratoses. Arch Dermatol. 2003;139(10):1313–20.
40. Alexiades-Armenakas M. Long-pulsed dye laser-mediated photodynamic therapy combined with topical therapy for mild to severe comedonal, inflammatory, or cystic acne. J Drugs Dermatol. 2006;5(1):45–55.
41. Alexiades-Armenakas MR, Geronemus RG. Laser-mediated photodynamic therapy of actinic cheilitis. J Drugs Dermatol. 2004;3(5):548–51.
42. Alexiades-Armenakas M. Laser-mediated photodynamic therapy of lichen sclerosus. J Drugs Dermatol. 2004;3(6 Suppl):S25–7.
43. Dover JS, Bhatia AC, Stewart B, Arndt KA. Topical 5-aminolevulinic acid combined with intense pulsed light in the treatment of photoaging. Arch Dermatol. 2005;141(10):1247–52.
44. Oh SH, Ryu DJ, Han EC, Lee KH, Lee JH. A comparative study of topical 5-aminolevulinic acid incubation times in photodynamic therapy with intense pulsed light for the treatment of inflammatory acne. Dermatol Surg. 2009;35(12):1918–26.
45. Attili SK, Lesar A, McNeill A, Camacho-Lopez M, Moseley H, Ibbotson S, et al. An open pilot study of ambulatory photodynamic therapy using a wearable low-irradiance organic light-emitting diode light source in the treatment of nonmelanoma skin cancer. Br J Dermatol. 2009;161(1):170–3.
46. Babilas P, Travnik R, Werner A, Landthaler M, Szeimies RM. Split-face-study using two different light sources for topical PDT of actinic keratoses: non-inferiority of the LED system. J Dtsch Dermatol Ges. 2008;6(1):25–32.
47. Koek MB, Buskens E, van Weelden H, Steegmans PH, Bruijnzeel-Koomen CA, Sigurdsson V. Home versus outpatient ultraviolet B phototherapy for mild to severe psoriasis: pragmatic multicentre randomised controlled non-inferiority trial (PLUTO study). BMJ. 2009;338:b1542.
48. Lowe NJ. Home ultraviolet phototherapy. Semin Dermatol. 1992;11(4):284–6.
49. Sadick N. A study to determine the effect of combination blue (415 nm) and near-infrared (830 nm) light-emitting diode (LED) therapy for moderate acne vulgaris. J Cosmet Laser Ther. 2009;11(2):125–8.
50. Wiegell SR, Haedersdal M, Eriksen P, Wulf HC. Photodynamic therapy of actinic keratoses with 8% and 16% methyl aminolaevulinate and home-based daylight exposure: a double-blinded randomized clinical trial. Br J Dermatol. 2009;160(6):1308–14.
51. Riddle CC, Terrell SN, Menser MB, Aires DJ, Schweiger ES. A review of photodynamic therapy (PDT) for the treatment of acne vulgaris. J Drugs Dermatol. 2009;8(11):1010–9.
52. Alexiades-Armenakas M. Photodynamic therapy for acne, rejuvenation, and hair removal. In: Ahluwalia GS, editor. Cosmetic applications of laser and light-based systems. Norwich: William Andrew Inc; 2009. p. 399–414.
53. Divaris DX, Kennedy JC, Pottier RH. Phototoxic damage to sebaceous glands and hair follicles of mice after systemic administration of 5-aminolevulinic acid correlates with localized protoporphyrin IX fluorescence. Am J Pathol. 1990;136(4):891–7.
54. Van der Veen N, de Bruijn HS, Berg RJ, Star WM. Kinetics and localization of PpIX fluorescence after topical and systemic ALA application observed in skin and skin tumours of UVB-treated mice. Br J Cancer. 1996;73(7):925–30.
55. Han I, Jun MS, Kim SK, Kim M, Kim JC. Expression pattern and intensity of protoporphyrin IX induced by liposomal 5-aminolevulinic acid in rat pilosebaceous unit throughout hair cycle. Arch Dermatol Res. 2005;297(5):210–7.
56. Bissonnette R, Shapiro J, Zeng H, McLean DI, Lui H. Topical photodynamic therapy with 5-aminolevulinic acid does not induce hair regrowth in patients with extensive alopecia areata. Br J Dermatol. 2000;143(5): 1032–5.
57. Demidova TN, Hamblin MR. Photodynamic therapy targeted to pathogens. Int J Immunopathol Pharmacol. 2004;17(3):245–54.

58. Maisch T. Phototoxicity of a novel porphyrin photosensitizer against MRSA in an ex-vivo porcine skin model. In: Presented at the sixth annual euro-PDT meeting. Berne, Switzerland, March 31–April 1, 2006.
59. Lambrechts SA, Demidova TN, Aalders MC, Hasan T, Hamblin MR. Photodynamic therapy for *Staphylococcus aureus* infected burn wounds in mice. Photochem Photobiol Sci. 2005;4(7):503–9.
60. Bisland SK, Chien C, Wilson BC, et al. Pre-clinical in vitro and in vivo studies to examine the potential use of photodynamic therapy in the treatment of osteomyelitis. Photochem Photobiol Sci. 2006;5(1):31–8.
61. Wong TW, Wang YY, Sheu HM, et al. Bactericidal effects of toluidine blue-mediated photodynamic action on *Vibrio vulnificus*. Antimicrob Agents Chemother. 2005;49(3):895–902.
62. Millson CE, Wilson M, MacRobert AJ, et al. Exvivo treatment of gastric Helicobacter infection by photodynamic therapy. J Photochem Photobiol. 1996; 32(1–2):59–65.
63. Darras-Vercambre S, Carpentier O, Vincent P, Bonnevalle A, Thomas P. Photodynamic action of red light for treatment of erythrasma: preliminary results. Photodermatol Photoimmunol Photomed. 2006; 22(3):153–6.
64. O'Riordan K, Sharlin DS, Gross J, Chang S, Errabelli D, Akilov OE, et al. Photoinactivation of Mycobacteria in vitro and in a new murine model of localized *Mycobacterium bovis* BCG-induced granulomatous infection. Antimicrob Agents Chemother. 2006;50(5): 1828–34.
65. O'Riordan K, Akilov OE, Chang SK, Foley JW, Hasan T. Real-time fluorescence monitoring of phenothiazinium photosensitizers and their antimycobacterial photodynamic activity against Mycobacterium bovis BCG in in vitro and in vivo models of localized infection. Photochem Photobiol Sci. 2007;6(10):1117–23.
66. Chabrier-Roselló Y, Foster TH, Pérez-Nazario N, Mitra S, Haidaris CG. Sensitivity of *Candida albicans* germ tubes and biofilms to photofrin-mediated phototoxicity. Antimicrob Agents Chemother. 2005;49(10):4288–95.
67. Teichert MC, Jones JW, Usacheva MN, Biel MA. Treatment of oral candidiasis with methylene blue-mediated photodynamic therapy in an immunodeficient murine model. Oral Surg Oral Med Oral Pathol Oral Radiol Endod. 2002;93:155–60.
68. Kamp H, Tietz HJ, Lutz M, Piazena H, Sowyrda P, Lademann J, et al. Antifungal effect of 5-aminolevulinic acid PDT in *Trichophyton rubrum*. Mycoses. 2005; 48:101–7.
69. Kamp H, Tietz HJ, Lutz M, et al. Antifungal effect of 5-aminolevulinic acid PDT in *Trichophyton rubrum*. Mycoses. 2005;48(2):101–7.
70. Watanabe D, Kawamura C, Masuda Y, Akita Y, Tamada Y, Matsumoto Y. Successful treatment of toenail onychomycosis with photodynamic therapy. Arch Dermatol. 2008;144(1):19–21.
71. Piraccini BM, Rech G, Tosti A. Photodynamic therapy of onychomycosis caused by *Trichophyton rubrum*. J Am Acad Dermatol. 2008;59:S75–6.
72. Donnelly RF, McCarron PA, Tunney MM. Antifungal photodynamic therapy. Microbiol Res. 2008;163(1): 1–12.

Index

M.H. Gold (ed.), *Photodynamic Therapy in Dermatology*,
DOI 10.1007/978-1-4419-1298-5, © Springer Science+Business Media, LLC 2011

Q

Z

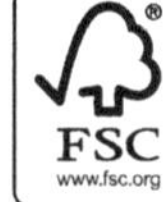

MIX
Papier aus verantwortungsvollen Quellen
Paper from responsible sources
FSC® C105338

If you have any concerns about our products,
you can contact us on
ProductSafety@springernature.com

In case Publisher is established outside the EU,
the EU authorized representative is:
Springer Nature Customer Service Center GmbH
Europaplatz 3, 69115 Heidelberg, Germany

Printed by Libri Plureos GmbH
in Hamburg, Germany